# Minor Illness or Major Disease?

# Minor Illness or Major Disease?

## FIFTH EDITION

**Brian Addison**  MPharm(Hons), MSc (Prescribing Sciences), PgCert (HELT), FHEA, MRPharmS

**Alyson Brown**  MPharm(Hons), PgDip (Prescribing Sciences), MRPharmS

**Ruth Edwards**  BSc(Hons), MSc (Clinical Pharmacy), PgCert (HELT), MRPharmS

**Gwen Gray**  BSc(Hons), PgDip (Clinical Pharmacy), MRPharmS

Robert Gordon University, Aberdeen, Scotland

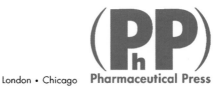

London • Chicago  **Pharmaceutical Press**

**Published by Pharmaceutical Press**

1 Lambeth High Street, London SE1 7JN, UK

© Royal Pharmaceutical Society of Great Britain 2012

(**PₕP**) is a trade mark of Pharmaceutical Press

Pharmaceutical Press is the publishing division of the Royal Pharmaceutical Society

First edition published 1982
Fourth edition published 2006
Fifth edition published 2012

Typeset by Newgen Imaging Systems, Chennai, India
Printed in Great Britain by Butler, Tanner & Dennis, Frome
Index provided by Indexing Specialists, Hove, UK

ISBN 978 0 85369 961 3

Suggestions and comments from readers are most welcome and should
be sent to Commissioning Editor, Pharmaceutical Press, 1 Lambeth
High Street, London SE1 7JN, UK.

A catalogue record for this book is available from the British Library.

# Contents

# Foreword

Across the UK community pharmacists provide a range of healthcare and well-being services and advice from locations in the heart of the community. These are not new roles; they have always been provided by community pharmacists and have their roots in the foundation of the profession. However, it was not until the 1970s and 1980s, when articles started to appear in professional journals, that the knowledge and skills to differentiate minor illness from major disease were systematically addressed and formed the basis of what was to become the first edition of this book. Now in its fifth edition, the need for pharmacists to master the required knowledge and skills to satisfactorily resolve a range of healthcare problems without the intervention of a doctor has never been greater.

Differentiation between a minor illness and a major disease is a key skill to ensure members of the public receive care from the most appropriate healthcare professional. This publication explores the range of illnesses that are encountered in community pharmacy and which can be managed effectively by the ever increasing range of medicines that can be counter-prescribed by a pharmacist without a prescription.

This edition has a new structure and the content has been updated and revised accordingly. For the first time the management of minor illnesses is placed within the broader context of healthcare. The reader is encouraged to adopt a reflective approach to their practice, and a framework is provided that can be readily adapted as new medicines become available, old products are discontinued and knowledge of disease management changes.

We hope that the publication of the fifth edition of *Minor Illness or Major Disease?* continues to support pharmacists, as well as pharmacy support staff in providing this important service to the communities they serve.

Dr Norman Morrow
Chief Pharmaceutical Officer for Northern Ireland
Dr Keith Ridge
Chief Pharmaceutical Officer for England
Professor Bill Scott
Chief Pharmaceutical Officer for Scotland
Professor Roger Walker
Chief Pharmaceutical Officer for Wales

# Preface

The title of this book originates from a series of articles written by Clive Edwards and Paul Stillman that were published in *The Pharmaceutical Journal* between 1979 and 1981 and then subsequently published as a book by the Pharmaceutical Press in 1982. A further series of articles in *The Pharmaceutical Journal* followed, as well as four editions of the book.

The present book is the fifth edition of *Minor Illness or Major Disease?* and this latest edition, like the first, is written at a time of continuing change in the role of the pharmacist. The new changing community pharmacy contracts, the appearance of Minor Ailments Schemes and the continuing reclassification of prescription-only medicines to pharmacy medicine status continues to give the pharmacist new opportunities to advise on self-treatment of self-limiting illnesses, to reduce health risks and foster healthy lifestyles in an expanding public health arena. This current edition is also written at a time when the evidence for the use of various products that have been available from pharmacies for the treatment of minor illnesses is being examined and in some cases products are being withdrawn from supply.

This new edition provides a fresh approach to the management of minor illnesses. The most obvious difference from the previous editions is the re-structuring of the book to mirror the structure of the *British National Formulary* (BNF). Illnesses are primarily considered under the BNF chapter heading where the majority of the drugs used to manage those illnesses can be found. However, there are exceptions to this based on the cross-referencing that occurs in the *BNF*. It is hoped that this approach will facilitate easy cross-reference to the more detailed drug monographs provided in the *BNF*.

This edition also draws on the theoretical underpinnings of problem-based learning. As many healthcare professionals will recognise, the information that is gained from a patient is vital to ensuring that any illness is managed safely and appropriately. The first step in this process is normally establishing the symptom picture that you are dealing with. Therefore, in this edition the management of minor illnesses will be discussed in the context of a case study.

Each section will begin with a case, which will then be followed by a discussion of the presenting symptoms, accompanying symptoms that may need to be considered, and then the various management options that could be utilised. This will then be followed by a discussion of the case study from two differing healthcare professional perspectives. This approach still presents the signs and symptoms of minor illnesses and major diseases but at the same time allows the reader to consider how they would deal with the case presented and ultimately make a decision whether the patient has a minor illness and can self-treat, or whether there is a need to seek a medical opinion.

A small bibliography appears at the end of most chapters focusing particularly on reviews and evidence of the efficacy of over-the-counter medicines. These bibliographies are merely tasters for a larger library of publications but they give some useful background to the enthusiast who may wish to pursue a particular topic. Unlike in previous editions, there is no chapter on Travel Health as this is not a minor illness and this topic is covered in more depth in *Travel Medicine for Health Professionals* by Larry I. Goodyer (Pharmaceutical Press, 2004). Also, for those who wish to find more details about herbal remedies, we recommend *Herbal Medicines* by Joanne Barnes, Linda A. Anderson and J. David Phillipson (Pharmaceutical Press, 2007).

Brian Addison
Alyson Brown
RuthEdwards
GwenGray
2011

# Acknowledgements

We would like to thank Clive Edwards and Paul Stillman for providing the initial publication on which this edition is based. We hope that we have done it justice and continue to provide a useful text that supports all members of the pharmacy team in responding to symptoms and providing advice to those who require treatment for minor illnesses.

Our thanks go to the Pharmaceutical Press for trusting us with writing this fifth edition of *Minor Illness or Major Disease?*, and especially to Louise McIndoe for help with this edition. Our thanks also go to various colleagues who have given us the benefit of their wisdom and to family and friends who have 'put up' with us during the process of writing this fifth edition.

We are indebted to the following for photographs: Science Photo Library; GlaxoWellcome; Wellcome Trust Medical Photographic Library; the Newcastle Dental School; and the Department of Dermatology, Royal Victoria Infirmary, Newcastle upon Tyne.

# About the authors

**Brian Addison** studied pharmacy at the School of Pharmacy, Robert Gordon University. He has worked as a hospital pharmacist in the United Kingdom and Australia and obtained an MSc Prescribing Sciences from the Robert Gordon University in 2004. He has been a Lecturer in Pharmacy Practice at the Robert Gordon University since 2002.

**Alyson Brown** studied pharmacy at the School of Pharmacy, Robert Gordon University. She has worked in various different sectors of pharmacy including community, prison service and training and education before joining the Robert Gordon University as a Lecturer in Pharmacy Practice in 2007.

**Ruth Edwards** studied pharmacy at the School of Pharmacy, Robert Gordon Institute of Technology. She worked in community pharmacy before becoming a Lloyds pharmacy Teacher Practitioner in 1996 and gained an MSc Clinical Pharmacy from Robert Gordon University in 2001. She has been a Lecturer in Pharmacy Practice at the School since.

**Gwen Gray** studied pharmacy at the School of Pharmacy, Robert Gordon University. She worked as a hospital pharmacist before moving to community pharmacy. She then became a Lloyds pharmacy Teacher Practitioner in 1999 and gained a diploma in Clinical Pharmacy from Robert Gordon University in 2000. She has been a Lecturer in Pharmacy Practice at the school since 2005.

The authors work together at the Robert Gordon University, Aberdeen, and all teach pharmacy practice on the Master of Pharmacy course as well as postgraduate courses. All four authors maintain their practice by undertaking locum work in community pharmacy. In 2010 they adopted a Problem Based Learning (PBL) approach to facilitate undergraduate Master of Pharmacy students learning about Minor Illnesses and Major Disease. This approach facilitates the development of a thorough grounding in this subject area and in developing a systematic approach to dealing effectively with new and unfamiliar situations.

# About the contributors

**Clare Leeds** studied Medicine at Leeds University, graduating in 1999. She started her medical career in Bradford and enjoyed posts in acute medicine, palliative care and general practice. She commenced GP vocational training in 2001, qualifying as a GP and gaining membership of the Royal College of General Practitioners in 2008. Clare has worked as a salaried GP and since her relocation to Aberdeen has been working as a GP locum.

**Susan Lennie** studied Dietetics at Queen Margaret College, Edinburgh. She worked as a clinical dietician in hospitals in the Midlands and north east England, specialising in both critical care and paediatrics, until 2002 when she joined Robert Gordon University as a lecturer in Nutrition and Dietetics. She maintains her clinical skills through a regular clinical attachment within the NHS.

# 1

# Introduction

*Brian Addison*

Community pharmacy remains the most accessible route for the public to access healthcare advice. The NHS Plan published by the Department of Health in 2000 stated that '*the frontline in healthcare is in the home*', therefore arguably the backup or second line in healthcare is in the pharmacy. A Department of Health report in 2008 estimated that there were 1.6 million visits per day to community pharmacies and around 1.2 million of those visits were for health-related reasons. The public can also access more health advice information on-line, with NHS Direct and NHS 24 websites both providing information on specific symptoms to help guide individuals to the appropriate level of care, whether that be self-care, seeking advice from a pharmacy, or seeking urgent medical attention.

## Self-care

Self-care is the action taken by an individual to optimise his or her health and wellbeing, both physical and mental. The term embraces both the prevention of illness and the self-treatment of minor ailments, as well as long-term conditions that have been diagnosed by a doctor.

Society is changing: people want more information, choice and control over their health. Self-care can lead to improved health and quality of life and a reduction in visits to general medical practitioners (GPs) and hospitals.

The promotion of good health and the prevention of ill health includes measures such as treating symptoms and preventing disease by reducing cigarette smoking and alcohol intake and encouraging exercise and healthy eating. Dealing with minor illness presents an opportunity to provide advice on all of these during consultations with the public based on the topics included in this book.

### The motivation for self-care

With so many people eligible for free prescriptions in the United Kingdom it is often argued that there is little motivation for self-care. This gives no credit to the wealth of non-prescription medicines available from a pharmacy without the need for a prescription from a doctor. It may be that doctors' knowledge of compound non-prescription medicines is limited, and that they therefore cannot recommend them with confidence for particular symptom complexes. Recent studies also suggest that the traditional medicalisation of presenting symptoms, with closed questions leading the enquirer to a conclusion, leaves the person still feeling unable to contribute to their own care. More patient-centred approaches have helped, sharing ideas and expectations and moving towards an agreed strategy, but the promotion of self-care needs to take this still further. Many people will have thought about their symptoms before presenting them to a professional, and it may be useful to elicit their previous experiences in some detail. What have they done both in this episode and in similar ones in the past? Has it helped, and what were the expectations that prompted it? Then, for example, reassurance that their actions are appropriate but need a little more time may offer them more support than reaffirming that the diagnosis is not serious.

For most, the obstructions to self-care go beyond the financial. Many people will spend money on medication if they feel confident and in control of minor illness. Our task is to support the decision-making process as well as to reassure, and to simplify the complexities of the pharmacology available.

Members of the public can turn to various health professionals, including pharmacists and members of the pharmacy team, for advice on self-care. In most cases they will rely on the skills of the health professional in addressing a current problem, but part of the treatment provided should, where possible, include education to deal with or prevent problems and symptoms in the future. This is where some simplified explanation of the background of the condition, the mode of action of any recommended medicine, and any monitoring required are useful to the sufferer. Also, if referral is appropriate, an explanation of what the doctor might do next or what possible diagnoses need to be excluded is also important.

### Partnership with medical practitioners

A good working relationship between community pharmacy and local medical practices is to be encouraged, so that local protocols and guidelines, where they exist, are observed. Where such protocols do not already exist, then the two professions should work together to produce new ones. The skills of pharmacists and doctors are complementary and, used appropriately, will enhance the care of individual members of the public.

## Non-prescription medicines

Self-medication with non-prescription medicines empowers the individual to take care of his or her own health and saves public expenditure for prescription drugs as well as releasing valuable doctor time. A commonly quoted statistic tells us that up to 40% of a GP's time is taken up by consultations for minor, self-remitting illnesses and GPs are increasingly recommending self-care. In the UK this is unacceptable to some people, because the majority of prescriptions are obtained free of charge and many people will object to having to pay for non-prescription medicines. Increasingly, self-care or minor ailment schemes operate in which certain non-prescription medicines for defined minor illnesses can be obtained free of charge from pharmacies by those individuals who fulfil the conditions to obtain free prescriptions. These schemes operate in the UK and allow pharmacies to be reimbursed for the cost of providing these medicines. Thus the payment barrier is overcome, and it has been shown that such schemes do reduce the workload of the general practitioner. However, following the abolition of prescription charges in Scotland and Wales, it remains to be seen whether this trend will be reversed and whether individuals will return to consulting their GP for minor, self-remitting illnesses in order to obtain medicines free of charge on prescription.

In terms of consumer choice, cost, convenience and previous experience are probably the main factors that determine whether a person obtains a drug from a pharmacy or on prescription. Advertising has a major influence on the purchase of a particular brand of a non-prescription medicine. People have the right to choose what they want, and thanks to increasing consumer demand and limited resources it has been necessary to use the skills and expertise of all health professionals. For pharmacy, this potential in supporting self-care has been outlined in various documents, such as *The NHS Plan* (Department of Health 2000), *The Right Medicine: A Strategy for Pharmaceutical Care in Scotland* (Scottish Executive, 2002), and *Pharmacy in England: Building on Strengths – Delivering the Future* (Department of Health, 2008).

## Reclassification of prescription-only medicines (POM) to pharmacy (P) medicines

The availability of drugs without a prescription from a doctor varies from country to country, and indeed in the United States it even varies from state to state. In the UK the variation in control of non-prescription medicines ranges from those products whose sale must be supervised by a pharmacist (pharmacy-only, or P medicine) to those whose sale is unrestricted and can occur in retail outlets other than pharmacies (general sales list, or GSL medicines). In recent years an increasing number of prescription-only medicines (POM) have been reclassified by the Medicines and Healthcare products Regulatory Agency (MHRA) following wide consultation and are now available to buy from pharmacies under specific restrictions.

Generally drugs will be accorded P medicine status if they fulfil various criteria:

- The condition for which they are used can be reliably self-diagnosed. However, there are exceptions to this, as for example the sale of antifungal agents for vaginal candidiasis, which are only licensed for use after an initial diagnosis has been made by a doctor. There are some more remote exceptions, such as theophylline (for asthma), glyceryl trinitrate and isosorbide (for angina), which are available legally without prescription.
- Where there is no evidence of irreversible or serious adverse reactions, even in high doses.
- In the UK drugs should have had a long use as prescription-only medicines before being reclassified to P medicine status, to ensure safety. However, some non-prescription medicines may not be innocuous and side effects may not become obvious until later

(e.g. phenylpropanolamine in cold remedies, and herbal medicines such as St John's Wort).
- Where the delay in obtaining a prescription for a drug may cause harm. Examples of such cases are levonorgestrel for emergency contraception.
- Where their use does not require medical supervision or monitoring by a doctor.

There may be other hidden criteria, often of a political or marketing nature.

There have been several high-profile switches of medicines from PoM to P medicine status in the UK, including omeprazole, simvastatin, chloramphenicol and sumatriptan. There have also been applications made for drugs that after consultation were not reclassified, e.g. trimethoprim and nitrofurantoin.

## Evidence-based medicine

Evidence-based medicine (EBM) should be used to inform clinical decisions, but it should be considered with all the available information about an individual before making a decision. Thus products may be recommended for use when there is no evidence base but still acknowledging the expectation of the individual member of the public who is requesting treatment.

In recent years it has become apparent that many non-prescription medicines do not have a research evidence base to support their effectiveness. However, this should not be interpreted to mean that members of the public should be denied particular treatments, but rather that health professionals need to use their training to ensure that no harm befalls them.

The maxim 'do no harm' is a prerequisite for care given by any healthcare professional, and all practitioners should be mindful of it. However, pharmacists are in an ideal position to offer advice on self-medication, particularly in at-risk groups such as the elderly, who may be taking many prescription drugs and will need advice to avoid drug interactions and duplication of medications.

Increasingly, with the medical revolution of the last half-century, we are in a culture where the public believes that there is 'a pill for every ill'. The placebo effect is huge, and often people come into a pharmacy with a desire or expectation that they will be given a remedy, as well as pertinent advice, to relieve their symptoms.

A parallel situation often occurs in the doctor's consulting room. In the first place it should be remembered that even prescription medicines are not effective to the same extent in every person. The term 'numbers needed to treat' (NNT) is well known to health professionals and is in effect an admission of this fact. Secondly, an individual's expectations, whether real or perceived, often influence the outcome of a consultation, not least the writing of a prescription. Doctors often make clinically inappropriate, non-evidence-based decisions for the sake of maintaining a good relationship.

## Complementary and alternative medicine

Complementary medicine is very popular with the public. Although in many cases remedies are not supported by placebo-controlled randomised clinical trials, individual choice and experience are important here, just as with more orthodox medicines. Not everyone responds to these remedies, and it may be that responders are those in whom we are seeing a large placebo effect or who have high expectations. Again, medicine is not a perfect science and individuals often respond in unexpected or inconsistent ways to all kinds of remedies.

There is much to be said for a holistic approach, and health professionals must make an effort to empathise with individuals who ask for their advice. A sympathetic reaction, a caring attitude and a genuine interest in an individual's problems will contribute to a significant placebo effect, regardless of whatever medicine may be recommended.

## Herbal medicines

Herbal medicines are becoming increasingly popular. There are two major issues to be borne in mind: efficacy and safety. Herbal products that are available from a variety of commercial sources will vary in composition. It is therefore difficult to confirm the efficacy of all products, as the amount of active ingredient will vary, often widely, from product to product. Added to this, the identity of the active ingredient may be in doubt. An example of this is

St John's Wort, where there is conflict as to whether the antidepressant activity is due to the hypericins or to hyperforin, and which ingredient causes liver enzyme induction.

Like conventional medicines, herbal medicines often have a controversial evidence base. St John's Wort, for example, has been the subject of many clinical trials and analyses, often with conflicting conclusions.

There is a myth among the public that herbal medicines are safe. Increasingly this is being found not to be the case, as for example in the case of St John's Wort, which is a liver enzyme inducer and can cause many interactions with prescription drugs. There have been other reports, such as tea tree oil causing severe skin irritation, cranberry juice potentiating the anticoagulant effects of warfarin, and kava causing liver reactions. These conflicting reports and evidence may be caused by the variation in composition between commercial brands referred to above.

In April 2011 the European Traditional Herbal Medicinal Products Directive (THMPD) 2004/24/EC came into effect. This directive requires each European Union Member State to set up a traditional herbal registration scheme for manufactured traditional herbal medicines suitable for use without medical supervision.

Further details of how this scheme will operate in the UK can be obtained from the MHRA, but its introduction means that companies can no longer sell manufactured unlicensed herbal medicines without a full marketing authorisation or a traditional herbal registration.

## Consultation and diagnosis

All members of the pharmacy team require training in the recognition and treatment of minor illnesses, but this should recognise the differing levels of expertise within the team, ensuring that individuals are triaged effectively and receive the appropriate level of care. Pharmacists need to be trained in the differential diagnosis of common minor ailments and should not be distracted or feel pressured by other elements of their work, such as dispensing, when consulting with a member of the public about a health issue. An effective consultation demands time, empathy and privacy, regardless of what else remains to be done in the pharmacy.

Because of their open availability, pharmacists have been the subject of various covert research activities, particularly by consumer associations over the years, with regard to the advice they give to the public. The publication of such investigations has inevitably highlighted the shortcomings of pharmacists' ability to ask the right questions and give the correct advice. Undoubtedly such research among other professions would produce a range of competencies from practice to practice. The methodology of such research studies is difficult and therefore sometimes of dubious value, but the studies do serve to highlight the fact that care is always necessary in taking a history from an individual who presents with symptoms in the pharmacy. History taking at this level is an important but not difficult skill to learn, and with experience and practice, proficiency can be achieved quickly.

## Diagnosis and history taking

Pharmacists have advised members of the public about the treatment of minor illnesses for as long as the profession has existed. Before embarking on any form of advice or treatment, some initial diagnosis is necessary to exclude any potentially serious cause that may require a medical consultation. This diagnosis of exclusion is one that should be able to be made in the vast majority of cases. It may be thought of as a screening or sieving process that can be achieved by gathering information from individuals in a careful and intelligent manner. It is a process many individuals perform themselves before self-medicating, and generally they are very competent at it. It is also commonly the modus operandi for GPs when someone presents with symptoms for the first time.

Clearly, this sort of diagnosis can take on various degrees of sophistication, and there is a suitable level at which the pharmacist can participate in the process. At this level it is not difficult, and with a structured approach, which closely follows that taught to doctors, valuable judgements as to whether referral for medical investigation or a recommendation for self-treatment is the more appropriate course of action can be made.

The suggested format that follows is one approach that can be used to elicit a comprehensive history.

## General rules

Almost too obvious to mention, but crucially important, is the question of who is seeking the advice? Is it the person relating the story, or are they a representative? It is difficult to obtain a satisfactory history from a third party, and if the person requiring advice is not present it is useful to establish whether their absence is due to the severity of the symptoms. Parents of young children will give good histories of a child's illness; if the child is present, the severity of the illness and other signs can be observed. In the absence of the individual experiencing the illness, practitioners should reassure themselves that they are in no doubt as to the severity and nature of the disease. If there is any uncertainty, it is unwise to recommend self-treatment.

To encourage a patient-centred consultation, the patient should be encouraged to provide an opening statement in which they explain the illness or presenting complaint in their own words. If necessary, this can be prompted by a general open question such as 'How can I help you?', 'What is the problem?' or 'How do you feel?' This allows them to relax and encourages them to talk and provide clues that can be followed up by more specific questions later. During this phase of the interview their demeanour or attitude can be observed so that the interviewer can consider the question 'Do they look ill?' Some people can articulate the severity of their illness adequately, but in others non-verbal signs (such as body language) must be observed to distinguish a very sick person from a relatively healthy one. This is particularly relevant in babies, who can indicate their discomfort by refusing to eat, by crying or screaming (even after being picked up), or by being irritable or behaving in some abnormal fashion.

The mnemonic, SIT DOWN SIR, is a useful tool to ensure that a full description of the illness or presenting complaint is obtained (see Table 1.1). It provides a structure to ensure that all features of a symptom are established and can be used as a prompt for the use of specific, focused questioning for information that has not been provided in the

| Table 1.1 | A mnemonic for the establishment of symptom features: SIT DOWN SIR |
|---|---|
| S | Site or location |
| I | Intensity or severity |
| T | Type or nature |
| D | Duration |
| O | Onset |
| W | With (other symptoms) |
| N | aNnoyed or aggravated by |
| S | Spread or radiation |
| I | Incidence or frequency pattern |
| R | Relieved by |

opening statement. Use of the mnemonic can ensure that a thorough history of the presenting complaint is taken. Although perhaps not standard practice, it might also be beneficial to take notes of the history provided as a means of later analysing efficiency in history taking, as well as with a view to the future when, like doctors, they may be challenged about what they have said.

## Symptom features

### Site or location

The site or location of a symptom can be helpful in diagnosis in some instances, for example where pain is the main symptom. For instance, a pain in the abdomen could be caused by appendicitis (central pain, moving to the right iliac fossa), renal colic (pain in right or left loin or iliac fossa), peptic ulcer (central or epigastric) or biliary colic (right hypochondrium). Similarly, headaches can be unilateral (migraine), frontal (migraine, sinusitis or tension) or occipital (tension, muscle spasm or subarachnoid haemorrhage). The site of a skin rash can distinguish a localised reaction, for example to a watchstrap, from the allergy to an antibiotic in which the whole body may be involved.

### Intensity or severity

The intensity or severity of a symptom, such as pain, a skin rash or bleeding from a wound, gives information not only about the likely diagnosis but also

about the urgency of a situation. This is essential when considering whether to temporise and monitor the course of a symptom or illness for a little longer, to give an non-prescription medicine, or to recommend referral for medical appraisal.

### Type or nature

Description of the type and/or nature of a symptom can help to differentiate certain conditions. For example, an abdominal pain that is cramp-like or colicky indicates the involvement of a hollow organ, such as the bowel or ureter, which contracts as a result of spasm of smooth muscle in the organ wall. On the other hand, the pain of a peptic ulcer is often described as 'gnawing'. Similarly, the appearance of a rash as flat or raised, single or multiple, or blistering or dry lesions can help to differentiate various skin conditions.

### Duration

The duration of any symptom must always be established. This information can be helpful to distinguish, say, the headache of migraine (which may last 4–72 hours) from a tension headache (which may persist for several days or weeks). The duration will also help to decide whether to refer in certain situations. For example, a toddler who has suffered from diarrhoea for three days requires referral for a medical assessment, whereas a toddler with diarrhoea of only a few hours' duration may respond adequately to hydration with a simple electrolyte mixture.

### Onset

The history of onset of a symptom or illness can provide clues to its likely cause. Thus, abdominal pain and diarrhoea that starts soon after overindulgence in a restaurant, or headache that occurs on awakening after an alcoholic binge are likely to require little more than reassurance, sympathy and simple non-prescription medicines.

### With (other symptoms)

Accompanying symptoms may not always be volunteered, especially if it is felt that they are not important or not related to the presenting complaint. Such information is, however, crucial to differentiating many disorders. For example, someone who complains of a productive cough or of diarrhoea should be asked whether there is blood in the sputum or motions, to distinguish between potentially serious disease and a more trivial illness. Someone with a red eye that is itching and watery may have a simple allergy, whereas a red eye that is painful or accompanied by some disturbance of vision will require immediate medical attention.

Thus, any symptom should be submitted to a systematic review, inquiring first about other symptomatology within the same body system and then, either by direct questioning or by more general open questions (depending on the problem), about any symptoms in other systems.

### Annoyed or aggravated by

Although not always relevant, there are some conditions for which inquiry about any factors that worsen the symptom can be valuable. The pain of a peptic ulcer, for example, can be worsened by a heavy meal, or alternatively by fasting, whereas that caused by gallstones will be particularly exacerbated by a fatty meal.

Headaches associated with a raised intracranial pressure will be worse after lying down and hence worse in the mornings, whereas tension headaches may be better in the mornings but worsen as the day goes on.

### Spread or radiation

There are several examples of where a sensation – usually pain – spreads characteristically and almost predictably to another part of the body. In the case of pain, this is known as referred pain. The diagnosis of appendicitis is classically made by the description of a pain that starts in the central region of the abdomen and then spreads to the right iliac fossa. The pain of angina often radiates to the left arm or jaw, and biliary colic occurs as pain in the upper abdomen that is referred to the back and felt between the shoulder blades. Some skin conditions begin as single discrete lesions in one part of the body before spreading elsewhere, whereas others present in a more generalised way.

### Incidence or frequency

If a symptom recurs, then in some circumstances the pattern of recurrence or relapse is characteristic. For example, classic migraine will rarely occur twice in the same week, whereas another form of migraine, known as cluster headache, occurs every day at the same time of day for several weeks. The 'hayfever' syndrome may often be difficult to distinguish from symptoms of the common cold, except that it is notable for its appearance in particular months of the year.

### Factors that relieve the condition

Just as some conditions are made worse by particular factors, there are some that can be characterised by factors that relieve them. The pain of peptic ulcer, for instance, is often relieved by small snacks (as opposed to large meals, which tend to aggravate it), and a migraine attack may be terminated by vomiting. Medicines are often useful to relieve and at the same time diagnose a condition. Thus, an anginal attack may be relieved by glyceryl trinitrate, and reflux dyspepsia alleviated by a large dose of antacid, but not vice versa.

It is also important to establish a drug history of any current or recent medicines that may have been taken. This will help in eliciting any drug-induced symptoms that the patient may be experiencing as a result of any prescribed or non-prescription medicines. This will also help establish whether there are other medical conditions that have not been mentioned (highlighted by the use of some prescribed medicines) and whether they have already tried a remedy for the present complaint.

At some point in the consultation, any relevant past history can be inquired after, such as personal or family history, together with occupation and social habits, for example smoking, drinking and exercise.

In many cases the cause of a symptom will be obvious, whereas in others a precise diagnosis, at least prospectively, will be impossible, and then the practitioner will depend on the exclusion of serious pathology.

At the same time, when the possibility of serious pathology cannot be eliminated it is essential that the message is delivered appropriately, depending on the demeanour of the person they are advising. People often have selective hearing and overreact to emotive words such as 'cancer' or 'tumour', perhaps in such a way that they will then avoid seeing the doctor in case the diagnosis is confirmed. It is necessary to avoid the use of such words, and to remember that statistically only a very small number of people who seek help about their symptoms will prove to have a serious disease, and an even smaller proportion of symptoms will be due to malignancy. However, there will always be a few instances where there is a degree of uncertainty, or where individuals fall into a certain category, in which case it is good professional practice to advise them to see their GP. The same process occurs daily in the doctor's consulting room, where he or she will refer for specialist opinion for similar reasons, to either confirm or exclude a specific diagnosis.

It is important that practitioners do not inadvertently raise fears in the minds of those who seek their advice, especially when recommending referral to a doctor. Obviously it is both educative and consoling to be able to explain to someone exactly why they should seek a medical opinion, and there is no doubt that a sympathetic ear and a comprehensible explanation of both symptoms and their management is appreciated. However, at the same time someone who needs urgent medical attention should be dealt with in a way that conveys the urgency without causing undue anxiety.

To complete the skill of diagnosis, even at this level, the practitioner needs to rely on two further attributes. Firstly, to have in mind the serious diagnoses when considering the symptoms that are presented. Secondly, but no less importantly, to be alert to that unpleasant feeling that develops in a diagnostician's mind when no satisfactory explanation can be reached. This is a developed skill that many call experience. If any of the serious diagnoses cannot be reasonably excluded and their remains an uncomfortable uncertainty about the best of course of action for a given situation, there should be no hesitation in directing the person seeking advice to more suitable assistance, e.g. referring to the general practitioner for a medical opinion.

The intelligent use of a standard format such as the one we have suggested for establishing a full history of the presenting complaint will ensure that the most important areas are covered and relevant information is obtained. The format we have used here will be applied as appropriate in the topics to be covered in this book, but as all practitioners will be aware, not every question is always applicable to every circumstance, and the answer to one question often obviates the need for another.

With practice, a standard approach allows a consultation to be conducted quickly and efficiently. It also provides a degree of reassurance that the relevant information for a symptom under consideration is established, and allows the practitioner to be confident that they have acted in the best possible faith and with acceptable profession competency to distinguish between minor illness and major disease.

# How to use this book

This book is divided into nine chapters (including this first chapter) and the conditions included in this book are arranged into chapters based on the chapters of the *British National Formulary (BNF)*. For example all the products that are used to treat minor illnesses that are included in the respiratory chapter of the *BNF* are dicussed in the respiratory chapter of this book. Therefore, products such as paracetamol that are used to treat a number of different conditions are included in the Central Nervous System chapter of this book beside all other analgesics, although a passing mention will be made to them in other chapters.

## Structure of chapters

At the start of each chapter there is a short introduction and a table that outlines the conditions and drugs that will be dealt with in that chapter. Each chapter is then split into sections that deal with different symptom complexes. The number of sections in each chapter varies depending on how these symptom complexes are commonly encountered.

### Case study and trigger questions

Each section begins by presenting a case study and some trigger questions. The reader is invited to consider their initial response to this case before continuing to read the subsequent text. However, it is not necessary to consider the case and the reader can skip this step and continue reading the remainder of the chapter. The intention of the case study is to encourage a reflective approach and to act as an aid to illustrate the complexity of differentiating between minor illness and major disease.

### Assessing symptoms

Following the case study there will be a section that discusses the assessment of the symptoms presented in the case study. In discussing the symptoms we use the mnemonic SIT DOWN SIR (described earlier) as a tool to illustrate how an assessment of the symptoms can help with the differentiation between minor illness and major disease.

### Accompanying symptoms

In differentiating between minor illnesses and major diseases there are often accompanying symptoms whose presence needs to be confirmed or excluded. In this section we discuss other symptoms that, while not presented in the case study, could potentially be a feature of the conditions under review, e.g. in someone reporting chest pain and differentiating between a gastrointestinal cause or pain of cardiac origin.

### Management options

In this section the possible management options are presented and discussed. This includes any general advice or management options that are appropriate for the symptoms presented. In presenting the various drugs that can be used to treat the symptoms we have utilised the group names used in the *British National Formulary* and refer you to this publication for a more in-depth presentation on the use of these drugs, e.g. dosage, frequency, side effects, cautions, contraindications.

In some cases complementary therapies and herbal medicines will be highlighted, but given our acknowledgment of the conflicting evidence and reports that exist in this area we refer you to other publications for more detail, e.g. *Herbal Medicines* by Joanne Barnes, Linda A. Anderson and J. David Phillipson (Pharmaceutical Press, 2007).

### Re-consider the case

At this point the case study and trigger questions are repeated and the reader is invited to re-consider their initial response to the case after reading the chapter. The case is then followed by a pharmacist response to the case and by a response from a general practitioner or dietitian. These responses aim to illustrate a more in-depth discussion of the thought process of dealing with the cases and to illustrate the similarities and differences in approach by two different healthcare professionals.

### Summary of key points and key referral criteria

Each section is completed by a table summarising the key information presented in the particular section and clearly links together minor illnesses with their management options. This section also provides a summary of the situations where referral for medical appraisal would be necessary. This section should not be considered as a comprehensive account of when referral should happen and practitioners must always use their professional judgement in deciding what is in the best interests of the person requiring treatment.

## Bibliography

Department of Health (2000). *The NHS Plan.* London: Department of Health.

Department of Health (2008). *Pharmacy in England: Building on Strengths – Delivering the Future.* London: Department of Health.

National Prescribing Centre (2004). Community pharmacy minor ailments schemes. *MeReC Briefing* 27: 1–8.

Scottish Executive (2002). *The Right Medicine: A Strategy for Pharmaceutical Care in Scotland.* Edinburgh: Scottish Executive.

# 2

# Gastrointestinal Illnesses

*Alyson Brown*

| This chapter will cover the following conditions: | This chapter will cover the following groups of medicines: |
|---|---|
| • Dyspepsia<br>• Heartburn<br>• Constipation<br>• Haemorrhoids<br>• DiarrhoealBS | • Antacids<br>• Compound alginates and indigestion preparations<br>• Antispasmodics<br>• Antisecretory drugs<br>• Antimotility drugs<br>• Laxatives<br>• Local preparations for anal and rectal disorders |

In this chapter we will consider common minor illnesses that occur in the context of the gastrointestinal (GI) tract – both the upper and lower regions – and the major diseases that can also present. A reasonably accurate diagnosis can often be made on the basis of a clear history, although sometimes the precise cause will remain a mystery. In such cases it is sufficient to determine the severity of the symptoms and the need for referral.

The gastrointestinal (GI) tract is split into the upper and lower regions with different conditions affecting the different regions (Table 2.1).

| Table 2.1 The upper and lower regions of the gastrointestinal tract | |
| --- | --- |
| **Upper gastrointestinal tract comprises:** | **Lower gastrointestinal tract comprises:** |
| • Mouth | • Jejunum |
| • Oesophagus | • Ileum |
| • Stomach | • Colon |
| • Duodenum | • Rectum |
| | • Anus |

When considering gastrointestinal illnesses, alarm symptoms and accompanying symptoms are often the same, regardless of the area of the gastrointestinal tract that is affected. Some alarm symptoms will require immediate referral owing to the severity of the likely underlying pathology; however, this needs to be considered in the context of the presenting illness and duration of symptoms.

## Dyspepsia and heartburn

Before reading further, consider the following case and note your initial thoughts.

**Case study**

A 30-year-old man comes into the pharmacy and asks you for advice as he has been experiencing pains in his chest and stomach. On further questioning, he describes a burning feeling that is often worse after large meals and at night-time. He admits to smoking socially and has a few drinks after his dinner on a regular basis.

**Trigger questions**

● What additional information would you need before considering the appropriate management options in this case?
● What issues concern you about this case?
● Are any alarm symptoms being exhibited that require more urgent treatment or referral?

### Assessing symptoms

The term 'pain' is often used to describe all symptoms ranging from a mild or vague discomfort, such as indigestion, to the more commonly accepted lay definition of pain as a sensation that hurts.

It is therefore important to further investigate a person's unique understanding of what they mean by 'pain' and specifically to attempt to identify the location and severity of the pain, which will often lead to further information about the condition they may be suffering from and help determine appropriate treatment or referral.

#### Location of pain

Assessing the location of the pain is often helpful in considering the possible cause of the pain, although there will be variability between individuals and presentation. Abdominal pain is often not localised, but will often present as covering the entire abdomen. The symptom of abdominal pain can encompass a multitude of possible diagnoses relating to the gastrointestinal tract, the genitourinary tract, and sometimes to other body systems from which pain may be referred to the abdomen. Most commonly in community pharmacy, this pain will represent either a non-specific gastritis or enteritis with no known cause that will resolve spontaneously or, alternatively, the early presentation of a disorder that is not yet sufficiently advanced to show all of its typical features. Thus, the rest of the history must be considered along with questions about the site of pain.

People may give a clue to the diagnosis by the manner in which they show the location of their pain. In answer to the prompt 'Show me where the pain is', someone with a peptic ulcer or other distinct lesion may point with a finger to an exact spot on the abdomen, whereas someone with a less-specific symptom may place a whole hand over the area where the discomfort is felt. Epigastric pain, pain above the umbilicus and located centrally and pain behind the breastbone is likely to indicate dyspepsia, whereas pain further down is more likely to indicate a bowel condition or occasionally a musculoskeletal condition. Pain that occurs in the chest may arise from the GI tract owing to acid reflux. In this situation further questioning is required to rule out any serious underlying pathology, as cardiac pain can present in a similar manner.

### Intensity and duration of pain

Severe pain that is continuous for more than a few hours may indicate serious pathology and possibly a medical emergency. If there is no previous history and the pain is sudden in onset, this would be described clinically as an acute abdomen. It may be caused by conditions such as pancreatitis, peritonitis, an active or perforated peptic ulcer, abdominal aortic aneurysm or gynaecological emergencies. The severity of abdominal pain will influence the decision on how soon a doctor should be seen.

Milder pain that occurs at some time during every day and persists for 2 weeks despite a course of treatment requires referral if it is troublesome. Obviously, the presence of certain accompanying symptoms may shorten the period before a doctor should be seen.

Symptoms that do not occur on a daily basis may be left for a little longer – up to 4 weeks – to assess the effect of symptomatic treatment before referring to the doctor.

### Type of pain

A description of the pain can be useful, but it should be remembered that this will often be dependent on the individual's experience of pain.

Abdominal pain will sometimes be described as a vague discomfort. This is typical of, but not exclusive to, the common indigestion seen with a non-specific gastritis. The condition is self-limiting, its cause usually being dietary overindulgence or poor eating habits. Various words can be used to describe indigestion or dyspepsia: reflux, trapped wind, burping, a bloated feeling or a grumbling stomach.

A sharp burning sensation in the epigastric region or behind the sternum is typical of oesophagitis due to reflux of stomach contents, and is referred to by the lay person as heartburn. This acid reflux occurs in everyone, particularly after or during meals, and is quite normal, although usually asymptomatic. When it causes symptoms, indicating damage to the lower oesophagus, it is referred to as gastro-oesophageal reflux disease (GORD). Such a sensation may also be caused by a peptic ulcer, although sometimes someone with an ulcer will complain of a more specific gnawing pain that can be pointed to with a finger.

The pain of angina or a myocardial infarction can mimic oesophagitis and other causes of abdominal pain. Although these conditions will be seen relatively rarely in the pharmacy, care should be taken to rule out underlying or more serious pathology.

An inflammatory process in any organ in the abdomen may result in a sensation of tenderness over the affected area. It is therefore important to ask not only about pain but also about any tenderness, particularly when light pressure is applied with a finger or when the person bends or stretches.

Colic is a term used to describe waves of severe pain superimposed on a more constant duller pain, and occurs when a hollow muscular organ is in spasm. Thus, a colicky or griping pain is most likely to indicate involvement of the stomach or bowel, the genitourinary system (such as the ureter, bladder, uterus or Fallopian tubes) or the bile duct system.

### Onset of pain

Factors surrounding the onset of abdominal pain can provide some useful clues about the diagnosis. Pain related to meals generally indicates a lesion in the stomach or bowel and is a classic symptom of a peptic ulcer (as well as non-ulcerative inflammatory conditions of the gastric and bowel mucosa). Epigastric or central pain that occurs a few minutes after a meal is typical of gastric ulcer, and pain that occurs 1–2 hours after a meal is more typical of duodenal ulcer. The pain of a duodenal ulcer is usually worse during the night. Both of these types of pain may respond to antacids, $H_2$-antagonists or proton pump inhibitors, but pain that persists despite such treatment requires referral.

Pain or other abdominal symptoms following a single incident of overeating or excess alcohol may represent either a non-specific (or non-ulcer) gastritis or indigestion, which will resolve quickly without the need for referral. However, if symptoms become severe or persist, they could represent some underlying pathological cause, such as food poisoning.

Any pain or discomfort that starts immediately on eating could represent oesophagitis or reflux, or even nervous dyspepsia. If treatment with non-prescription medicines is not successful, this condition requires attention and it is best to refer the individual for reassurance or investigation.

Gastrointestinal symptoms can be caused by aspirin and other non-steroidal anti-inflammatory drugs (NSAIDs) and iron, whereas oesophageal symptoms may be caused by bulking agents, potassium salts, NSAIDs, tetracyclines, bisphosphonates and steroids, especially if the person is lying in bed. Calcium channel blocking drugs are also associated with dyspepsia.

### Factors that aggravate or relieve pain

Pain from a peptic ulcer is not always aggravated by food: sometimes food acts as a buffer to the acid attacking the damaged mucosa and hence provides some relief. Classically, a gastric ulcer is said to be aggravated by food and a duodenal ulcer to be relieved by it. Food will trigger heartburn, and sufferers will often complain of a sensation of obstruction at the gastro-oesophageal junction if a stricture is present.

The pain of oesophagitis or acid reflux may be aggravated by lying down (and is therefore a problem at night) or bending. Sometimes smoking, alcohol, chocolate or coffee can lower the pressure in the oesophageal sphincter and allow reflux to take place.

Antacids, $H_2$-antagonists and proton pump inhibitors (PPIs) usually provide some relief in peptic ulceration and oesophagitis, but do not help in nervous dyspepsia or in biliary colic due to gallstones. Pain in biliary colic due to gallstones will be exacerbated by fatty foods, and a reduction in the amount of fat eaten will relieve or prevent the pain to some degree. This is not always diagnostic, however, as the pain of peptic ulcer may be affected in the same way.

The colicky pain of colitis or gastroenteritis will often be temporarily relieved by passing a stool, which differentiates these conditions from appendicitis, in which no such relief will usually occur.

Pain caused by non-specific gastritis, peptic ulcer, oesophagitis or hiatus hernia is normally relieved temporarily by antacids, $H_2$-antagonists or PPIs. This may be helpful in distinguishing these conditions from angina. The pain of angina usually responds to sublingual glyceryl trinitrate, which may have been prescribed for the individual. Chest pain not responding to either type of drug should be evaluated in terms of the possibility of a myocardial infarction.

## Accompanying symptoms

A great many other symptoms may accompany abdominal pain or discomfort. If any alarm signals are present, then a referral to the doctor is appropriate. Box 2.1 lists alarm symptoms as defined by The National Institute for Health and Clinical Excellence (NICE) in 2004.

Where treatment has been tried and failed in people over the age of 55 years, the following cases should be referred:

- Previous gastric ulcer
- Previous gastric surgery
- Pernicious anaemia
- NSAID use
- Family history of gastric cancer.

### Weight loss

Weight loss, particularly unexplained and unintentional, is a significant sign in anyone with abdominal

| Box 2.1 Alarm symptoms as defined by (NICE) |
| --- |
| - Significant gastrointestinal bleeding |
| - Progressive dysphagia |
| - Unintentional weight loss |
| - Epigastric mass |
| - Suspicious barium meal |
| - Iron deficiency anaemia |
| - Persistent vomiting |

symptoms, and becomes more so from middle age onwards. It may be caused by a peptic ulcer, but it could signify a sinister pathology, such as a carcinoma, and should always be referred.

### Blood in the stool

Melaena (blood in the stool) is a warning symptom that needs referral for either reassurance or investigation, particularly in the older population. If there is a past history of haemorrhoids, it may be possible to differentiate spotting of blood on toilet tissue due to haemorrhoids from a black, tarry stool containing blood from a lesion further up the bowel. However, if the symptoms have changed in someone with previously diagnosed haemorrhoids, or if there is any doubt whatsoever, then it is wise to refer them for a medical opinion.

Fresh (bright red) blood smearing the stool in a young person, associated with symptoms of haemorrhoids (see Haemorrhoids below), is probably acceptable in the short term. However, in those over the age of 40 years any type of blood in the stool requires investigation.

### Anaemia

The most common cause of anaemia in people admitted to hospital is a gastrointestinal bleed, and it is therefore necessary to refer anyone with signs of anaemia, with or without abdominal symptoms, to the doctor.

Signs of anaemia are tiredness, facial pallor, pale conjunctiva (seen by everting the lower eyelid and comparing with the red/pink conjunctiva lining the lower lid of a healthy person) and pale palms of the hands (again observed by comparing with the pink palms of a healthy individual). Severe anaemia can cause shortness of breath.

### Menstrual disorders

(Refer to Chapter 6.)

Abdominal symptoms associated with specific times in the menstrual cycle, such as mid-cycle, premenstrual or perimenstrual pains, suggest that the problem relates to the genital tract. Where involvement of the genital tract is suspected or requires exclusion, any irregularity should be inquired for,

such as a missed period, vaginal discharge, abnormal bleeding, and particularly any symptoms associated with early pregnancy, such as nausea, breast changes and nocturia. Individuals with pain associated with any of these features will generally require referral to exclude serious conditions such as a tubal pregnancy, salpingitis or endometriosis.

### Jaundice

Frank jaundice can be recognised by a yellow discoloration of the skin. More subtle signs can be detected by inspecting the sclera of the eye, which will have a yellow colour or tinge compared to the white of a normal eye. Jaundice suggests liver or biliary involvement and requires referral.

### Dysphagia

A genuine difficulty in swallowing food or drink requires referral to exclude oesophageal obstruction. People with GORD may complain of this symptom, which is due to a narrowing of the oesophagus caused by a stricture created by the irritant reflux. This may improve with symptomatic treatment. A feeling of a lump in the throat that does not affect swallowing should also be followed up, although perhaps not as urgently as genuine dysphagia.

### Swelling

Localised swelling in the abdomen is associated with hernias. General abdominal distension may be real or imagined, and can occur with relatively benign dyspepsia as well as with more serious diagnoses. However, referral is necessary if there is a real change in the abdominal girth measurement together with abdominal symptoms.

More often the individual will complain of feeling bloated, usually with flatulence. This is a common symptom of many abdominal disorders and is not really helpful in making a differential diagnosis.

### Vomiting

Vomiting that persists for more than 1 or 2 days requires a medical opinion. Usually the cause will be food or alcohol intolerance or gastrointestinal infection, but it can occur as a result of severe pain (as in renal or biliary colic and appendicitis), in reflux oesophagitis and in nervous dyspepsia. In the presence of severe abdominal pain, vomiting may be a sign of obstruction. Vomiting can also arise from extra-abdominal causes, such as migraine or a raised intracranial pressure.

In children, vomiting may be caused by fever, unassociated with other abdominal symptoms. This is common in acute systemic viral infections in the young. It is usually of no consequence, unless frequent enough to raise the possibility of dehydration or an alternative cause.

### Dysuria/frequency

Pain or a burning sensation on passing urine, frequency and urgency may suggest a urinary tract infection or a renal stone. Inflammation of other organs in the abdomen, such as the bowel or appendix, can also irritate the urinary tract, causing these symptoms.

### Rash

Severe pain on one side of the trunk is characteristic of herpes zoster infection (shingles), and often precedes the appearance of a rash. The rash follows the course of sensory nerves and may be seen across the front of the upper abdomen or chest, around the side of the trunk and on the back. The rash looks like that of chickenpox (flat at first, then forming pustules and vesicles). Immediate referral is necessary for the doctor to consider treatment with antiviral drugs, which should be started as early as possible after the diagnosis has been made.

### Cough

Sometimes people with acid reflux may have a cough. This is thought to be due to stimulation of the vagus nerve by the reflux of acid into the oesophagus.

### Special considerations in children

Abdominal pain in babies from the age of 2 weeks to 4 months may indicate colic. This usually occurs in the evenings. The baby will draw up its knees and cry, despite being picked up. The condition resolves spontaneously by the age of 4 months.

One serious cause of abdominal pain in babies aged between 4 months and 2 years is intussusception. In this condition, two adjacent sections of bowel telescope together, causing obstruction and an acute abdomen. The condition is a medical emergency.

Projectile vomiting in babies at about 6–8 weeks of age is a possible indicator of obstruction, such as pyloric stenosis. Referral is necessary.

Viral conditions can cause enlargement of the mesenteric lymph glands (in the abdomen) in children. This may produce a non-specific abdominal pain, usually associated with fever, which may be confused with other potentially more serious conditions. It usually resolves spontaneously.

## Management options

Normally, excessive reflux is prevented by tone in the lower oesophageal sphincter and by oesophageal peristalsis. Lifestyle measures can be advised that might help to reduce the symptoms caused by a failure of the former mechanism. Small, regular and frequent meals are better than hurried greasy food binges, and eating late at night should be avoided. Fat in food lowers the tone of the lower oesophageal sphincter, which is undesirable in acid reflux. Sphincter pressure may also be lowered by smoking, alcohol, chocolate, coffee, or even peppermint, which is present in some antacid preparations. Heartburn can often be relieved by raising the head of the bed and by avoiding bending and stooping. Weight reduction may be helpful in relieving symptoms in people who are overweight. Box 2.2 describes some general lifestyle advice that can be given.

Gastric acid suppression can be achieved by traditional antacids such as aluminium and magnesium

---

**Box 2.2  General lifestyle advice**

- Eat small, frequent meals
- Reduce weight if overweight
- Stop smoking
- Reduce alcohol intake
- Reduce caffeine intake
- Reduce chocolate intake
- Reduce fat intake
- Raise the head of the bed when sleeping
- Avoid bending or stooping
- Don't eat a main meal directly before bedtime

salts; by H$_2$-receptor antagonists such as raniti-dine, cimetidine and famotidine; and by PPIs such as omeprazole. Additional agents such as alginates, which form a protective cover over the oesophageal endothelium, can also be used either alone or in combination with acid-suppressant therapy. The most appropriate class of agent can be chosen according to the severity or frequency of the symptoms.

### Antacids (BNF section 1.1.1)

Traditional antacids are perceived to be the least potent of the three classes, but large doses may be as effective as the H$_2$-receptor antagonists. Individual choice and convenience and the type of formulation will often determine which to use. Antacids are relatively fast-acting in suppressing symptoms (about 1 hour) and are particularly suitable for isolated episodes of dyspepsia.

Antacid preparations should be taken either 1 hour before or 1 hour after meals for maximum efficacy. Earlier administration after meals will result in the antacid being ejected from the stomach into the duodenum by gastric emptying, which normally occurs within an hour of eating. Also, food acts as a good buffer against acid attack on the gastric mucosa. Care should be taken in recommending antacids as a number of drugs are known to interact with these (Table 2.2).

**Table 2.2  Major drug interactions with antacids**

| Drug | Effect |
| --- | --- |
| Chlorpromazine | Reduced absorption |
| Ciprofloxacin, norfloxacin | Reduced absorption |
| Digoxin | Reduced absorption |
| Enteric-coated tablets | Coating disrupted in stomach |
| Iron | Reduced absorption |
| Lithium | Serum levels reduced by sodium (bicarbonate) |
| Penicillamine | Reduced absorption |
| Rifampicin | Reduced absorption |
| Sucralfate | Efficacy reduced as pH increases |
| Tetracyclines | Reduced absorption |
| Warfarin and phenindione | Reduced absorption |

### Magnesium salts

Magnesium salts are effective antacids, but in doses required to give symptomatic relief they can cause diarrhoea. Many products, for example magnesium carbonate mixture and magnesium trisilicate mixture, contain a relatively high sodium content, which may be unsuitable for people with heart failure or hypertension.

### Aluminium salts

Antacids containing aluminium are also effective. They are considered by some to be longer-acting than magnesium salts because of a slowing effect on gut transit time. This in turn can lead to constipation. For this reason, they may be considered less suitable than magnesium salts for older people. Many proprietary antacids contain a mixture of aluminium and magnesium.

### Calcium salts

Calcium salts have the reputation of being fast-acting. They can lead to constipation and, theoretically at least, may cause acid rebound by stimulating the secretion of gastrin, which in turn causes more acid to be secreted by the stomach. The clinical significance of this is unclear.

### Bismuth salts

Bismuth is an old-established antacid that is effective but that can cause constipation.

### Sodium bicarbonate

Sodium bicarbonate is a fast-acting antacid but should be avoided in people whose sodium intake needs to be limited. It should not be used on a long-term basis, as it is absorbed and may cause metabolic alkalosis.

### H$_2$-receptor antagonists (BNF section 1.3.1)

H$_2$-receptor antagonists are also relatively fast-acting (about 1 hour) and can be taken once a day and if, for example, they are taken at night, they will provide relief over a period of about 12 hours.

The H$_2$-receptor antagonists should not be taken continuously for longer than 2 weeks without consulting a doctor, to avoid masking symptoms of serious disease.

### Proton pump inhibitors (BNF section 1.3.5)

Proton pump inhibitors such as omeprazole tend to be more potent acid suppressants, but there can be a delay of up to 2 days before maximum symptom relief is felt. They are thus appropriate for treating recurrent symptoms, which may occur several times a week, rather than the isolated episode following a dietary extravagance the night before, although this may be a theoretical strategy rather than a proven practical difference with respect to their use as a non-prescription medicine. The licence for omeprazole in the UK permits its occasional use for longer periods, provided there is symptomatic relief within 2 weeks and that symptoms are controlled by 4 weeks.

### Alginate (BNF section 1.1.2)

Alginates are present in some proprietary medicines and are useful for relieving symptoms of GORD. They are said to form a floating viscous gel on top of the stomach contents. This protects the vulnerable mucous membrane of the oesophagus when the gastric contents are forced up into it. Such medicines are suitable for hiatus hernia and other causes of reflux.

### Domperidone (BNF section 4.6)

Domperidone is a prokinetic agent that stimulates gastrointestinal peristalsis and is licensed as a non-prescription medicine for the relief of postprandial symptoms of dyspepsia, heartburn and nausea. It is thus a useful agent to consider when acid suppressants have been tried without success, or when nausea is an accompanying symptom of indigestion.

### Simeticone (BNF section 1.1.1)

Simeticone reduces the surface tension of the mucus-coated gas bubbles in the stomach and small bowel so that small bubbles coalesce. It is claimed to act as a defoaming agent, allowing gas to be eliminated. It is included in many proprietary antacid mixtures.

 **Re-consider the case**

Before reading further, re-consider the following questions and your initial thoughts on this case.

**Trigger questions**

- What additional information would you need before considering the appropriate management options in this case?
- What issues concern you about this case?
- Are any alarm symptoms being exhibited that require more urgent treatment or referral?

**Case study**

A 30-year-old man comes into the pharmacy and asks you for advice as he has been experiencing pains in his chest and stomach. On further questioning he describes a burning feeling that is often worse after large meals and at night-time. He admits to smoking socially and has a few drinks after his dinner on a regular basis.

 Pharmacist opinion

Anyone presenting with symptoms of chest pain needs careful consideration. In the first instance, cardiac conditions need to be ruled out as the cause of the pain. Although unlikely in a young man, lifestyle factors should also be considered in identifying the potential cause of the presenting symptoms, such as smoking, alcohol intake, diet and working life, including stress. He would also need to be

Pharmacist opinion (*continued*)

asked about the specific location of the pain as pain in the chest radiating to the jaw or left arm would require immediate referral.

He has described a burning feeling, which is a classic symptom of heartburn or GORD, where the acid from the stomach contents causes inflammation of the oesophagus. This burning sensation is common after meals and at night-time. An alginate preparation can give relief to these symptoms if taken after meals and at bedtime; however, a PPI could also be suggested and a review after 2 weeks to ensure that symptoms are controlled. If symptoms persist, a referral to the GP would be appropriate.

General lifestyle advice would also be important for this man as factors such as stress, smoking, alcohol and large meals can exacerbate the condition. He can also consider raising the head of the bed at night to reduce the occurrence of night-time symptoms.

General practitioner opinion

In people with chest symptoms it is important to rule out cardiac causes. The symptoms described by this man relate to meal times, they are not precipitated by exercise and do not radiate to the left arm or neck. Cardiac causes of chest pain in a 30-year-old man would be uncommon.

These symptoms sound like gastro-oesophageal reflux disease. Characteristic features are burning sensations and night-time symptoms. Symptoms are caused by backflow of gastric contents up onto the oesophagus causing inflammation. This can occur with no symptoms and can also present with a dry cough; if left untreated it can lead to problems swallowing. Precipitating factors include smoking, alcohol, caffeine and obesity.

Lifestyle issues need to be addressed here, smoking and alcohol will be making the symptoms worse. Appropriate weight loss should be encouraged, and symptoms may be resolved by weight loss alone. Changing posture at night to an upright position will help to reduce night-time symptoms.

Initial use of a PPI for 1 month often leads to resolution of symptoms. Some people will need long-term treatment. Sodium alginate preparations can also be used for symptom relief. Prokinetic agents that lead to faster passage of food through the stomach into the duodenum are often also prescribed, e.g. domperidone.

Summary of key points

| Condition | Management |
|---|---|
| Dyspepsia is characterised by epigastric pain and heartburn is characterised by a burning sensation in the epigastric region. It occurs commonly after meals and at night. | General lifestyle measures should be addressed such as smoking cessation, losing weight and avoiding aggravating foods. Antacids, $H_2$-receptor antagonists and proton pump inhibitors can be used in management of symptoms. If there is no resolution or improvement of symptoms within 2–4 weeks, sufferer should be referred. |

## When to refer

- Sudden onset of intense pain with no relief
- Symptoms related to medication
- Pain unrelated to meals
- Persistent symptoms not responding to non-prescription medicines
- Age over 55 years with recent onset of dyspepsia
- Blood in stool
- Unexplained weight loss
- Dysphagia
- Swelling (not bloating)
- Vomiting for more than 1–2 days
- Diarrhoea or constipation for more than 1 week
- Dysuria
- Symptoms aggravated by exercise
- Pain radiates to arm, neck or jaw

## Constipation, diarrhoea, IBS

Before reading further, consider the following case and note your initial thoughts.

## Case study

A 23-year-old woman comes into your pharmacy and asks for advice on treating stomach cramps and a change in bowel habit.

**Trigger questions**

- What additional information would you need before considering the appropriate management options in this case?
- What issues concern you about this case?
- Are any alarm symptoms being exhibited that require more urgent treatment or referral?

### Assessing symptoms

#### Change in bowel habit

The normal bowel habit can vary between individuals, from twice daily to once every 2 or 3 days. The normal pattern for the individual should be considered prior to further questioning around symptoms to allow for comparison of any changes.

#### Constipation

Constipation may mean different things to different people and it is important to ask an individual what they mean when they complain of constipation, to ensure that the problem is real in the clinical sense and not imagined. Generally, the following two criteria should be fulfilled: first, there is a change in bowel frequency from the norm for that individual and, second, hard stools are passed, often with difficulty and straining. There are often other symptoms present, such as a feeling of incomplete defecation and abdominal pain and bloating.

The causes of constipation range from simple changes in lifestyle and daily routine to major bowel or systemic disease. If it is persistent and inadequately treated, constipation can lead to some unpleasant complications, such as haemorrhoids, faecal impaction in the colon or rectum, intestinal obstruction or urinary tract complications.

### Duration

Simple transient constipation will resolve spontaneously within a few days. As a general rule it is not necessary to treat acute constipation until the symptom has lasted for 4 days, provided no other symptoms are present. The actual timescale will obviously depend on the individual's previous frequency of bowel movement. If constipation has persisted for up to 14 days then a laxative that is available as a non-prescription medicine should be tried for 4 days. Should there be no bowel movement within this period, a referral is recommended.

In some people, particularly young children and the elderly, constipation may arise from a failure to respond to the desire to defecate. Over a period of months or years this may lead to chronic habitual constipation. If untreated, this may lead to stasis and loss of tone in the muscle of the colon, which in turn may progress to megacolon (permanent dilatation of the large bowel), thus making peristalsis difficult without resort to stimulant laxatives. Bowel habit may be less than once weekly.

### Onset

Possible causes of constipation may be elicited by asking about recent events and changes in lifestyle that may have coincided with the onset of symptoms. For example, changes in the diet, such as reduced fibre intake (in particular insoluble fibre such as wholegrain cereals) or a reduced overall intake (as in dieting or illness), will change the frequency of defecation.

Dehydration caused either by a reduced fluid intake or by prescribing of diuretics will lower the water content of the large bowel and result in hard faeces, which may be difficult to pass. Older people with a low fluid intake are particularly susceptible.

Changes in lifestyle, such as a change in job, shift work, a change in eating patterns or a lack of exercise (e.g. in people confined to bed or those on holiday from an active job), can all contribute to a reduced bowel frequency.

Concurrent disease (see below) and certain drugs may be the cause of constipation in some cases. Also, various physiological changes to the body that occur in old age and in pregnancy cause constipation. Sometimes, constipation-dominant irritable bowel syndrome starts after a gastrointestinal illness.

### Diarrhoea

Diarrhoea is a symptom that requires a clear, quantitative description by the sufferer, as its definition will vary considerably between individuals. A general definition would be a change in normal bowel habit resulting in increased frequency of bowel movements and the passage of soft or watery motions. It is often – but not always – accompanied by colicky pain. Thus, at one end of the spectrum diarrhoea may present as frequent, formed, small stools and at the other as frequent, voluminous watery motions. The difference may sometimes be useful in assessing the severity of the individual's condition.

The most common type of diarrhoea presenting in the pharmacy is acute, and the most likely causes are dietary insults or bacterial or viral infection. The vast majority of these cases will resolve spontaneously in 2 or 3 days without any specific treatment.

Chronic diarrhoea that lasts for weeks rather than days may indicate a pathological cause. It may represent the recurrence or flare-up of a previously diagnosed disorder, such as irritable bowel syndrome, or a problem that requires medical referral for investigation and diagnosis.

About 10 litres of fluid each day pass through the lumen of the intestines of a healthy adult. Some 2–3 litres of this is ingested orally, and the rest is secreted into the lumen along the course of the alimentary tract; 8 or 9 litres of this is reabsorbed from the small intestine, so that about 1 or 2 litres reach the colon. Absorption from the colon or large bowel results in about 200 mL remaining, and this is excreted in the stool. Both the small and large intestines have spare absorptive capacity to cope with more fluid, but it can be appreciated that, with such huge volumes involved, small changes in either the absorptive or the secretory function of the gut can result in a major loss of fluid. This piece of physiology may be educative for a person who is suffering from diarrhoea and will help them to understand how the condition should be managed.

### Severity and type

The severity of diarrhoea may be graded arbitrarily in terms of frequency, volume, duration, and the presence of particular accompanying symptoms.

Any person who suffers severe malaise or pain with diarrhoea for more than 1 or 2 days, without any sign of improvement, should be referred.

### Duration

The common acute types of diarrhoea caused by viruses or bacteria (the latter usually from contaminated food or water) generally resolve spontaneously in 2–3 days, but may take up to 5 days. A simple 'stomach upset' – the result of ingestion of toxins but without living organisms – may resolve in only 12–24 hours. It is therefore reasonable to wait to see whether improvement occurs before making any decision to refer, unless concomitant symptoms dictate otherwise.

Persistent night-time diarrhoea requires medical appraisal for the presence of inflammatory bowel disease, such as Crohn disease or ulcerative colitis.

In young children with diarrhoea the timescale for referral should be shorter than for older children or adults (see 'Special considerations' below).

Chronic diarrhoea, i.e. lasting for weeks, or longer or recurrent episodes usually indicate major pathology, requiring referral. However, in many instances the sufferer will have a known diagnosis, such as irritable bowel syndrome, inflammatory bowel disease, diverticular disease or some malabsorption syndrome, and they will have been advised how to treat the symptoms by their doctor.

### Onset

It should be established whether the onset of symptoms was associated with any particular event. Symptoms occurring within 72 hours of eating food, particularly dairy products, poultry or meat, and especially if others who ate the same food have the same symptoms, suggest a bacterial cause. Onset within 6 hours of eating those foods, together with vomiting, and again, if the symptoms are shared with others who ate the same food, suggests infection with preformed toxins from bacteria.

Association with drug therapy or particular foods should be inquired about. It may be possible to identify an intolerance to particular food items, such as mushrooms, milk or alcohol (usually beer in large amounts). Recent travel to tropical or sub-tropical countries may indicate diarrhoea related to contamination of food or water (so-called travellers' diarrhoea). This is usually of short duration. Persistent symptoms might signify more serious infection, such as bacterial or protozoal dysentery, cholera (bacterial) or giardiasis (protozoal).

### Irritable bowel syndrome (IBS)

Irritable bowel syndrome is an increasingly common condition in individuals who present to their GPs with bowel symptoms. It is characterised by abdominal colicky pain and a change in bowel habit, which may be constipation or diarrhoea or alternate between the two. In so-called constipation-dominant IBS, sufferers often describe bowel movements as inadequate. There is often abdominal bloating and pain.

On investigation, there is no detectable pathology or evidence of organic disease. The condition is common in young adults, and emotion and stress are aggravating factors. Treatment should be tailored to individual symptoms with spasmolytics, analgesics, high-fibre diet and bulk-forming laxatives.

If this has not previously been diagnosed by a doctor, then the individual should be referred to their GP for investigation as treatment with a non-prescription medicine is not licensed and cannot be provided.

Irritable bowel syndrome is a relatively common condition, affecting about 15% of the population and often commencing in the under-40 age group. It is often a diagnosis of exclusion, as there is no specific disease marker. Symptoms vary among sufferers, but characteristically there is recurrent abdominal pain that is relieved by emptying the bowel, urgency, diarrhoea that sometimes alternates with episodes of constipation, abdominal distension and bloating, a feeling of rectal fullness and incomplete evacuation. The diagnosis is often by exclusion of other conditions after the individual has had thorough tests and investigations.

### Stomach cramps

The sufferer should be asked to clarify what they mean by stomach cramps. Similarly to 'pain', stomach cramps can have a variety of meanings for different people, and the specific location and type of cramp should be investigated. These should be considered alongside other symptoms that are being experienced in order to aid the diagnosis.

## Accompanying symptoms

### General malaise

If the individual feels ill or unable to work while having constipation this should be regarded as unusual and a referral to the doctor made to exclude any underlying organic cause. The same applies to any fever or night sweats that may also be experienced.

### Blood and mucus in the stool

In the vast majority of cases, blood noticed on defecation will have a perfectly innocent explanation. Blood noticed as specks or as a light smear on the toilet paper after a bowel movement is most likely to be due to haemorrhoids or a fissure in the anal canal or the skin surrounding it. Straining to defecate can cause or exacerbate haemorrhoids. Fresh blood present only on the surface of the stool has most likely come from the anus or the most distal part of the colon. Blood that is mixed with the faeces, giving a dark colour, often described as tarry, may have a more serious cause, such as diverticulosis, a bleeding peptic ulcer or, rarely, a carcinoma. People taking iron tablets often have a darkened stool, which is of no consequence.

Unless a previous diagnosis of haemorrhoids or a similar condition has been made by a doctor, and there has been no change in the severity of bleeding, it is wise to recommend anyone with rectal bleeding to visit their GP for assessment. If small amounts of blood are seen, as described above, which fit a known diagnosis, the constipation may be treated in the normal way for a few days.

Mucus in the stool is a sign of acute inflammation of the large bowel lining and may present either when there is serious pathology or when there is an acute episode of a less serious, self-remitting condition. It is therefore neither diagnostic nor worrying on its own, but should be considered as a sign for referral if it persists, or if it is accompanied by other worrying symptoms, such as blood in the stool.

### Pain

Continuous or severe abdominal pain accompanying constipation, which has been present for 2 days or more, requires a medical opinion, as the possibility of obstruction in the bowel (possibly caused by a tumour) must be borne in mind. In such cases colicky pain, abdominal distension and vomiting may be present, in addition to constipation that is total, i.e. neither stool nor gas is passed.

Abdominal discomfort is common in diarrhoea. It may present as a sharp, colicky or griping pain, produced by spasm of the smooth muscles of the gut wall and usually felt in the central region of the abdomen, and is generally of no significance. However, severe abdominal pain that is not resolving requires referral.

Rarely, abdominal pain with diarrhoea may represent irritation of the bowel by an inflamed appendix. In such cases the stools are usually not watery or profuse but merely unformed. Acute appendicitis usually begins with pain in the central abdominal region or right flank and there is right-sided tenderness. The pain is continuous, except when perforation occurs, when the pain suddenly stops for 1 or 2 hours and then starts again. The pain of appendicitis wakes the individual at night. Left-sided pain or tenderness, accompanied either by diarrhoea alone or sometimes by alternating episodes of diarrhoea and constipation, may be a sign of diverticular disease.

### Nausea or vomiting

The presence of nausea or vomiting with constipation should be regarded as an unusual sign and the individual should be referred for a medical opinion to eliminate the possibility of intestinal obstruction.

Vomiting with diarrhoea suggests an infective gastroenteritis caused by a virus or bacteria, the latter often from a food source. When vomiting and diarrhoea occur together there is an increased risk that the sufferer will become dehydrated if the condition does not resolve within a few days. Individuals require appropriate advice, especially the young and the elderly. Generally babies with vomiting and diarrhoea require same-day referral, and young children and the elderly should be referred if there is no significant improvement after 48 hours.

Early signs of mild dehydration in adults include increased thirst and a dry mouth, which will respond to increased fluid intake. In babies and young children, more serious signs may be a lack of alertness, and limpness. In adults, lethargy, confusion, tachycardia and cold, clammy skin and a loss of skin elasticity or retraction of the orbit of the eye (sunken eyes) will indicate dehydration, which requires same-day referral.

### Weight loss

Sudden weight loss for no obvious reason is a suspicious sign that requires referral for the doctor to exclude malignancy. Significant weight loss over a few weeks may be a symptom of a previously diagnosed illness causing chronic diarrhoea. However, in all cases where a diagnosis has not been made, referral is necessary to exclude tumours (particularly in the elderly) or malabsorption syndromes.

### Diarrhoea

In young adults, alternating bouts of diarrhoea and constipation, together with abdominal pain, are typical of the irritable bowel syndrome. In older people such symptoms are suggestive of spurious (overflow) diarrhoea. If irritable bowel syndrome has been previously diagnosed by the doctor, bulk-forming laxatives are useful when constipation is the predominant symptom. Failure to control symptoms in this way requires referral. Suspicion of spurious diarrhoea in older people requires investigation and treatment by the doctor.

### Concurrent disease

Hypothyroidism can manifest as constipation, together with lethargy and slowness of movement and mental activity. Depression has been said to cause constipation, although in some cases this may be related to treatment with tricyclic antidepressants.

People who have angina or have recently suffered a myocardial infarction may require laxatives if straining at stool causes chest pain. In addition to previously diagnosed disorders of the bowel, other conditions may cause secondary diarrhoea. For example, hyperthyroidism and diabetes can cause diarrhoea, the latter as a result either of disease of the autonomic nerves in the bowel in long-standing and poorly controlled diabetes, or of the effect of drug treatment.

### Frequency and urgency of micturition

Frequency and urgency of urination are commonly present when there is diarrhoea, which is essentially frequency and urgency of defecation. This is caused by the proximity of the colon and the urinary tract, and the general reflex irritability of smooth muscle in the walls of these hollow organs.

### Dyspareunia (painful intercourse)

In women, dyspareunia is sometimes complained of by sufferers of irritable bowel syndrome. It may be due to proximity to an inflamed or distended colon, although it can be exacerbated by stress.

### Upper respiratory symptoms

Symptoms of the common cold occurring at the same time as diarrhoea suggest a viral infection.

### Fever

A fever, with or without malaise, suggests infection. In adults this may be monitored for a few days, unless the individual has recently returned from a tropical or subtropical country, in which case referral is necessary to exclude diagnoses such as dysentery and malaria.

### Other chronic symptoms

As mentioned above, people with a diagnosed chronic condition will often suffer from other long-term symptoms apart from their chronic diarrhoea, and the majority will be familiar with these and able to cope with them. Such symptoms may include abdominal pain, bloating and abdominal distension, nausea and fatigue. Unless there is a sudden change in the severity of these accompanying symptoms or an otherwise unexpected occurrence, reassurance and, if appropriate, simple symptomatic treatment are all that is required.

## Aggravating factors

Various food intolerances have been shown to cause symptoms in some sufferers of irritable bowel syndrome. These include wheat, dairy products, coffee, potatoes and onions. It is well known that stress or anxiety can induce or exacerbate diarrhoea. Although this is typical of the history of irritable bowel syndrome, which is seen particularly in young adults, it is not exclusive to the condition. Apart from any causative agent involved, diarrhoea may be worsened by dietary changes, such as an increase in fibre or fat content, spices, alcohol, or even an excess of tea or coffee.

## Special considerations

### Pregnancy

During the second and third trimesters of pregnancy an increased amount of circulating progesterone causes relaxation of the smooth muscle of the bowel. This, together with physical compression of the bowel by the growing uterus and the effects of iron therapy, often results in constipation. Other changes in lifestyle in pregnancy, such as reduced exercise and eating fads, increase the tendency to develop constipation. Women can be reassured that the symptom is a natural response of the bowel to pregnancy. If dietary management is not successful, treatment is necessary with non-prescription laxatives, such as bulking agents or senna, because haemorrhoids may develop if constipation is allowed to persist. Although the risk of inducing uterine contraction is theoretical, stimulant laxatives are often avoided in the late stages of pregnancy.

### Children

Babies who are being breast-fed normally produce fewer stools than bottle-fed babies. This is perfectly normal and does not require any intervention. Constipation in a bottle-fed baby may be caused by insufficient water being added to the milk powder, resulting in osmotic diarrhoea. Lactose intolerance can also lead to osmotic diarrhoea. Babies or older children who become irritable, feverish or drowsy, or who scream, have pain, feed or eat less or vomit, should be referred.

As in adults, the frequency of bowel movement in children varies, but the majority pass stools at least once per day. Most children with constipation have ways of withholding the passage of stools. Attempts to defecate are frequently accompanied by pain, causing screaming. The stools become hard, leading to straining and painful defecation, which leads to retention of stools. Common causes in children often relate to unsuitable toilet facilities at school or on holiday, or to teasing by classmates.

Older children may develop phobias about toileting, or may refuse to respond to the call to defecate in order to attract attention. This has the subconscious but desired effect of producing anxiety in the parent, who may become obsessive about the child's bowel habit.

In babies the cause of diarrhoea may be infection, and parents should be advised to take special care when sterilising bottles. Very young children are at increased risk of dehydration. Babies under 6 months old with stools that are loose and more frequent than normal should be referred after 24 hours if the condition is not improving.

Children under 2 years who have diarrhoea for more than 48 hours should be referred if they seem unwell or are not drinking normally. Dehydration can be difficult to judge, but a limp, non-alert baby should be referred as soon as possible. The important fact to remember is that diarrhoea causes water and electrolyte loss, which must be checked, particularly in young children, by giving adequate fluids and, if possible, electrolyte mixtures. Traditionally, treatment of children has also involved restricting food until the diarrhoea improves, but a more modern approach is described below (see 'Management of diarrhoea').

### Older people

Constipation that is more than transient should be viewed with suspicion the older the person is, as bowel cancer becomes increasingly more common above the age of about 50 years.

With increasing age, muscle tone in the bowel is reduced and faecal stasis can occur. In older people regularity of the bowel habit can be an obsession, and they will use laxatives not only to restore the habit to normal but also as a prophylaxis against any future possibility of constipation. This can lead to chronic laxative abuse, causing further reduction in bowel muscle tone and chronic constipation.

Constipation in older people should be taken seriously, as it may reflect a state of dehydration that requires rectifying. A bowel filled with impacted faeces may compress adjacent structures such as the urinary tract and cause urinary retention.

Some older people with impacted faeces may have concomitant diarrhoea. This is caused by small amounts of liquid stool being forced past the impacted stool in the rectum, causing so-called spurious or overflow diarrhoea. In this condition hard faeces obstruct most of the diameter of the bowel lumen. However, some fluid faeces can seep past the impacted mass, leading to a loose, unformed stool that is produced in relatively small amounts. It is most common in the immobile, frail elderly. Treating this condition as diarrhoea will only cause more constipation. The individual should instead be referred for a rectal examination and disimpaction of the faeces.

Older people, like children, are susceptible to the dehydrating effect of diarrhoea, especially those who are taking diuretics and those whose fluid and food intake is poor. It is wise to operate guidelines for referral similar to those described for children under 2 years of age.

### Travellers' diarrhoea

Travellers' diarrhoea is an acute diarrhoea that may be caused by a change in diet (e.g. an increase in oily or spicy food), in climate, or in the mineral content of drinking water. It is usually self-limiting but can be disruptive to holidays or business trips. If it persists, it may be due to infection, often with bacterial toxins such as from *Escherichia coli*, *Campylobacter* or *Shigella*. In some cases the infection may be viral. Infection usually occurs in a country where sanitary conditions are poor or drinking water is contaminated. Persistent cases require further investigation and referral. Box 2.3 provides some advice for travellers abroad.

## Management of constipation

### Laxatives (BNF section 1.6)

For people who have constipation of short duration (less than 14 days), the short-term relief of symptoms should be obtained by a laxative. Stimulant laxatives provide the most rapid effect, whereas osmotic laxatives and bulking agents usually have an onset of action of 2–3 days.

The cornerstone of long-term management is dietary advice, emphasising the value of fibre and

| **Box 2.3 Advice for travellers abroad** |
|---|
| • Drink bottled water or water sterilised with purification tablets |
| • Avoid ice (unless made personally using bottled water) and ice cream |
| • Avoid salads and uncooked vegetables (which may have been washed in contaminated water) |
| • Avoid fruits that cannot be peeled |
| • Avoid unpasteurised milk |
| • Avoid murky swimming pools |

fluid intake. Second-line treatment is the use of bulk laxatives. Insufficiencies in the diet, particularly a lack of insoluble fibre (e.g. wholegrain cereals) or an inadequate fluid intake, are often responsible for bouts of constipation. Reduced intake of refined carbohydrates, such as sugar, cakes and pastry, and education regarding a healthy diet, fluid and exercise, will often solve the problem without resort to laxatives.

As already stated, with the standard Western diet some people will have a bowel movement only once every 2–3 days. There is, however, evidence that such patterns are associated with an increased incidence of bowel problems, such as diverticular disease, and even more sinister problems, including cancer. There is a school of thought that everyone should have a bowel movement at least once per day, and that the diet should be changed – or at least extra fibre added – until this occurs.

Laxatives may be divided into four categories: bulk, stimulant, osmotic and stool softeners. However, some laxatives previously thought to belong to one category only, now appear to have dual modes of action. Liquid paraffin, a lubricant laxative, was popular in the past, but its use is now deprecated because of its many potential adverse effects. These include seepage from the oesophagus into the airways and lungs with devastating effects, and a tendency to reduce the absorption of fat-soluble vitamins.

Although guidance is given for the appropriate use of various classes of laxative, sometimes individual preference and experience, as well as side effects and cost, are important factors to take into consideration when choosing a laxative.

As for the vast majority of conditions and symptoms treated with non-prescription medicines, a failure to produce relief within 7–14 days indicates that the person should seek a medical opinion. This is not only to exclude any significant cause for the constipation, but also to prevent chronic use, leading to laxative abuse, particularly of the stimulant type.

Generally, the approach to simple, acute constipation should be to use stimulant or bulk laxatives. Bulk laxatives are particularly useful in older people, but fluid intake should be adequate too. Dry, hard faeces should be softened with docusate before using a stimulant laxative. People with neurological disorders, such as multiple sclerosis, Parkinson disease, etc., require specialist referral when bowel problems become evident. Treatment of acute constipation in children should be essentially the same as for adults. However, NICE guidance suggests polyethylene glycol and electrolytes as first line treatment options followed by a stimulant laxative if required. Diet and lifestyle advice should also be routinely given to all individuals presenting with constipation.

### Bulk-forming laxatives (BNF section 1.6.1)

Bulking agents act by retaining water in the large bowel, thus increasing stool bulk and stimulating bowel movement and shortening bowel transit time, resulting in a soft stool. They often take 1 or 2 days to exert a significant effect. Examples include methylcellulose, sterculia, ispaghula husk and bran. Wheat bran can cause pain and bloating in some individuals, particularly in those with irritable bowel syndrome, but soluble products such as ispaghula and sterculia appear not to cause the same problems. They are relatively safe to use and are popular because they are inert substances that mimic the natural action of fibrous food in the bowel. They can be recommended to both young and elderly, and are safe for use in pregnancy.

Bulk-forming laxatives should be taken with plenty of fluid to speed transit along the alimentary tract, as cases of oesophageal and bowel obstruction have been reported. This is particularly important in the elderly, who may have a reduced fluid intake or difficulty in swallowing. People who take these agents with inadequate amounts of water immediately before retiring to bed will be prone to oesophageal obstruction.

### Stimulant laxatives (BNF section 1.6.2)

Where bulking agents are inappropriate or ineffective, the stimulant laxatives (irritant or contact laxatives) may be considered, particularly for short-term or infrequent use. They are believed to stimulate nerve endings in the nerve plexuses of the bowel wall causing increased peristalsis. They are faster-acting than the bulk laxatives, and a bowel movement can be expected within 8–12 hours of taking them. They are commonly given at night to provoke a bowel movement the next morning. Examples include senna and bisacodyl. Both of these drugs are safe and effective. Traditional agents in this category, such as castor oil, which is hydrolysed in the bowel to form ricinoleic acid, and phenolphthalein, should not be recommended because of the possibility of unpleasant adverse effects. Senna is safe to use in pregnancy after the first trimester and bisacodyl suppositories (adult and paediatric dosage forms) can produce a bowel movement within 1 or 2 hours of insertion and are therefore useful when a rapid result is desired.

The chronic use of stimulant laxatives has in the past been associated with tolerance and bowel atony, but there is no strong evidence to support this.

People with irritable bowel disease and diverticulosis may take these drugs in combination with bulk laxatives under medical advice. It should be noted that ispaghula, referred to above under 'bulk-forming laxatives', is also sometimes classified as a stimulant laxative, presumably because the increased bulk stimulates bowel movement.

### Osmotic laxatives (BNF section 1.6.4)

Like bulking agents, osmotic laxatives retain fluid within the bowel to stimulate peristalsis and the formation of a soft stool. They tend to be more powerful than the bulk-forming laxatives. The most common agents in this category are magnesium salts, such as magnesium sulphate (Epsom salts), and lactulose.

Magnesium sulphate has a rapid effect, whereas the onset of action of lactulose is generally 2 or 3 days. Magnesium salts are absorbed to some extent and chronic use is not recommended. In people with chronic renal disease they are best avoided, except as a single treatment.

Glycerin suppositories are believed to act by both a local osmotic action and a local stimulant effect. They should not be recommended for children unless all oral medications have been tried and failed.

### Stool softeners

The term 'stool softener' generally refers to those agents that act like detergents by reducing the surface tension of hard faeces in the bowel, allowing water to penetrate the stool. The only drug in this category in common use is docusate sodium. It is useful in people with haemorrhoids who are constipated, and may be valuable in the elderly or for constipation induced by codeine or prescribed opioids. In opioid-induced constipation it should be combined with a stimulant laxative, such as senna, to promote peristalsis.

## Management of diarrhoea

By the time symptoms occur, the bowel mucosa will already have been damaged by bacteria or toxins. It then becomes inflamed and cannot function normally to absorb fluids and electrolytes. Instead, there is a net secretion of fluids into the gut, and although the inflammation will normally subside within a few days, extra fluids are often needed to counteract the fluid loss. The cornerstone of treatment of acute diarrhoea is therefore to maintain an adequate fluid balance (Chapter 8 provides further information on oral preparations for fluid and electrolyte imbalance). This is particularly important in young children and the elderly. If the sufferer complains of thirst, this should be satisfied so that lost body water can be replaced. In adults, bland sugarless drinks, such as water or tea, should be given.

Fasting is generally not necessary if the sufferer wants to eat. This is also true for babies and children. Sufferers will, however, often report that food – even a small amount – goes right through them. Some authorities argue that fasting deprives the infecting bacteria of nutrients in the bowel and thus shortens the illness. More recently, others have argued that it makes no difference to the outcome. It is difficult to give definitive guidelines on this issue.

Breast-fed babies should continue to feed, as there is no evidence that this is deleterious. Although there is no evidence to show that fasting in bottle-fed babies is of any benefit, it is traditional to stop milk feeding for 24 hours, during which time a proprietary oral rehydration solution should be given instead. The next day, the milk feed can be diluted to a quarter of the normal concentration with water, followed by a 50% dilution the next day, three-quarter strength the next day, and finally upgrading to full strength. Fluids or diluted milk feeds should be offered at least every 3 hours. This will maintain nutrition and fluids at the desired level.

### Antimotility drugs (BNF section 1.4.2)

Some authorities decry the use of antidiarrhoeals on the basis that they do not appear to shorten the duration of illness and any benefit is symptomatic. However, for social reasons people will often insist that symptomatic treatment is desirable, and antidiarrhoeal medicines have an obvious placebo effect. All the spasmolytic drugs discussed below are useful for the diarrhoeal phase of irritable bowel syndrome. They can relieve the urgency of defecation and help with the sensation of incomplete evacuation of which people complain.

Loperamide is available from pharmacies and is an effective symptomatic treatment suitable for adults and children over 12 years old. It decreases bowel motility through its action on opioid receptors in the gut and increases bowel transit time, thus permitting the absorption of fluid and electrolytes. It does not possess the potential adverse effects of anticholinergic drugs such as hyoscine and dicyclomine (dicycloverine), and because it does not cross the blood–brain barrier it has no central effects. In addition to its antimotility action, loperamide also exhibits some antisecretory properties. Like other antidiarrhoeal agents, it is not recommended for people with inflammatory bowel disease except under medical supervision, as it may cause constipation, obstruction and dilatation of the bowel (megacolon).

Traditional medicines, such as kaolin and morphine mixture, as well as a number of proprietary products containing morphine, have been popular for the treatment of acute diarrhoea, although there is little objective evidence of their efficacy. However, they can lead to addiction if overused. Kaolin and morphine mixture has been reported to cause hypo-kalaemia because of the liquorice extract it contains, but this is unlikely unless there is chronic usage of large doses.

Codeine, an opioid, like morphine, is available in low dosage in some products available without prescription, but, like morphine, its efficacy at such doses is dubious and may be outweighed by its abuse potential.

### Antispasmodics (BNF section 1.2)

Mebeverine is a direct-acting spasmolytic drug that has no anticholinergic activity. It has been used for many years for the symptomatic treatment of irritable bowel syndrome, and as such it appears to be effective in relieving the abdominal cramps and hypermotility of the large bowel, with few adverse effects.

Like mebeverine, alverine has no anticholinergic activity, but exerts a direct relaxant effect on the bowel smooth muscle and is also an acceptable treatment for the symptoms of irritable bowel syndrome.

Formulations of peppermint oil have been designed to release the oil in the distal small bowel to avoid potential irritable effects in the mouth and oesophagus. Dispersion of the oil in the small bowel allows transport to the large bowel, where the active ingredient, menthol, exerts a direct spasmolytic effect. It has been a popular prescribable treatment for irritable bowel syndrome for many years and is an acceptable addition to, or replacement for, other spasmolytic agents

### Antimuscarinics (BNF section 1.2)

Hyoscine N-butylbromide is an anticholinergic drug licensed for intestinal spasm and irritable bowel syndrome.

### Adsorbents and bulk forming drugs (BNF section 1.4.1)

Adsorbents, such as kaolin, pectin and charcoal, have a traditional place in the mind of the public for the treatment of diarrhoea, although in practice they serve little useful therapeutic purpose. Use of these agents is likely to add bulk to the stool, as they are not absorbed from the gastrointestinal tract. This may, however, lull sufferers into a false sense of security because they could still be losing large quantities of fluid from the bowel, but this will be less readily apparent because of the cosmetic effect of the adsorbent agent.

Bulking agents are usually used to treat constipation, but they can be useful in conditions that produce chronic diarrhoea by absorbing water in the bowel and creating a formed stool. In irritable bowel syndrome, for instance, small doses of ispaghula or sterculia have been used to treat the diarrhoeal phase, but this should be tried carefully because the effect in some people may be to worsen the flatus and bloating. There is some evidence that bran, in contrast to other types of fibre, may worsen the symptoms of irritable bowel syndrome, but this is controversial.

### Bismuth subsalicylate

This agent has been successfully marketed because of its dual site of action in the upper and lower bowel. It is promoted for the treatment of heartburn and nausea as well as diarrhoea. It decreases intestinal motility and permits the absorption of fluids to take place. Because it is converted to salicylate, it should not be given to those with sensitivity to aspirin, nor to children under 16 years.

### Re-consider the case

Before reading further, re-consider the following questions and your initial thoughts on this case.

#### Trigger questions

- What additional information would you need before considering the appropriate management options in this case?
- What issues concern you about this case?
- Are any alarm symptoms being exhibited that require more urgent treatment or referral?

**! Re-consider the case** (*continued*)

**Case study**

A 23-year-old woman comes into your pharmacy and asks for advice on treating stomach cramps and a change in bowel habit.

Pharmacist opinion

This patient would need to be asked further questions about the symptoms she is presenting with. Firstly, she has mentioned a 'change in bowel habit'. This needs to be investigated further to find out what she means by this. It is also important to ask what her normal bowel habit is as it is then easier to compare any changes to what is 'normal' for her. People will often describe diarrhoea or constipation as a change in bowel habit, and in a person of this age, alternating diarrhoea and constipation could be an indication that she is suffering from irritable bowel syndrome. It would also be important to consider whether she has any alarm symptoms such as blood in the stools, nausea or vomiting or weight loss as these would require referral to a GP for investigation.

If IBS has never been diagnosed, then she would need to be referred to the GP for diagnosis as appropriate non-prescription medicines are only licensed in previously diagnosed IBS. If IBS has previously been diagnosed, then treatments available as non-prescription medicines are hyoscine and peppermint oil along with symptomatic relief for both the symptoms of diarrhoea and constipation if necessary. Lifestyle and dietary advice are also important in the management of IBS, especially as both can exacerbate the condition.

General practitioner opinion

These symptoms could be caused by an array of different conditions. Further questioning is needed here to distinguish between the following differential diagnoses:

- Inflammatory bowel disease
- Coeliac disease
- Irritable bowel syndrome
- Gastroenteritis
- Constipation

If the patient was older, bowel cancer would also be on the list. A change in bowel habit may mean many different things and details here are important. A 6-week history of diarrhoea 5 to 10 times a day associated with weight loss would lead to suspicions of inflammatory bowel disease and require specialist input. A history of changing from opening bowels every day to once or twice a week with the occasional stomach cramp would suggest constipation and simple changes to her diet may be all that are needed.

It is clear that a detailed history in this case is extremely important. One of the most common problems in this age group would be irritable bowel syndrome. Typically, symptoms are worse during times of stress. Loose stool and stomach cramps are common symptoms, but the bowels can react to

General practitioner opinion (*continued*)

become more constipated also; other features include abdominal bloating. Part of treatment would be to recognise the symptoms as stress related. Anxiety that the symptoms are caused by something more serious only exacerbates original symptoms. Diarrhoea-predominant IBS can be treated with dietary changes, peppermint preparations, antispasmodics and use of tricyclic antidepressants. Sufferers are usually able to self-manage with a combination of dietary change and intermittent use of medication.

 Summary of key points

| Condition | Management |
|---|---|
| Constipation is defined as a change in bowel frequency from the norm, where hard stools are passed often with difficulty and straining. | Consider use of laxatives for constipation of up to 14 days' duration. If no improvement or symptoms last longer than 14 days, then individual requires referral.<br>Lifestyle advice is also important. |
| Diarrhoea is defined as a change in bowel habit resulting in increased frequency of bowel movements and passage of soft or watery motions. | Dietary and hygiene advice is important and rehydration solutions may be advised to ensure dehydration does not occur. Antidiarrhoeal drugs such as loperamide may also be advised. |
| Irritable bowel syndrome is characterised by alternating constipation and diarrhoea alongside abdominal pain. | Requires referral if not previously diagnosed. |

 When to refer

- Returned from recent travel abroad
- Severe abdominal pain
- Duration longer than 14 days without improvement, particularly in older people and individuals with diabetes, hypothyroidism, haemorrhoids or Parkinson disease, and those who have had strokes or are aged over 40 who present with a sudden change in bowel habit for the first time
- Taking long-term laxatives, unless prescribed by the doctor
- Constipation and not passing flatus
- Fluctuating constipation and diarrhoea, unless already investigated by the doctor
- Showing signs of dehydration
- Where symptoms do not improve with time or where symptoms get worse
- Blood in stools
- Nausea of longer than 3–4 days in duration
- Loss of appetite for longer than 3–4 days
- Unexplained weight loss
- Fatigue
- Fever
- Pregnancy or breastfeeding
- Diarrhoea waking sufferer at night for more than 2–3 nights
- Special care for children suffering constipation or diarrhoea and referral after 48–72 hours depending on symptoms

# Haemorrhoids

Before reading further, consider the following case and note your initial thoughts.

 **Case study**

A 50-year-old woman comes into your pharmacy. She mentions that she has recently been experiencing pain when defecating and is worried that it is something serious as she has noticed some spots of blood when she has been cleaning herself.

**Trigger questions**

- What additional information would you need before considering the appropriate management options in this case?
- What issues concern you about this case?
- Are any alarm symptoms being exhibited that require more urgent treatment or referral?

## Assessing symptoms

### Pain

It is important to establish the nature of any reported pain. Pain associated with haemorrhoids can also be described as a pressure and may be treated symptomatically without referral to a GP for further investigation.

More severely affected individuals, especially those with external haemorrhoids, may suffer intense pain. Anal fistulae or fissures in the anal canal are also painful. Anyone complaining of severe pain should be referred for examination and an accurate diagnosis.

### Blood in stools

Ideally, any rectal bleeding requires a diagnosis by a doctor, especially in middle-aged and older people, to exclude any serious cause. Blood in the stool is common in people with haemorrhoids; if bleeding is noted just as spotting or streaks on the toilet paper after defecation, a non-prescription medicine and advice will usually be appropriate, at least for a short time, particularly if the individual is reticent about seeing a doctor.

Because the vast majority of people will not consult their GP about mild cases of haemorrhoids, it is easy for them to become blasé about the presence of blood. Although the correct advice is to refer everyone with rectal bleeding who has not received a diagnosis from a doctor, some people with mild haemorrhoids will prefer to self-diagnose.

As blood present in the stools is one of the classic alarm symptoms, all of the presenting symptoms must be taken into account before recommending treatment, as the presence of symptoms such as loss of weight, or nausea and vomiting would suggest that referral would be more appropriate for investigation of the underlying cause. The duration of symptoms must also be taken into account, as symptoms persisting for a longer duration and particularly if non-prescription treatment is not relieving symptoms would require referral.

Fresh blood coating the stool is typical of lesions in the descending colon and rectum, and individuals with this symptom should be referred to exclude serious pathology. Similarly, any blood that is evident in the flush water in the toilet requires referral. Blood mixed in the stool, giving a dark red or black tarry appearance, suggests that the source is higher in the gastrointestinal tract. This is typical of bleeding gastric or duodenal ulcers, or lesions such as polyps or cancers in the colon. Such cases should be referred for further investigation.

## Accompanying symptoms

### Itching

People with mild cases of haemorrhoids, or in the early stages of the condition, will complain of itching in the perianal region. This is common and thought to be due to irritation caused by the haemorrhoids and also due to a discharge that may occur.

### Constipation

Constipation is one of the contributing factors to development of haemorrhoids and in itself must be treated if it occurs. Constipation can cause the passing of large stools and straining while attempting to defecate. Both of these can cause an increase in the pressure of the veins around the anal area and can be a contributing factor in the development of haemorrhoids. The symptoms of haemorrhoids can also be worse directly after a bowel motion.

## Aggravating symptoms

Someone with haemorrhoids may relate their onset to a cough, sneeze, or episode of physical exertion. They may first appear when straining at stool, or during episodes of constipation. Haemorrhoids can often recur. Aggravating factors, such as constipation, can sometimes be identified and it is important that these are dealt with as well as the haemorrhoids themselves.

Haemorrhoids are common in pregnancy and are thought to be due to the increase in pressure due to the location of the baby and hormonal changes.

## Management

### Soothing and compound haemorrhoidal preparations (BNF sections 1.7.1 and 1.7.2)

Non-prescription treatments for haemorrhoids are available as suppositories, creams and ointments. Most contain mixtures of astringents (bismuth salts), local anaesthetics, antiseptics, antipruritics, zinc and other miscellaneous substances. However, the most effective preparation is likely to be one that contains hydrocortisone, a proven anti-inflammatory agent. Care should be taken against protracted use, because the perianal skin can become steroid dependent if topical steroids are used for a prolonged period. Preparations containing local anaesthetics should only be used for short periods because of the risk of sensitisation of the skin.

People with haemorrhoids should be advised that constipation will exacerbate the symptoms of haemorrhoids. They should be recommended a laxative for the short term and counselled about adding more roughage (or bran) to the diet and increasing fluid intake. Bulking agents, such as ispaghula and sterculia, are suitable, but if constipation has been present for some time, or is particularly stubborn, a stimulant laxative such as senna may be appropriate to obtain the first motion. They should be advised not to put off the call to defecate and to avoid prolonged straining.

Pregnant women who suffer from haemorrhoids should be advised to increase the fibre content of their diet, as the high progesterone levels in pregnancy have the effect of relaxing the smooth muscle of the bowel.

The cornerstone of relieving the symptoms of haemorrhoids is perianal hygiene. The perianal skin should be washed at least once daily and then patted dry, to prevent irritation by faecal matter in the perianal folds.

### Re-consider the case

Before reading further, re-consider the following questions and your initial thoughts on this case.

**Trigger questions**

- What additional information would you need before considering the appropriate management options in this case?
- What issues concern you about this case?
- Are any alarm symptoms being exhibited that require more urgent treatment or referral?

**Case study**

A 50-year-old woman comes into your pharmacy. She mentions that she has recently been experiencing pain when defecating and is worried that it is something serious as she has noticed some spots of blood when she has been cleaning herself.

Pharmacist opinion

The symptoms that this patient has described are common in people who suffer from haemorrhoids. Although the presence of blood is considered to be an alarm symptom, if the blood appears as bright red spots it is suggestive of a condition such as haemorrhoids as the blood is produced as a result of straining to defecate. Haemorrhoids are often caused by constipation, and so as well as symptomatic treatment, lifestyle advice and laxatives may also be advisable if constipation is found to be a contributing factor.

Further conversation would need to be had with the patient to determine whether the haemorrhoids were external or internal and a suitable local anaesthetic preparation advised such as suppositories or an external cream or ointment. In some cases where symptoms are severe and the individual has already tried some treatment and it has failed, it would be appropriate to refer to the GP as surgical intervention may be appropriate. The presence of any alarm symptoms such as weight loss, blood (other than what has previously been described), nausea or vomiting would also need to be referred for further investigation.

 General practitioner opinion

The presence of blood usually does cause alarm; however, the history here is suggestive of haemorrhoids.

This woman is in an age group where the possibility of more serious causes of bleeding would need serious consideration. A clear history of constipation, hard stools and straining to defecate would support a diagnosis of haemorrhoids. The blood is usually bright red, found on the toilet paper or in the toilet bowl. There may be an associated anal fissure, which is caused as the anal canal stretches during passage of large hard stool.

Symptoms of weight loss, diarrhoea, blood mixed in with stool or vomiting would need further investigation.

Treatment of haemorrhoids involves tackling the cause, which is normally constipation. Pressure in the abdomen puts strain on the blood vessels within the rectal mucosa leading to varicosity, exactly the same as varicose veins that are common in the legs.

Local anaesthetic creams will relieve symptoms in the short term. Dietary changes may be needed to resolve constipation, and faecal softeners are also helpful. Stimulant laxatives can be used, but if stool is still hard it can cause cramping pain.

Persistent symptoms warrant examination of the rectum as anal cancer can mimic symptoms of haemorrhoids. Occasionally, haemorrhoids do not respond to medical treatment, symptoms can become intolerable and surgical intervention is required.

 Summary of key points

| Condition | Management |
| --- | --- |
| Haemorrhoids are characterised by pain or an uncomfortable feeling when defecating and blood often appears either on the outside of the stools or on toilet paper when cleaning. Constipation is a common pre-disposing and aggravating factor. | Symptomatic treatment containing local anaesthetics and antipruritics are available as both internal and external preparations. |

**When to refer**

- Severe pain
- Presence of thrombosed haemorrhoid
- Infection present, e.g. perianal abscess
- Anal fissure or fistula

## Bibliography

Banks M, Farthing M (2003). Acute diarrhoea: guide to acute management. *Prescriber* 19 Oct: 48–59.

British Society of Gastroenterology (2007). *Guidelines on the Irritable Bowel Syndrome: Mechanisms and Practical Management*. Available at: http://www.bsg.org.uk/clinical-guidelines/small-bowel-nutrition/guidelines-on-the-irritable-bowel-syndrome-mechanisms-and-practical-management.html (accessed 26 July 2011).

Douglas G *et al.*, eds (2005). *MacLeod's Clinical Examination*. Edinburgh: Churchill Livingstone.

Kumar P, Clark M, eds (2005). *Clinical Medicine*. London: Elsevier Saunders.

Drug and Therapeutics Bulletin (2004). Probiotics for gastro-intestinal disorders. *Drug Ther Bull* 42(11): 85–88.

Kamm MA (2003). Constipation and its management. *Br Med J* 327: 459–460.

National Institute for Health and Clinical Excellence (2004). *Dyspepsia: Managing Dyspepsia in Adults in Primary Care*. London: National Institute for Health and Clinical Excellence.

National Institute for Health and Clinical Excellence (2009). *Diarrhoea and Vomiting in Children Under 5*. London: National Institute for Health and Clinical Excellence.

National Institute for Health and Clinical Excellence (2010). *Constipation in Children and Young People*. London: National Institute for Health and Clinical Excellence.

National Prescribing Centre (2004). The management of constipation. *MeReC Bulletin*, 14: 1–4.

Scottish Intercollegiate Guidelines Network (2003). *Dyspepsia an Evidence Based Approach to Investigation and Management*. Edinburgh: Scottish Intercollegiate Guidelines Network.

## Self-assessment questions

The following questions are provided to test the information presented in this chapter.

*For questions 1–7 select the best answer in each case.*

1. Select which of the following is a correct definition of heartburn:
   a. Pain in the epigastric region which radiates to the left arm
   b. Pain in the epigastric region which occurs after meals
   c. Epigastric pain and sensitivity in the abdominal area
   d. Pain in the abdominal area which is worse at night
   e. Epigastric pain which has occurred after ibuprofen use

2. Select which of the following is not a referral criterion for gastrointestinal symptoms:
   a. Dysphagia
   b. Regular use of ibuprofen
   c. Unintentional weight loss
   d. Malaise
   e. Gastrointestinal bleeding

3. Select which of the following does not interact with antacids:
   a. Amoxicillin
   b. Digoxin
   c. Oxytetracycline
   d. Enteric-coated aspirin
   e. Iron sulphate

4. Select which of the following is not a common presenting symptom for constipation:
   a. Hard stools
   b. Bloating
   c. Infrequent defecating compared to normal habit
   d. Straining to defecate
   e. Presence of blood in stools

5. Select which of the following is considered to be the most effective treatment for haemorrhoids:
   a. Lidocaine
   b. Hydrocortisone
   c. Bismuth oxide
   d. Zinc oxide
   e. Benzyl benzoate

6. Select which of the following is not a common symptom associated with haemorrhoids:
   a. Itch
   b. Fresh blood coating the stool
   c. Discomfort when defecating
   d. Constipation
   e. Dark red blood incorporated in the stool

7. Select which of the following people would be suitable for treatment with senna:
   a. An elderly woman with symptoms of constipation who has been taking paracetamol and codeine regularly for 2 days
   b. A man who has been experiencing symptoms of constipation for 3 weeks
   c. A 55-year-old man who has had constipation for 2 days following 3 days of diarrhoea
   d. A woman who is 8 weeks pregnant and starting to experience symptoms of constipation
   e. A 45-year-old woman who is experiencing constipation and who has been taking lactulose for 2 weeks

*For questions 8–10 select from the list below one lettered option which is most closely related to it. Each lettered option may be used once, more than once, or not at all.*
   a. 1 hour
   b. 12 hours
   c. 1–2 days
   d. 2 weeks
   e. 4 weeks

8. Is the of onset of action for antacids.

9. Anyone who has symptoms of persistent vomiting should be referred after this point.

10. Is the duration of action of an $H_2$-antagonist.

*For questions 11–12 select from the list below one lettered option which is most closely related to it. Each lettered option may be used once, more than once, or not at all.*
   a. ranitidine
   b. magnesium salts
   c. sodium bicarbonate
   d. omeprazole
   e. dimeticone

11. Diarrhoea is a very common side effect

12. Is a proton pump inhibitor

*Questions 13–16: Each of the questions or incomplete statements in this section is followed by three responses. For each question one or more of the responses is/are correct. Decide which of the responses is/are correct and then choose a–e as indicated in the table below.*

| Directions summarised | | | | |
|---|---|---|---|---|
| a | b | c | d | e |
| If 1, 2 and 3 are correct | If 1 and 2 only are correct | If 2 and 3 only are correct | If 1 only is correct | If 3 only is correct |

13. The following medicines can be supplied from a pharmacy without a prescription to treat symptoms of dyspepsia:
    1 – ranitidine tablets
    2 – sodium alginate and potassium bicarbonate suspension
    3 – pantoprazole tablets

14. The following medicines can be supplied from a pharmacy without a prescription to treat symptoms of IBS in someone who is 15 years old and has previously been diagnosed with IBS:
    1 – domperidone tablets
    2 – mebeverine hydrochloride tablets
    3 – peppermint oil capsules

15. The following are common presenting symptoms of diarrhoea:
    1 – defecating more frequently than normal
    2 – passing watery stool
    3 – a colicky type pain

16. Diarrhoea
    1 – requires antibiotic treatment
    2 – should always be referred for investigation
    3 – is most commonly caused by a bacterial or viral infection

*Questions 17–20 consist of two statements linked by the word* because; *decide whether each statement is true or false. If both statements are true then decide whether the second statement is a correct explanation of the first statement. Choose a–e as your answer as indicated in the table below.*

| Directions summarised | | | |
|---|---|---|---|
| | First statement | Second statement | |
| a | True | True | Second statement is a correct explanation of the first statement |
| b | True | True | Second statement is not a correct explanation of the first statement |
| c | True | False | |
| d | False | True | |
| e | False | False | |

17.

| | | |
|---|---|---|
| Epigastric pain radiating to the jaw and left arm should be referred immediately for investigation | BECAUSE | Cardiac illnesses present with similar symptoms to dyspepsia and should always be investigated if cardiac symptoms are present |

**18.**

| A person who has symptoms of reflux should be advised to stop smoking | BECAUSE | Nicotine interacts with possible pharmacological treatments used in reflux |
|---|---|---|

**19.**

| Magnesium salts are effective in treating the symptoms of heartburn | BECAUSE | Alginates form a 'raft' effect on top of the stomach contents. |
|---|---|---|

**20.**

| Individuals with haemorrhoids should only be offered dietary advice | BECAUSE | Constipation is a pre-disposing factor to developing haemorrhoids |
|---|---|---|

## Answers

1-b; 2-d; 3-a; 4-e; 5-b; 6-e; 7-a; 8-a; 9-c; 10-b; 11-b; 12-d; 13-b; 14-c; 15-a; 16-e; 17-a; 18-c; 19-b; 20-d

# 3

# Respiratory System

*Brian Addison*

| **This chapter will cover the following conditions:** | **This chapter will cover the following groups of medicines:** |
|---|---|
| • Cough<br>• Sinusitis<br>• Hay fever/allergic rhinitis<br>• Flu/influenza<br>• Common cold<br>• Sore throat<br>• Tonsillitis<br>• Croup<br>• Whooping cough | • Demulcents<br>• Expectorants<br>• Cough suppressants<br>• Antihistamines<br>• Decongestants (topical and oral)<br>• Nasal corticosteroids<br>• Sodium cromoglicate |

In this chapter we will consider the symptoms of common minor illnesses of the respiratory tract that are encountered in pharmacies and the major diseases that these need to be differentiated from. This chapter will also consider general approaches to dealing with these conditions and the specific groups of drugs that can be used to manage these conditions.

The respiratory system's main role is to absorb oxygen from the atmosphere and to remove waste gases from the body, primarily carbon dioxide. The respiratory tract can be separated into the upper respiratory tract comprising the nasal cavity, pharynx and larynx, and the lower respiratory tract comprising the trachea, bronchi and lungs. The respiratory tract is also connected to the ears via the Eustachian tubes and thus conditions that affect the respiratory tract can also produce symptoms in the ear.

The symptoms that manifest in the respiratory tract can often occur in a number of different conditions/disease states and it is important to view the complete symptom picture that is presented; for example, viral infections are a common cause of both colds and sore throats and both can occur at the same time. A runny nose can be caused by a cold but also occurs in hay fever. Similarly, a cough can be caused by a cold but can also be a symptom of asthma.

## Sneezing, congestion, rhinorrhoea, fever

Before reading further, consider the following case and note your initial thoughts.

### ? Case study

A fit 25-year-old man comes into the pharmacy. 'Nothing serious', he explains, 'certainly nothing to keep me off work.' He describes experiencing sneezing, nasal congestion and a runny nose. He also complains of a little wheeze on exertion and a fever. But he feels that it is nothing to worry his doctor about.

**Trigger questions**

- What additional information would you need before considering the appropriate management options in this case?
- What issues concern you about this case?
- Are any alarm symptoms being exhibited that require more urgent treatment or referral?

## Assessing symptoms

### Sneezing

Sneezing is an expulsion of air from the lungs through the nose and mouth, usually in response to irritation of the nasal mucosa by foreign particles. It can be a feature of the common cold and of hay fever.

The common cold is caused by infection with rhinoviruses, the majority of them belonging to a group called the picornaviruses. The common cold

is highly infectious and spread by close personal contact and by nasal droplets produced by sneezing.

The influenza virus is also spread by close personal contact and sneezing but produces a much more serious and potentially life-threatening condition in some at-risk groups, e.g. in the elderly, those with respiratory conditions, and those with chronic diseases. There are two main forms of the influenza virus, influenza A and influenza B, but both belong to the orthomyxovirus group (see Table 3.1).

The common cold produces a mildly systemic upset characterised by tiredness, slight pyrexia, malaise, sore nose and a watery nasal discharge. Influenza, however, causes a fever, shivering and generalised aching in the limbs that usually starts abruptly.

If nasal symptoms are the result of the common cold then they would be expected to last for only a few days and not longer than 2 weeks. If sneezing has lasted for this duration, it should be re-assessed bearing in mind the possibility of hay fever.

Hay fever is better described as seasonal allergic rhinitis and is defined by the presence of sneezing attacks and nasal discharge or blockage for more than an hour on most days. If this occurs for a limited period of the year it is described as seasonal; however, if it is present throughout the year it is described as perennial. Nasal irritation, sneezing and watery rhinorrhoea are the most troublesome symptoms.

In allergic rhinitis, sneezing is likely to be paroxysmal (occurring as a bout or fit of repetitive sneezing) and accompanied by itchiness in the nose and/or palate, which some sufferers experience before the onset of nasal symptoms. It is also useful to consider the existence of a family or personal history of asthma and/or eczema, which raises the suspicion of allergy. Considering the presence or absence of these

| Table 3.1 | Forms of influenza virus |
|---|---|
| **Form** | **Description** |
| Influenza A | Causes worldwide pandemics and has capacity to develop new antigenic variants |
| Influenza B | Is associated with localised outbreaks of a milder nature |

| Table 3.2 | Classification of allergic rhinitis |
|-----------|-------------------------------------|
| **Classification** | **Definition** |
| Intermittent | Symptoms occur at the same time each year. When seasonal allergic rhinitis is caused by grass and tree pollen allergens, it is also known as hay fever. It lasts for less than 4 weeks or less than 4 days per week, although because of multisensitisation hay fever sufferers may have a longer season. |
| Perennial | Symptoms last more than 4 weeks or more than 4 days per week, typically because of allergens from house dust mites and pets. There is sensitivity to various components in the atmosphere, such as pollen, mould spores, dust and pollutants. |
| Occupational | Symptoms are due to exposure to allergens at work, for example, flour allergy in a baker. |

symptoms will help to distinguish an allergic cause from a viral infection.

In the summer months in the United Kingdom, allergic rhinitis is most likely to be caused by pollen allergy. In the UK 90% of 'hay fever' sufferers are allergic to grass pollen (most prolific from May to July) and 25% have an allergy to tree pollen (March to May). At other times of the year allergy may be due to hypersensitivity to antigens found in dust, the spores of some fungi (late summer to early autumn), animal dander, feathers and other materials in the home or workplace. This type of allergy may persist throughout the year and is termed perennial rhinitis, producing symptoms either continuously or in irregular episodes when the allergen in the atmosphere is particularly high. Table 3.2 describes a historical classification of allergic rhinitis; more recently allergic rhinitis has been classified by severity and persistence of symptoms. Such classifications, although reported in the literature, are limited in their usefulness in determining an appropriate treatment for an individual.

## Nasal congestion

Nasal congestion is caused by an inflammatory reaction in the lining of the nose, causing dilatation and engorgement of blood vessels and oedema of the mucous membrane. Nasal congestion is the most unpleasant and inconvenient symptom of the common cold but it can be caused by some drugs, in particular antihypertensive agents, that inhibit the sympathetic nervous system (e.g. alpha- and beta-blocking drugs) and oral contraceptives. Excess mucus may or may not be a feature of nasal congestion but if it is present and is clear and watery this may indicate allergic rhinitis, although this may also be the case with the common cold, at least initially.

## Rhinorrhoea (runny nose)

Rhinorrhoea is a discharge from the nasal mucous membrane. Mucus is produced by the membrane as a protective measure of the airways and its production may be increased as a defensive mechanism to protect the nasal cavity and airways. Rhinorrhoea can often accompany nasal congestion as the dilatation and engorgement of blood vessels that occur in nasal congestion stimulate the mucus-secreting glands in the mucosa. Rhinorrhoea can be a symptom of allergic rhinitis and the common cold. In allergic rhinitis the mucus will probably be clear and watery; this may also be the case, at least initially, in someone suffering from the common cold, although the mucus can be thicker and yellowish green in the common cold. However, excess mucus, particularly if it is purulent, would be suggestive of a possible bacterial infection.

## Fever

Fever is when the body temperature is raised above the normal temperature of 37°C. A fever in adults with headache, especially with aching muscles, aching joints and/or general malaise, is common in viral infections and sometimes accompanies other symptoms of upper respiratory tract infection. A raised temperature may be a common accompaniment to a viral or bacterial throat infection and as such is of no great significance. However, someone with a persistent sore throat who complains of heavy sweats at night should be advised to see a doctor for a check-up, especially if the lymph nodes in the neck are enlarged, as in rare cases this might reflect a neoplastic disease such as lymphoma. A high temperature in children raises the rare possibility of a convulsion and so should be treated. It is a sudden rise in temperature rather than a persistently elevated temperature that is thought to cause these convulsions.

## Accompanying symptoms

Often nasal symptoms can be accompanied by a host of other symptoms such as shivering, sweating, headaches, sore throat and sometimes earache, the latter especially in children. Other symptoms also include those detailed below.

### Conjunctivitis (red eye)

Conjunctivitis is an inflammation of the anterior eye and is a common cause of red eye. It may be a sign of a common viral infection such as the common cold as it is possible for infections of the nasal mucosa to extend through the nasolacrimal duct to the conjunctiva of the eye. But red eyes are probably better known as an accompaniment to allergic rhinitis. In allergic rhinitis the eyes usually itch and the sufferer will rub them, whereas in the common cold this is not a predominant feature. Eye conditions are considered in more depth in Chapter 7.

### Myalgia

Myalgia (aching muscles and joints) can commonly accompany a viral respiratory infection, when the diagnosis is often known as flu or influenza and unless persistent it is of no consequence provided the sufferer feels relatively well. Influenza is a viral infection that produces upper and sometimes also lower respiratory symptoms accompanied by systemic symptoms such as malaise, myalgia and fever. True influenza can only be diagnosed during epidemics, and confirmation of an epidemic is given by public health teams. In the absence of this official label, the majority of such cases are labelled 'flu-like'. The distinction clinically can be less clear. At-risk groups, such as the elderly and those with chronic diseases, especially respiratory conditions but also cardiovascular disease and diabetes, should be advised to inquire from their local medical practice about their suitability for vaccination against influenza.

### Sinusitis

Sinusitis is an infection of the paranasal sinuses (Figure 3.1) that is most commonly associated with upper respiratory tract infection. *Streptococcus pneumoniae* and *Haemophilus influenzae* are the main causative organisms of sinusitis, although

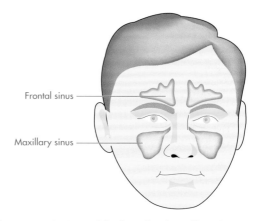

**Figure 3.1**  Position of the frontal and maxillary sinuses.

occasionally a fungal infection can also be the cause. Sufferers experience tender sinuses and headache (which may be unilateral or bilateral) and this can be accompanied by the common cold and nasal congestion. A green, purulent nasal discharge may also be a feature. The skin over the sinuses (around the orbit of the eye) is sensitive to pressure applied by the fingers.

In most cases sinusitis can be managed by providing symptomatic relief such as simple analgesia with paracetamol or ibuprofen and/or a nasal decongestant. Antibiotics are not normally required as sinusitis is usually caused by a virus. It is important that the sufferer understands that it can take around 2½ weeks for symptoms to resolve, which is longer than for the common cold.

## Management options

The best approach is to provide symptomatic relief for the specific symptoms that have been reported. Traditional advice for the common cold has been to take some aspirin or paracetamol, to keep warm and to drink plenty of fluids; this is generally sound advice. A high fluid intake maintains adequate hydration of the body to counteract excessive fluid loss caused by fever. It also increases hydration of the mucous membranes. Steam inhalation provides local hydration of the tissues of the upper respiratory tract and may work by diluting the secretion of mucus, making it less viscous and tenacious. Although the use of steam inhalation is based on folklore and anecdote, it is harmless and can be safely included in any supportive advice given in

---

**Box 3.1   Allergen avoidance advice**

- Stay indoors when the pollen count is high.
- Keep windows closed.
- Avoid parks and fields and obvious areas where pollen count will be high.
- Use sunglasses when going outside.
- Wash hands and face on returning indoors.
- If there is a pet in the house, its fur should be wiped down after it has been outside.
- A filter mask that covers the nose and mouth can be effective, especially if someone's activities cannot be confined indoors.

---

addition to recommending an appropriate non-prescription medicine. It is important when steam inhalation is recommended that the sufferer is cautioned about the potential for scalding the nasal passages if the water used is too hot; boiling water should not be used.

Some relief of allergic rhinitis can be obtained by allergen avoidance, provided the allergen is known. Box 3.1 describes some measures that can be taken; these are no more than common sense but are worth pointing out to sufferers, who may be too focused on hoping that a medicine is going to provide total relief.

In recent years the UK government has promoted a campaign to encourage members of the public to adopt appropriate hygiene measures. These measures include always carrying a tissue to catch a sneeze or cough, disposing of the tissue as soon as possible, and washing hands as soon as possible after sneezing or coughing. These measures aim to minimise the transmission of the viruses that cause upper respiratory tract infections, particularly during the cold and flu season.

### Aromatic inhalations (BNF section 3.8)

Menthol and other oils, such as eucalyptus, are present in many formulations that alleviate the symptoms of the common cold. These include inhalations, pastilles and nasal sprays. As well as having a great placebo effect, these oils do appear to relieve nasal congestion by a cooling effect on the mucous membranes. They are also useful in the relief of nasal obstruction in acute rhinitis or sinusitis. The use of strong aromatic inhalations in children under the age of 3 months is not advised. These oils should not be used regularly for long periods as they may damage the cilia in the respiratory mucosa.

### Antihistamines (BNF section 3.4)

Antihistamines are effective in nasal symptoms because of their intrinsic anticholinergic properties, although there is less evidence to support their use in upper respiratory tract infections in comparison with symptoms of an allergic origin. The drugs suppress the production of mucus in the nasal mucosa and thus give symptomatic relief in rhinorrhoea, as well as reducing the postnasal drip that irritates the pharynx and causes coughing. They also reduce the cholinergic transmission of impulses in the nervous pathway of the cough reflex and thus can act as a cough suppressant. Because of their anticholinergic effects, antihistamines should not be recommended to anyone with narrow-angle glaucoma or prostatism. They can also cause dry mouth, constipation and palpitations, and can interfere with accommodation in the eye.

The first-generation antihistamines such as chlorphenamine, diphenhydramine and promethazine are well known for their sedative and anticholinergic effects, but have been largely superseded by the second-generation drugs such as loratadine, cetirizine and acrivastine, which are less likely to cause sedation. The second-generation antihistamines are more effective in relieving sneezing, itching and rhinorrhoea than nasal congestion.

Nasal sprays and eye drops are available containing azelastine and levocabastine. They have a rapid onset of action compared with oral antihistamines (15 minutes, compared with 1–3 hours). The nasal sprays are effective in relieving nasal itchiness, runny nose and sneezing, but not so effective for nasal congestion. This is because they have some anticholinergic activity and dry up secretions. Nasal decongestants or intranasal steroids can be used with the antihistamine if necessary to relieve congestion. A combination of the antihistamine antazoline and sympathomimetic xylometazoline is available as eye drops for the relief of itchy, allergic conjunctivitis. Antihistamine eye drops can cause temporary local irritation and this is important advice to impart when supplying these products.

### Intranasal steroids (BNF section 12.2.1)

Nasal sprays containing steroids, such as beclometasone, budesonide and fluticasone, are effective in alleviating rhinorrhoea, itchiness and sneezing as well as nasal congestion in allergic rhinitis via a local anti-inflammatory effect. They may take several days to exert maximum effect and should be used regularly as a prophylactic measure. They can be used as combination therapy with an oral or topical antihistamine – the latter used for intermittent flare-ups and the steroid spray for the persistent symptoms. However, they are licensed for supply without a prescription only for the prevention and treatment of allergic rhinitis in adults over 18 years subject to a maximum single and daily dose. The use of higher doses or use in individuals under the age of 18 requires these products to be prescribed and supplied via a prescription.

### Sodium cromoglicate (BNF section 12.2.1)

The mast cell stabiliser sodium cromoglicate can be sold to the public as eye drops for the treatment of acute seasonal and perennial allergic conjunctivitis, subject to a maximum pack size. The eye drops require to be administered four times a day and provide relief from the symptoms of allergic conjunctivitis, such as itchy and runny eyes. Mast cell stabilisers prevent the release of histamine from mast cells and therefore should be considered as a prophylactic treatment and will only be effective with continued administration.

### Systemic nasal decongestants (BNF section 3.10)

Phenylephrine, ephedrine and pseudoephedrine are the most commonly used oral sympathomimetic agents. Sympathomimetics stimulate alpha-adrenoceptors, causing vasoconstriction in the nasal mucosa, resulting in shrinkage of the inflamed tissue and an increase in the lumen of the nasal passages, facilitating breathing and drainage of mucus. They also possess some beta-agonist activity, which confers some bronchodilator effects and hence they can be found in combination remedies for coughs and colds, although this beta-activity has the potential to disturb blood glucose control by an anti-insulin effect, and hence they should be used with caution in diabetes. Their use is also cautioned in hypertension, hyperthyroidism, pregnancy and ischaemic heart disease because of their ability to increase blood pressure. Products containing sympathomimetics should be avoided in anyone taking monoamine oxidase inhibitors.

Systemic effects of sympathomimetics can be minimised by using a locally acting formulation such as nasal drops or spray, providing rapid and effective relief from nasal congestion when applied to the nasal membranes. The most commonly used are phenylephrine, which is relatively short acting, and oxymetazolone and xylometazolone, which are claimed to have duration of action of up to 8 hours. They produce relatively few systemic side effects because the local vasoconstriction reduces drug absorption from the site of application. However, the use of local decongestants is associated with a phenomenon known as rhinitis medicamentosa, which is a rebound effect whereby congestion follows the vasoconstriction. The phenomenon can be avoided by reducing use to no more than 7 days.

Owing to the potential for misuse of these agents, their supply to the public from a pharmacy without a prescription has been limited to a maximum of 720 mg of pseudoephedrine salts. It is also a requirement of this restriction that pseudoephedrine salts and ephedrine base (or salts) cannot be supplied at the same time.

### Echinacea

Echinacea has been promoted as a herb that stimulates the immune system and is a popular remedy for treating the common cold. Reports of its effectiveness are largely anecdotal and several clinical trials have shown it to be ineffective, both in reducing the severity of symptoms and in shortening the duration of the cold. For further information on the use of echinacea we refer you to *Herbal Medicines* by Joanne Barnes, Linda A. Anderson and J. David Phillipson (Pharmaceutical Press, 2007).

Table 3.3 describes some important interactions between drugs that are available as non-prescription medicines that are included in various products used to treat the common cold and some prescribed drugs.

**Table 3.3** Interactions between non-prescription medicines for colds and prescribed drugs

| Non-prescription medicines | Interacting drug | Consequence |
| --- | --- | --- |
| Antihistamines | Anxiolytics<br>Hypnotics<br>Sedatives<br>Alcohol | Enhanced sedation and CNS depressant effects |
| Antihistamines (because of intrinsic anticholinergic properties) | Anticholinergic drugs, including tricyclic antidepressants<br>Phenothiazines | Enhanced anticholinergic effect, e.g. dry mouth, blurred vision, constipation and urinary retention |
| Sympathomimetics (particularly oral formulations) | Anticholinergic drugs<br>Antihypertensive therapy | Reduced antihypertensive effects |
| | Monoamine oxidase inhibitors (MAOIs) | Hypertensive crisis |
| | Tricyclic antidepressants | Hypertension is possible with phenylephrine (less likely with ephedrine and pseudoephedrine) |

 **Re-consider the case**

Before reading further, re-consider the following questions and your initial thoughts on this case.

**Trigger questions**

- What additional information would you need before considering the appropriate management options in this case?
- What issues concern you about this case?
- Are any alarm symptoms being exhibited that require more urgent treatment or referral?

**Case study**

A fit 25-year-old man comes into the pharmacy. 'Nothing serious', he explains, 'certainly nothing to keep me off work.' He describes experiencing nasal congestion, a runny nose and sneezing. He also complains of a little wheeze on exertion and a fever. But he feels that it is nothing to worry his doctor about.

 Pharmacist opinion

A history of this illness needs to be determined, including its duration, progression and the presence of other features that may not have been revealed. Considering the initial symptoms of nasal congestion, runny nose and sneezing presented in this case, it would be possible to use a combination of an antihistamine and sympathomimetic to treat these symptoms. Based on the information provided, there are no contraindications to the use of any of these products in this case. The use of sympathomimetics is cautioned in diabetes, hypertension and hyperthyroidism. However, the presence of wheeze on exertion and a fever, does suggest that this is not just the common cold. Establishing a medical history for this man would be important to rule out pre-existing asthma, particularly in relation to the wheeze on exertion.

Asthma is characterised by wheezing, caused by bronchoconstriction, hypersecretion of mucus and inflammation of the bronchi, it must be noted that although wheezing is classically present, asthma can sometimes present solely as a cough without wheezing.

Pharmacist opinion (*continued*)

In asthma there is difficulty in breathing, particularly on expiration, such that sufferers feel that they cannot remove all the air from their lungs. Asthma may be caused by allergens (extrinsic asthma) or may show no relation to obvious allergens (intrinsic asthma). It may be triggered by respiratory infection, air pollution, or drugs such as beta-blockers. Acute attacks are sudden in onset, common during the night, and in children may present as a persistent dry cough.

The presence of fever is also of concern and is suggestive of an infectious process. Fever is not uncommon in viral upper respiratory tract infections and therefore it would be important to consider whether there was a medical need for this to be further investigated. It would also be important to establish the absence of any recent foreign travel as this would certainly warrant a further medical investigation of his symptoms.

 General practitioner opinion

In dealing with this patient it is helpful to understand why he has come: does he want something to help him feel better, or does he just want some reassurance that it is indeed 'nothing serious'? An initial assessment of systemic symptoms and signs will be very useful. Symptoms such as sweating, rigors, racing heartbeat would suggest this illness is affecting him systemically and may need further investigation. Objective signs of temperature, pulse and respiratory rate would also be helpful. Anyone who cannot speak in full sentences at rest requires immediate medical attention.

His chest symptoms warrant a little exploration. Does he smoke? Does he have a pre-existing respiratory condition, e.g. asthma? Has he been on any recent foreign trips? Wheeze on exertion may be a sign of asthma. This man may already have a diagnosis of asthma, whether current or in childhood. The wheeze could be the first presentation of asthma or a worsening of pre-existing symptoms. The wheeze may be a sign of lung damage caused by smoking and it is worth remembering that some people with asthma do choose to smoke.

There can also be the presence of wheeze during a chest infection; the presence of systemic symptoms and signs would suggest this as a possible cause. Very rarely in adults a wheeze can be a sign of an inhaled foreign body. This is unlikely in this case, but worth consideration.

It may be appropriate to discuss infection control issues if he decides to stay at work. The type of work he does will have a bearing on how appropriate it is for him to continue to work and his employers may have their own policy regarding this.

 Summary of key points

| Condition | Management |
| --- | --- |
| Allergic rhinitis (hay fever) is characterised by an itchy nose, sneezing, rhinorrhoea, nasal congestion, red and itching eyes. | Avoidance of known allergen or measures that reduce exposure to allergen. Antihistamines can be used to provide symptomatic relief. Intranasal steroids and sodium cromoglicate eye drops can be used for prophylaxis of symptoms. Intranasal decongestants can be used if nasal congestion is present. |

### Summary of key points (*continued*)

| Condition | Management |
|---|---|
| Sinusitis is characterised by tender sinuses, headache and often accompanied by common cold and nasal congestion. | Symptomatic relief can be provided with oral analgesics such as paracetamol or ibuprofen at an appropriate dose for the sufferer.<br>Nasal decongestants can be useful in relieving the symptoms of sinusitis.<br>Antibiotics are not normally required as sinusitis is usually caused by a virus.<br>Symptoms can take around 2½ weeks to resolve. |
| Common cold is characterised by nasal symptoms of sneezing, rhinorrhoea, congestion and other symptoms such as sore throat, headache, coughing. | Symptomatic relief can be provided with oral analgesics such as paracetamol or aspirin at an appropriate does for the sufferer.<br>Systemic or topical decongestants may provide relief if nasal congestion is present.<br>Oral antihistamines may provide relief from rhinorrhoea by drying nasal secretions. |
| Influenza is characterised by a sudden onset of fever, shivering and generalised aching of the limbs. | Bed rest.<br>Maintain fluid intake.<br>Symptomatic relief can be provided with oral analgesics such as paracetamol or aspirin at an appropriate dose for the sufferer. |

### When to refer

- Production of purulent mucus for several days
- Sinus or ear pain that does not resolve after 7 days
- Any concurrent illness or history where infection may be a risk, depending on the severity of symptoms, e.g. chronic respiratory conditions, heart failure or immunosuppression
- Suspected influenza infection in at-risk groups such as people with long-term underlying health conditions, e.g. diabetes, asthma, pregnant women, children under 1 year
- Where symptoms do not improve with time or where symptoms get worse

## Cough and sore throat

Before reading further, consider the following case and note your initial thoughts.

### Case study

One Saturday afternoon a man in his late 20s comes into the pharmacy and asks to speak to the pharmacist. He is smartly and fashionably dressed and is suffering from a sore throat. He has been using regular paracetamol for around 8 days so that he could continue to work. But after a few days a cough developed. It is productive, with some white or yellow phlegm. His past history reveals that he has had throat infections before, and received antibiotics on several occasions from his GP. He believed they worked, as he started improving a few days later. He has contacted his surgery, which offered him a telephone call from a nurse, which he felt inappropriate. He has an important and busy job, and cannot afford any time off work.

**Case study** (*continued*)

**Trigger questions**

- What additional information would you need before considering the appropriate management options in this case?
- What issues concern you about this case?
- Are any alarm symptoms being exhibited that require more urgent treatment or referral?

## Assessing symptoms

### Sore throat

A sore throat is generally a self-limiting condition, with an estimated 50–80% of sore throats having a viral cause. Sore throats caused by either viral or bacterial infections will usually disappear spontaneously within a few days, and as such they are not serious and do not warrant treatment with antibiotics. Sore throats are often described by the sufferer as painful, and therefore pain alone is not always a cause for referral unless it is persistent and accompanied by other symptoms. A sore throat persisting for more than 1 week requires consideration for referral, and if it is persistent for 2 weeks it should be referred for medical appraisal.

The Centor criteria are a useful tool to help decide on the severity and need for referral for someone presenting with an acute sore throat. The criteria look for the following four clinical signs: presence of tonsillar exudate; presence of tender anterior cervical lymphadenopathy or lymphadenitis; history of fever; and absence of cough. The presence of three or four of these clinical signs may indicate that the individual has a bacterial throat infection and may benefit from antibiotic treatment. Conversely, the absence of three or four of these clinical signs suggests that the individual does not have an infection and therefore that antibiotic treatment is less appropriate.

Examining the back of the throat by getting the patient to open the mouth as wide as possible and then stick out the tongue (a tongue depressor and the light of an auriscope will help greatly with this examination) will reveal on each side of the throat the anterior and posterior pillars of the fauces, between which the tonsils are situated (Figure 3.2).

Tonsillitis (an acute inflammation of the tonsils) can be caused by a bacterial or viral infection and

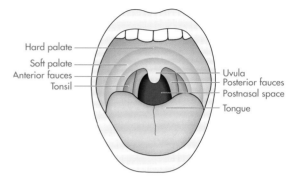

**Figure 3.2**   Diagram showing the position of the tonsils.

the tonsils will appear red and swollen; they can sometimes also have white flecks of pus (Figure 3.3). This can result in difficulty in swallowing and cause the lymph glands of the neck to become tender and enlarged.

Tonsillitis is generally self-limiting, but if there is no improvement after 3 days then the sufferer should be referred as it may be necessary to differentiate between tonsillitis and a streptococcal infection,

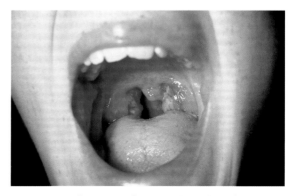

**Figure 3.3**   White spots of pus on enlarged tonsils.

(Reproduced with permission from Dr P. Marazzi/Science Photo Library, SPL M270.063).

which may require antibiotic therapy, as both conditions have a very similar presentation.

Quinsy (an abscess on the tonsils), may develop about 1 week after the onset of tonsillitis. The sufferer has a painful throat that may spread to the ear, feels ill, has difficulty in swallowing and experiences some obstruction to breathing. This is a rare condition and requires referral. Referral would also be appropriate if the lymph nodes in the neck (Figure 3.4) appear swollen, are tender and are extraordinarily painful or do not improve after 5–7 days, as antibiotic therapy may need to be considered.

The presence of enlarged, tender lymph nodes in the neck or elsewhere, in a teenager or young adult complaining of a persistent severe sore throat might suggest a diagnosis of glandular fever (infectious mononucleosis), particularly if they also feel ill and weak. The condition follows a series of attacks, with each attack becoming milder than the last. The first attack will resolve in 2–4 weeks but each subsequent attack occurs after a longer time. This process can take several months, rarely up to 2 years, and the fatigue persists between attacks. The diagnosis can be confirmed by a blood test and therefore would require referral for medical opinion.

Recurrent sore throats should be seen as a potential sign of various, but rare, causes such as immunosuppression caused by drugs or other conditions such as HIV (human immune deficiency virus) infection and AIDS (acquired immune deficiency syndrome). The drugs listed in Box 3.2 have the potential to cause bone marrow suppression, resulting in a deficiency of white blood cells and repeated infections of the throat and other organs. Ulcers or small petechial haemorrhages (purple or red spots)

| Box 3.2 Drugs with potential to cause immunosuppression |
| --- |
| • Carbimazole |
| • Cytotoxics |
| • Gold salts |
| • Tolbutamide |
| • Chlorpropamide |
| • Phenothiazines |
| • Antimalarials |
| • Some antibiotics |

on the palate or the mucosa of the mouth, or ulcers and blistering on the lips and inside the mouth are common symptoms of drug-induced bone marrow suppression, a situation that requires urgent referral for medical opinion as the consequences of a lowered white cell count can be extremely serious.

Sore throat caused by drug deposition during inhalation of steroids can be reduced by advising rinsing of the mouth with water after use of a steroid inhaler. People with undiagnosed or poorly controlled diabetes are susceptible to throat infections, especially those caused by fungi and yeasts, such as *Candida* (thrush). Oral thrush may be recognised by the appearance of white spots on the buccal mucosa and soft palate.

### Cough

The cough reflex is a protective mechanism that is stimulated by irritation of the respiratory mucosa in the lungs, the trachea or the pharynx. The reflex has three nervous components: (a) receptors in the mucosa of the respiratory tract are sensitive to chemical or mechanical stimulation and activate the discharge of afferent impulses along cholinergic (vagus) nerve fibres to (b) the cough centre in the brain stem; (c) efferent impulses from the cough centre are then transmitted along cholinergic nerves. This causes contraction of the diaphragm, abdominal and intercostal muscles, resulting in a rapid expulsion of air from the lungs, taking with it mucus and irritating particles on the surface of the respiratory mucosa. It is often a reaction to infection or contamination of the respiratory tract and is a protective mechanism to clear the airways of contaminants.

It may sometimes be desirable to encourage a cough and sometimes to suppress it, and in many

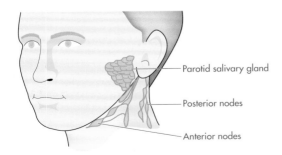

**Figure 3.4** Main group of lymph nodes in the neck.

Parotid salivary gland

Posterior nodes

Anterior nodes

**Table 3.4**   Comparison of non-productive and productive cough

| Non-productive cough | Productive cough |
|---|---|
| • No sputum production.<br>• Dry tickling sensation, irritating not only to sufferer but to those who work and live with them.<br>• Typical response to damage to the upper respiratory tract epithelium caused by:<br>  • viral infection<br>  • smoking (active and passive)a dry atmosphere<br>  • air pollution<br>  • a change in temperature.<br>• May also be a feature of some serious conditions such as asthma or lung cancer, or an adverse reaction to drugs, e.g. ACE inhibitors. Wait for 4 weeks before referring anyone who is taking an ACE inhibitor to a doctor to try and differentiate the cause of the cough. | • Sputum production, helpful in eliciting the severity of any underlying cause.<br>• In some circumstances sufferers will deny bringing up any sputum, although they will say that they can feel phlegm on their chest. In such cases, the cough is best regarded as productive rather than non-productive. |

cases interference with it may delay its disappearance or exacerbate the underlying disturbance that caused it. The most frequent cause of a cough in the developed world is an upper respiratory tract infection such as the common cold, but other common causes include allergies and exacerbations of chronic obstructive pulmonary disease.

A cough may be broadly described as either productive – i.e. producing sputum – or non-productive (dry), with no sputum, so obtaining an accurate history and description of the cough is critical to choosing the most appropriate management option. Sputum occurs when excess mucus is produced in the respiratory tract; the most common cause of excess mucus production is cigarette smoking. The production of sputum is a feature of chronic bronchitis and the classic definition of chronic bronchitis is the production of sputum on most days over at least 3 months for two consecutive years. This causes damage to the lungs and the development of permanent symptoms, such as breathing difficulties, wheezing and shortness of breath. Table 3.4 provides a comparison of the features of productive and non-productive cough.

Doctors often inquire about the colour of expectorated sputum and, although a crude judgement, it is still a useful observation to assist decision making in determining an appropriate course of action (Table 3.5).

**Table 3.5**   Types of sputum production

| Type | Description |
|---|---|
| Clear or white | Generally considered as being of little significance, unless produced in copious amounts. |
| Thick yellow, green or brown, or foul-smelling | Suggests a lower respiratory (i.e. lung) infection, such as bronchitis, but this is not always the case and sometimes may just represent cell debris being cleared from the airways. |
| Clear, straw-coloured | Seen in disorders of allergic origin, such as some forms of asthma, the yellow tinge being caused by the presence of large quantities of eosinophils from the blood as part of the allergic response. |
| Blood in the sputum (haemoptysis) | Seen as either copious fresh blood, spots or streaks, which may sometimes colour the sputum brown. It should be regarded with suspicion and referral for further investigation is suggested, as it may be a sign of pulmonary embolism, tuberculosis, bronchitis or lung cancer. Check that the blood does appear to be coming from the lung and not from the mouth, throat or nose (caused by trauma, such as nose blowing). |
| Pink and frothy | Seen in heart failure, where there is congestion of blood in the lungs and some leakage of plasma into the air spaces. Pneumonia typically produces rust-coloured sputum at first, which may progress to being bloodstained. |

| Table 3.6 | Duration and frequency of coughs | |
| --- | --- | --- |
| **Acute** | **Subacute** | **Chronic** |
| • Duration less than 3 weeks.<br>• Usually self-limiting.<br>• Most common cause is viral infections of the upper respiratory tract.<br>• Medical opinion should be considered if there is no improvement in cough after 2–3 weeks. | • Duration 3–8 weeks.<br>• A cough that started as a common cold but has persisted longer than 3 weeks is most likely due to persistent postnasal drip, which is self-limiting, bacterial sinusitis or asthma. | • Duration lasting more than 8 weeks.<br>• A long-standing or recurrent cough, especially in those over the age of 40 years, may be a sign of more sinister disease such as lung cancer.<br>• Persistent cough may also be an adverse effect of some drugs.<br>• Chronic coughs are best referred, as they may be due to chronic lung disease.<br>• Recurrent coughs may indicate a serious problem requiring referral. For instance, in chronic bronchitis a persistent cough is present for more than 3 months in the year, and in bronchiectasis recurrent chest infections occur that require treatment with antibiotics.<br>• Cigarette smokers often have a recurrent cough, which may be due to chronic bronchitis, and they should be examined by their doctor to exclude infection or lung damage. |

Obviously, at first appearance all coughs will be acute (Table 3.6), but sufferers will seek advice at different times after onset, and this makes it possible to decide whether self-treatment or referral is more appropriate. Although uncommon, gastro-oesophageal reflux disease (GORD) can be a cause of chronic cough and may present with a cough alone or together with heartburn, oesophageal reflux and oral regurgitation. It is usually diagnosed by various tests and a trial with antacid therapy such as a proton pump inhibitor.

## Accompanying symptoms

### Difficulty in swallowing (dysphagia)

Anyone with a sore throat will find it less easy than normal to swallow, but if there is more than the expected degree of difficulty then a referral should be considered. In children and teenagers with throat infections, especially tonsillitis, a sensation may develop of the throat 'closing over'. This is usually more apparent than real, but if drinking becomes very difficult or saliva cannot be swallowed, referral is advised. In extreme cases, such as quinsy, where there is an abscess on the tonsils, inflammation at the back of the throat may be so severe as potentially to restrict breathing.

In very rare cases, dysphagia may be related to an obstruction in the throat or a tumour pressing on the oesophagus. It should be remembered that the reason for asking about difficulty in swallowing is to exclude those rare, severe cases where either the pharynx is dangerously inflamed or there is additional pathology causing obstruction that requires a medical opinion. It is often difficult to distinguish between a genuine difficulty in swallowing (dysphagia) and pain on swallowing. The latter can be expected with a sore throat and will be commonly complained of. A pertinent question to ask is whether the sufferer can swallow liquids. If the answer is negative, then an urgent referral for medical investigation should definitely be made.

### Hoarseness

Some degree of hoarseness is to be expected with a sore throat, particularly when the larynx is involved. Inflammation of the larynx or laryngitis is characterised by hoarseness and can be a complication of an upper respiratory infection, such as a cold or sore throat, or due to the inhalation of irritants such as tobacco smoke. Hoarseness that does not resolve within 5 days requires a medical opinion regarding the value of starting antibiotics. Persistent and unusually severe hoarseness accompanied by difficulty in swallowing should also be referred for a medical opinion to allow more sinister but rarer causes such as laryngeal or pharyngeal tumours to be excluded.

### Earache

Infection in the pharynx can easily spread to the ear via the Eustachian tube. Earache should be referred if it has not improved after 72 hours or if there is a discharge, as it is not only unpleasant but may be caused by bacterial infection, which should be assessed for suitability for treatment with antibiotics.

### Skin rash

A sore throat and a skin rash occurring together may reflect a reaction to a drug, and if this is suspected referral for medical investigation and appraisal is necessary. A florid, itching rash all over the body can develop either during or shortly after finishing a course of ampicillin or amoxicillin in someone who has glandular fever (infectious mononucleosis). Therefore, phenoxymethylpenicillin should normally be the antibiotic of choice for streptococcal sore throats.

### Nasal congestion, sore throat, fever, myalgia, malaise

Cough is commonly associated with or preceded by symptoms of the common cold or influenza-like illnesses such as nasal congestion. In such cases it is invariably nothing more than a simple viral infection, which may be treated symptomatically with non-prescription drugs. If symptoms of a cold are either already present or developing, it is likely that the sore throat is part of the cold syndrome, caused by a viral infection. Viral infections cause sufferers to feel ill and run down, but if there is severe malaise, particularly in the presence of other symptoms, then they should be referred for medical investigation without delay. Fever and sweating in someone with a cough suggests infection.

### Shortness of breath, difficulty in breathing (dyspnoea), chest pain

These symptoms should be viewed as alarm symptoms that require further, urgent medical investigation. Such symptoms may be progressive over a number of months or years, indicating chronic bronchitis, emphysema, heart failure or other serious diseases, or they may be recurrent, as in asthma, when the characteristic wheeze may be heard.

The lung tissue itself has no sensory pain fibres. Pain felt in the chest caused by respiratory disease can arise from the pleura, trachea, bronchi, or the vascular supply. Such pain always requires immediate medical referral. Pain felt on deep inspiration or coughing may be caused by pleurisy or pulmonary embolism.

The lung is normally held against the thoracic wall by a relative negative pressure in the pleural space that 'sucks' it out to assume the shape of the thoracic cavity. If the pleural envelope is ruptured, air enters into the pleural cavity, neutralising the negative pressure, and as a result the lung collapses. This is a pneumothorax. It occurs without warning and for no apparent reason, particularly in healthy young men, as well as in bronchitis or emphysema. It gives rise to a severe, unilateral chest pain which may be either constant or pleuritic in nature, and there may be some dyspnoea. The pain may be felt over the shoulder or sternum and may resemble that of angina or myocardial infarction.

Pulmonary embolism is caused by a thrombus that has formed elsewhere and has detached itself from its primary site, such as a deep vein in the calf of the leg; where this is the case, it is likely that there will be pain in the calf muscle along with swelling in the calf or the ankle. Once detached, the thrombus is carried by the circulation to the lung, where it lodges in the pulmonary artery. The arterial lumen is then blocked, causing lung tissue supplied by the artery to die (pulmonary infarct). Chest pain associated with a pulmonary embolism will usually be of sudden onset and accompanied with some dyspnoea. Cough will be a minor feature of this picture, but these symptoms could also be produced by intercostal muscle strain following a coughing bout.

### Weight loss

An unintended dramatic loss of weight suggests the possibility of serious disease and therefore medical referral would be appropriate. In considering the respiratory system, two conditions that need to be considered are tuberculosis and lung cancer.

Tuberculosis is a disease of slow onset and in its early stages the symptoms are often mild. It is common in developing countries but does also occur in the UK. It is often overlooked in the elderly because of its insidious onset and its resemblance to bronchitis and congestive heart failure. Symptoms include a persistent cough, blood in the sputum (not always), fever or night sweats and weight loss. People at risk include the elderly, those who have contact with known cases, immigrants and alcoholics.

Lung cancer is more common in men than women, is seen more often in cigarette smokers, and usually appears between the ages of 50 and 70 years. These characteristics need to be considered when considering the cause of a cough. A cough may have been present for some time in smokers, but any change in its character is a signal to refer for further medical investigation.

## Management options

Like any other 'trivial' symptom, a cough with no serious underlying cause will be self-limiting and will disappear spontaneously within a few days. However, public expectations are high, and members of the public will still seek a 'cough bottle' even if the evidence suggests that it is little more than a placebo. A number of Cochrane reviews have shown insufficient evidence for or against the use of various preparations in the management of cough, although clinical studies have shown that some people will find a cough remedy helpful even if the actual clinical benefit may be questionable. Given the self-limiting nature of a cough with no serious underlying cause, it will remain difficult to establish an evidence base.

This still allows the option of a 'cough bottle' to be recommended if the sufferer wants to try it. Thus a form of words can be constructed that will acknowledge the awareness of the negative evidence base while not discouraging people who might want to try a cough medicine. This in turn should encourage a dialogue between the health professional and the sufferer, allowing the individual to retain some choice in managing their symptoms.

It should be borne in mind that many cough preparations do contain drugs with recognised pharmacological activity, even if the clinical significance is unproven. It is pertinent, therefore, that some logical rationale is considered when choosing a product containing a mixture of drugs to give symptomatic relief. Table 3.7 summarises some rational combinations.

**Table 3.7** Examples of pharmacologically rational cough mixtures marketed in the UK

| Suppressant | Bronchodilator/ decongestant | Antihistamine |
| --- | --- | --- |
| Dextromethorphan | | Triprolidine |
| Dextromethorphan | Ephedrine | |
| Dextromethorphan | Pseudoephedrine | Diphenhydramine |
| Dextromethorphan | Pseudoephedrine | Triprolidine |
| Codeine | Pseudoephedrine | Diphenhydramine |

Historically there have been some irrational combinations available in the UK. For example, combinations of expectorants and cough suppressants, or expectorants and antihistamines, are irrational. If a cough is productive and requires an expectorant, then it should not be suppressed at the same time. Similarly, antihistamine drugs will reduce bronchial secretions by an anticholinergic mechanism and this is pharmacologically antagonistic to the effect of an expectorant. Some combinations are entirely logical. For example, a mixture of a bronchodilator and an expectorant, or a bronchodilator and a cough suppressant/antihistamine does not present any obvious pharmacological antagonism.

In April 2009 following a review by the Medicines and Healthcare products Regulatory Agency (MHRA), the Commission on Human Medicines (CHM) advised that cough and cold remedies containing antitussives, expectorants, nasal decongestants and antihistamines no longer be used for the treatment of coughs and colds in children less than 6 years old. This recommendation reflected the lack of robust evidence that cough and cold remedies containing these ingredients are effective and that some reports of harm with these ingredients have been received. Therefore, the decision was made that the risks of such products in this age group outweigh the benefits given the increased incidence of coughs and colds in children under the age of 6.

### Lozenges and sprays (BNF section 12.3)

Lozenges have a traditional place in the treatment of sore throats. However, the clinical benefit of the antibacterial agents they contain is tenuous, especially given that around 50–80% of sore throats are viral in nature. These agents include dequalinium, tyrothricin, hexylresorcinol, amylmetacresol, benzalkonium and cetylpyridinium. Probably the most useful effect of the majority of lozenges lies in their ability to stimulate the flow of saliva, which acts as a demulcent and soothes the pharynx. Some lozenges contain a local anaesthetic such as benzocaine or lignocaine, but the amount is probably too small to offer any real benefit. These two local anaesthetics are also available in a spray preparation.

Lozenges containing the non-steroidal anti-inflammatory drug (NSAID) flurbiprofen give another dimension to the treatment of sore throats. Flurbiprofen has anti-inflammatory and analgesic properties that offer promising therapeutic potential and another option to sufferers. However, this promise has not been substantiated by any good evidence, as clinical trials have only been carried out against placebo. Nevertheless, trials have shown flurbiprofen to be better than placebo. The duration of flurbiprofen use is restricted to 3 days, and it is contraindicated in children under 12 years, in anyone already taking NSAIDs, in those with a history of asthma or peptic ulcer disease, and in those with a known allergy to aspirin or other NSAIDs.

If aspirin or NSAIDs are not contraindicated, another approach to the treatment of a painful throat is to dissolve one or two soluble aspirins and use the solution as a gargle. The effect is essentially the same as using flurbiprofen lozenges.

### Cough suppressants (antitussives) (BNF section 3.9.1)

Cough suppressants can usefully provide symptomatic relief of a dry, irritating or tickly cough that produces little or no sputum. Care should be taken in recommending a cough suppressant if chronic obstructive pulmonary disease is present, as the cough reflex is essential to clear the airways of mucus.

Centrally acting cough suppressants act on the cough centre in the brain and reduce the discharge of impulses down the efferent nerves to the muscles that produce coughing. Examples are codeine, pholcodine and dextromethorphan. All are capable of causing sedation (though allegedly less so with dextromethorphan), and long courses will give rise to constipation and may produce dependence. Thus, only short courses should be recommended.

Pholcodine and dextromethorphan reputedly have fewer adverse effects and less abuse potential than codeine, although this is unlikely to be of clinical significance in normal, short-term use.

In October 2010 an MHRA Public Assessment Report concluded that there was a lack of robust evidence for the efficacy of codeine in suppressing a cough in a child and the risks associated with the use of liquid codeine medicines for the suppression of a cough in children and young people under the age of 18 outweighed the benefits. Therefore, oral liquid medicines containing codeine should not be used to treat cough in children or young people less than 18 years of age.

### Expectorants (BNF section 3.9.2)

Expectorants have traditionally been used to increase bronchial secretions and thus reduce the tenacity of mucus, which can then be coughed up. They have a place in cough therapy, but their efficacy is controversial owing to the lack of strong supportive, objective data, although there is considerable subjective support for their use. Plugs of mucus and debris in the small airways can cause breathing difficulties and act as sites of infection, and sufferers who attempt to remove sputum they can 'feel' in their chests may become exhausted by coughing if the mucus is so viscous that it adheres to the mucosal lining of the lungs. There are therefore good reasons for trying to facilitate expectoration.

Hydration of the airways will facilitate adequate production of non-viscous mucus from the glands lining the lungs. This can be simply and effectively achieved by drinking plenty of fluid, so that the tissues remain hydrated, as well as by humidifying the inspired air with steam inhalations. The addition of substances such as menthol or compound tincture of benzoin (Friar's balsam) to the hot water providing the steam is probably of no extra value except for a psychological effect (which should not be undervalued). One theory of how expectorants have their effect is by irritating the gastric mucosa. This produces a reflex stimulation of the bronchial tree, which responds by secreting more mucus.

Various ammonium salts have been used over the years and the chloride is still used, albeit less commonly than previously. Guaifenesin is present in many proprietary cough medicines, although the dosage varies considerably. It would be logical to recommend doses of 100–200 mg for maximum effect. Ipecacuanha at subemetic doses stimulates the gastric mucosa and is used as an expectorant. Citric acid and sodium citrate have expectorant properties, but in the doses used these are probably weak. Squill is an old-established medicine that may be found in some proprietary cough remedies. Liquid extracts of liquorice, capsicum, terpin, menthol and eucalyptus oil also appear in proprietary cough medicines.

### Demulcents (BNF section 3.9.2)

Demulcents, such as honey, glycerin (glycerol) and syrup, are said to act by coating the pharyngeal mucosa, which may be inflamed, and offer some protection from irritants such as smoke or dust particles. Their efficacy probably relates largely to a soothing placebo effect, but the demulcent effect on the mucosa may be a real one and may also serve to hydrate the delicate mucosal tissues. Where postnasal drip occurs, demulcents may reduce irritation of the pharyngeal mucosa.

Demulcents are now the only option (alongside paracetamol for symptomatic relief) for the management of coughs and colds in children under the age of 6 years as antitussives, expectorants and decongestants are no longer licensed for this age group. Demulcents also remain useful for pregnant women, where again the combination of a self-limiting condition and lack of robust evidence of the efficacy of cough medicines makes the use of demulcents the safer option.

### Re-consider the case

Before reading further, re-consider the following questions and your initial thoughts on this case.

**Trigger questions**

- What additional information would you need before considering the appropriate management options in this case?
- What issues concern you about this case?
- Are any alarm symptoms being exhibited that require more urgent treatment or referral?

**Case study**

One Saturday afternoon a man in his late 20s comes into the pharmacy and asks to speak to the pharmacist. He is smartly and fashionably dressed and is suffering from a sore throat. He has been using paracetamol regularly for around 8 days so that he could continue to work. But after a few days a cough developed. It is productive, with some white or yellow phlegm. His past history reveals that he has had throat infections before, and received antibiotics on several occasions from his GP. He believed they worked, as he started improving a few days later. He has contacted his surgery, which offered him a telephone call from a nurse, which he felt inappropriate. He has an important and busy job, and cannot afford any time off work.

### Pharmacist opinion

Age is an important consideration in this case, as a persistent or recurrent sore throat in teenagers and young adults requires referral to exclude glandular fever. Age is also important when considering the development of the cough as a cough in a child needs to be considered carefully and a full history taken as a persistent irritant cough can indicate asthma in a child.

Pharmacist opinion (*continued*)

Cough is also a feature of croup and whooping cough (pertussis), both of which occur in children. The term 'croup' is used loosely by both medical and non-medical people to encompass a variety of symptoms associated with an irritant cough in children. Properly used, the term describes an infection (usually viral) of the larynx and trachea that leads to oedema and narrowing of the airway. There is a severe and violent cough, which is often paroxysmal (occurring in bouts) and the child often has difficulty in breathing between bouts, as well as exhibiting stridor (noisy inspiration).

Whooping cough, although now rare because of immunisation programmes, does still occur in children, usually those under 5 years of age. The condition may present initially as a cold, and after a few days a cough develops, occurring at around hourly intervals. After about a week a whoop is heard on inspiration following a spasm of explosive coughing. The cough produces a plug of thick sputum, and is accompanied sometimes by vomiting. The whoop may last for several weeks or months. In both situations referral for medical appraisal is necessary.

This man does not present any obvious alarm symptoms and although he reports a productive cough, the nature of the phlegm described is not an immediate cause for concern, especially considering the absence of any other alarm symptoms such as unintentional weight loss, dysphagia, or swollen cervical lymph nodes. If the man has an expectation that he needs antibiotic treatment then clearly he does need either to speak with his GP or accept the offer of a telephone call from the nurse as these do need to be supplied via a prescription. There is a general misconception within the general population that antibiotics are needed for sore throats, but considering that around 50–80% of sore throats have a viral cause and are self-limiting, the use of antibiotics is generally inappropriate unless a bacterial cause is established. In this case, advising on self-care and the use of analgesia whether oral or topical would be an appropriate course of action to adopt assuming that there were no reasons for referral.

General practitioner opinion

This man has some preconceptions regarding antibiotics and has already had contact with another health professional. It is important to bear in mind that there are associated emotions related to this man's symptoms; the initial focus on physical symptoms should direct discussion.

The aim here is to work out whether these symptoms are caused by viral or bacterial infection. He has continued to work and it would be helpful to know what kind of work he has been able to do while unwell. Has he had high temperatures associated with his symptoms? Has he been able to swallow fluids and solids? His temperature could be taken in the pharmacy. Does he look unwell? Is he sweating? Is there evidence of swollen lymph glands? Cervical lymph nodes run down the neck on both sides from the angle of the jaw. Using a pen torch to examine the back of the throat may reveal mild inflammation of the pharynx (a little red) or moderate inflammation with swollen tonsils.

Symptoms and signs to support a bacterial infection would be persistent high temperatures, inability to concentrate at work – particularly inability to do manual work – presence of tender swollen lymph nodes and moderate to severe inflammation of the pharynx.

The history in this case implies that this is a viral throat infection. Negative findings on examination would support this conclusion. He now needs gentle handling of his preconceptions. People normally appreciate thorough questioning and examination, so he should be appreciative of the time already spent with him. He should now be receptive to a clear explanation of the nature of viral throat

Reference

### General practitioner opinion (*continued*)

infection. He should understand that the condition is self-limiting and will not respond to antibiotics. Advice regarding supportive treatment including use of paracetamol and/or NSAIDs should be given. This could be supported by printed information.

### Summary of key points

| Condition | Management |
| --- | --- |
| Cough can be characterised as productive or non-productive and acute, subacute or chronic. | Depends on type and duration of cough but consider expectorants, cough suppressants and demulcents. Demulcents are the only option for children under 6 years. |
| Sore throat is usually self-limiting and can be seen alongside coughs and colds. | Consider the use of oral analgesics, throat lozenges and sprays. |
| Tonsillitis is characterised by red and swollen tonsils with or without flecks of white pus. | Oral analgesics, throat lozenges and sprays can be advised in the short-term. Refer for medical appraisal if there is no improvement after 3 days, as antibiotic treatment may need to be considered. |
| Whooping cough is characterised by malaise, anorexia, mucoid rhinorrhoea and conjunctivitis followed by paroxysms of cough. | Requires referral. |
| Croup is characterised by an irritant cough in children that occurs in bouts. | Requires referral because a child can sometimes experience difficulty in breathing between bouts of coughing. |

### When to refer

*If presenting with a sore throat:*

- Individuals who are immunosuppressed or taking medication such as carbimazole, phenothiazines, antibiotics, cytotoxic drugs, gold, chlorpropamide or steroids
- Accompanied by a skin rash
- History of endocarditis, rheumatic fever or artificial heart valves
- Accompanied by painful enlarged lymph glands in the neck, or enlarged glands that do not improve within 5–7 days
- Long-term or recurrent hoarseness or loss of voice
- Earache that does not resolve after 72 hours or is accompanied by a discharge
- Difficulty in swallowing
- Recurrent tonsillitis in children

*If presenting with a cough/cold:*

- Difficulty in breathing, wheezing (especially in young children), breathlessness
- Malaise in teenagers and young adults for more than 7 days
- Severe symptoms that do not improve within 7 days
- Dry night-time cough in children

**When to refer** (*continued*)

- Any concurrent illness or history where infection may be a risk, depending on the severity of symptoms, e.g. chronic respiratory conditions, heart failure or immunosuppression
- Recurrent cough or constant smoker's cough, except where the doctor has given specific guidance for action at a previous consultation
- Chest pain, either unilateral or bilateral, particularly if exacerbated on coughing or deep inspiration
- Sputum is bloodstained or purulent, i.e. unusual colour (green, brown) or foul smelling*
- Concurrent medication such as ACE inhibitors
- Weight loss, particularly in those over the age of 40
- Painful or red, inflamed calf
- General malaise, feeling systemically unwell, persisting sweats or fever
- No improvement of symptoms after 14–21 days, depending on severity, or a deterioration in the condition with time

*Note that green sputum is commonly present in viral infections and may sometimes not justify referral, provided there are no other referable signs or symptoms. Purulent postnasal drip may also be mistaken for sputum, which would not normally require referral.

## Bibliography

Arroll B, Kenealy T (2005). Antibiotics for the common cold and acute purulent rhinitis. *Cochrane Database Syst Rev* Jul 20; (3): CD0002473: CD000247. doi: 10.1002/14651858.CD000247.pub2.

Douglas G *et al.*, eds (2005). *MacLeod's Clinical Examination*. Edinburgh: Churchill Livingstone.

Kumar P, Clark M, eds (2005). *Clinical Medicine*. London: Elsevier Saunders.

Morice AH *et al.* (2006). British Thoracic Society Guidelines: Recommendations for the management of cough in adults. *Thorax* 61 (Suppl I): i1–i24.

Medicines and Healthcare Products Regulatory Agency (2010). *Oral Liquid Medicines Containing Codeine*. MHRA Public Assessment Report. London: MHRA.

Medicines and Healthcare Products Regulatory Agency (2010). *Children's Over-the-Counter Cough and Cold Medicines: New Advice*. London: MHRA. http://www.mhra.gov.uk/Safetyinformation/Safetywarning salertsandrecalls/Safetywarningsandmessagesfor medicines/CON038908 (accessed 27 March 2011).

National Institute for Health and Clinical Excellence (2008). *Prescribing of Antibiotics for Self-limiting Respiratory Tract Infections in Adults and Children in Primary Care*. London: NICE.

Oduwole O, *et al.* (2010). Honey for acute cough in children. *Cochrane Database Syst Rev* Jan 20; (1): CD007094. doi: 0.1002/14651858.CD007094.pub2.

Scottish Intercollegiate Guidelines Network (2010). *Management of Sore Throat and Indications for Tonsillectomy*. Edinburgh: Scottish Intercollegiate Guidelines Network.

Smith SM *et al.* (2008). Over-the-counter (OTC) medications for acute cough in children and adults in ambulatory settings. *Cochrane Database Syst Rev* Jan 23; (1): CD001831. doi: 10.1002/14651858.CD001831.pub3.

## Self-assessment questions

The following questions are provided to test the information presented in this chapter.

*For questions 1–7 select the best answer in each case.*

1. Select which of the following causes the common cold:
   a. Paramyxoviruses
   b. Rhabdoviruses
   c. Picornaviruses
   d. Togaviruses
   e. Orthomyxoviruses

2. Select which of the following is not normally considered a symptom of the common cold:
   a. Pyrexia
   b. Aching limbs
   c. Sore nose
   d. Malaise
   e. Rhinorrhoea

3. Select which of the following is the most common causative organism of sinusitis:
   a. *Mycoplasma pneumoniae*
   b. *Pseudomonas aeruginosa*
   c. *Escherichia coli*
   d. *Streptococcus pneumoniae*
   e. *Klebsiella pneumoniae*

4. Select which of the following is not a caution for the use of pseudoephedrine:
   a. Asthma
   b. Hypertension
   c. Pregnancy
   d. Hyperthyroidism
   e. Ischaemic heart disease

5. Select which of the following drugs interacts with antihistamines:
   a. Salbutamol
   b. Paracetamol
   c. Beclometasone
   d. Fluoxetine
   e. Diazepam

6. Select which of the following is not a feature of influenza:
   a. Fever
   b. Shivering
   c. Aching limbs
   d. Abrupt onset
   e. Sinusitis

7. Select which of the following best describes the symptoms of croup:
   a. Severe and violent paroxysmal cough with stridor
   b. Productive cough accompanied by vomiting
   c. Whoop on inspiration
   d. Stridor
   e. Productive cough with pink and frothy phlegm

*For questions 8–10 select from the list below one lettered option which is most closely related to it. Each lettered option may be used once, more than once, or not at all.*
   a. productive cough
   b. non-productive cough
   c. acute cough
   d. subacute cough
   e. chronic cough

8. Has a duration of less than 3 weeks.

9. Is a typical response to damage to the upper respiratory tract epithelium by air pollution.

10. Can be an adverse drug reaction to lisinopril.

*For questions 11–12 select from the list below one lettered option which is most closely related to it. Each lettered option may be used once, more than once, or not at all.*
   a. chlorphenamine
   b. loratadine
   c. pseudoephedrine
   d. acrivastine
   e. azelastine

11. Is available as a nasal spray and as eye drops.

12. Has a cough suppressant action.

*Questions 13–16: Each of the questions or incomplete statements in this section is followed by three responses. For each question one or more of the responses is/are correct. Decide which of the responses is/are correct and then choose a–e as indicated in the table below.*

| Directions summarised | | | | |
|---|---|---|---|---|
| a | b | c | d | e |
| If 1, 2 and 3 are correct | If 1 and 2 only are correct | If 2 and 3 only are correct | If 1 only is correct | If 3 only is correct |

13. The following medicines can be supplied from a pharmacy without a prescription to treat allergic rhinitis:
   1 – loratadine tablets
   2 – sodium cromoglicate eye drops
   3 – beclometasone nasal spray

14. The following medicines can be supplied from a pharmacy without a prescription to treat allergic rhinitis in someone who is 16 years old:
   1 – loratadine tablets
   2 – sodium cromoglicate eye drops
   3 – beclometasone nasal spray

15. A liquid cough medicine containing pholcodine can be used to treat:
   1 – a cough producing clear, straw coloured sputum
   2 – a dry, irritating cough in a 12 year old child
   3 – a dry, irritating cough that has lasted for 7 days in a non-smoking adult

16. Tonsillitis
   1 – causes the tonsils to appear red and swollen
   2 – can be caused by bacterial or viral infection
   3 – always requires treatment with antibiotics

*Questions 17–20 consist of two statements linked by the word* because; *decide whether each statement is true or false. If both statements are true then decide whether the second statement is a correct explanation of the first statement. Choose a–e as your answer as indicated in the table below.*

## Directions summarised

| | First statement | Second statement | |
|---|---|---|---|
| a | True | True | Second statement is a correct explanation of the first statement |
| b | True | True | Second statement is not a correct explanation of the first statement |
| c | True | False | |
| d | False | True | |
| e | False | False | |

**17.**

| Shortness of breath and dyspnoea are alarm symptoms that require referral for medical investigation | BECAUSE | Shortness of breath and dyspnoea can be indicative of chronic disease such as chronic bronchitis or cardiac failure |
|---|---|---|

**18.**

| Anyone who complains of a sore throat and is taking carbimazole does not need further investigation | BECAUSE | Carbimazole has the potential to cause neutropenia and agranulocytosis |
|---|---|---|

**19.**

| Earache that has not improved in 72 hours in someone complaining of a sore throat should be referred for medical investigation | BECAUSE | Infection in the pharynx can easily spread to the ear via the Eustachian tubes |
|---|---|---|

**20.**

| Hoarseness that does not resolve within 5 days requires referral for medical investigation | BECAUSE | Hoarseness that has persisted for more than 5 days will need antibiotic treatment |
|---|---|---|

## Answers

1-c; 2-b; 3-d; 4-a; 5-e; 6-e; 7-a; 8-c; 9-b; 10-b; 11-e; 12-a; 13-a; 14-b; 15-c; 16-b; 17-a; 18-d; 19-a; 20-c

# 4

# Central Nervous System

*Ruth Edwards, Brian Addison and Susan Lennie*

| **This chapter will cover the following conditions:** | **This chapter will cover the following groups of medicines** |
|---|---|
| • Analgesia<br>• Soft tissue Inflammation and Joint Disorders<br>• Headache and migraine<br>• Insomnia<br>• Nausea and vomiting<br>• Smoking cessation<br>• Obesity | • Non-opioid analgesics (paracetamol)<br>• Non-steroidal anti-Inflammatory drugs (oral and topical)<br>• Opioid analgesics<br>• Rubefacients<br>• Glucosamine<br>• Cod liver oil<br>• Antimigraine drugs (including sumatriptan)<br>• Anti-emetics<br>• Sedating antihistamines<br>• Nicotine replacement therapy products |

In this chapter we will consider the different illnesses that require the use of analgesia, including different causes of pain such as soft tissue inflammation, joint disorders and headache (including migraine). Nausea and vomiting will also be covered in this chapter as they may accompany migraine and the drugs used to treat nausea and vomiting are included in the Central Nervous System chapter of the *British National Formulary (BNF)*. Insomnia is included in this chapter for the same reasons. Although not specifically minor illnesses, obesity and smoking cessation will also be covered in this chapter as the drugs used in the management of obesity and smoking cessation are also included in the Central Nervous System chapter of the *BNF*.

## Pain, headache, migraine, nausea and vomiting, and insomnia

Although a seemingly disparate group of conditions, pain (including headache), nausea and vomiting, and insomnia can often occur together, with each being a possible cause of the other. Obviously each of these symptoms can occur independently, but the management options are usually the same whether or not they are associated with another symptom. In addition, there is some cross-over in the products used to manage these symptoms.

Individuals very commonly present with pain in community pharmacy including musculoskeletal pain, dental pain, period pain, aches and pains associated with colds and flu, and headache. Analgesics make up the biggest market share of non-prescription medicines in the United Kingdom.

Pain is a universal experience but a subjective, emotional symptom that is often difficult for individuals to define. Pain is commonly defined as an unpleasant sensory or emotional experience associated with actual or potential tissue damage, or described in terms of such damage. Pain is often classified into nociceptive (from the stimulation of specific pain receptors), somatic (often known as musculoskeletal pain), visceral (from the internal organs of the main body cavities) or neuropathic (from within the nervous system, either peripheral or central). Pain is also commonly divided into acute pain (usually with a definable cause and time of onset) and chronic pain (defined as pain lasting more than 3 months with appropriate treatment or beyond the time in which recovery might usually be expected).

Pain is often mistreated or undertreated and can lead to anxiety, depression, insomnia, lethargy and reduced physical and mental functioning. Pain control is more likely to be achieved if a proper history is taken and the elements of this are covered in Box 4.1.

Nausea alone or nausea and vomiting may present either along with or independently of pain. Insomnia and sleep disturbance are in the top ten symptoms presented in primary care to GPs and will often present in community pharmacy.

Before reading further, consider the following case and note your initial thoughts.

 **Case study**

A woman in her mid-40s reports 'tension headaches'. She has had them before, often premenstrually when she feels stressed. Recently they have become bad enough to need treatment. The headache is usually left sided and builds up over about an hour, and she senses when one is imminent. She often feels nauseated and has tried paracetamol without effect.

**Trigger questions**

- What additional information would you need before considering the appropriate management options in this case?
- What issues concern you about this case?
- Are any alarm symptoms being exhibited that require more urgent treatment or referral?

- Location of the pain.
- Speed of onset, duration and whether the pain is intermittent or constant.
- Intensity or severity (use of pain scales can make this more objective).
- Character of the pain (will indicate whether it is neuropathic or nociceptive, somatic or visceral).
- Any aggravating or relieving factors.
- Impact on daily living.
- Social, emotional and psychological aspects.

## Assessing symptoms

### Headache

Most people suffer from headaches from time to time and in the majority of cases the headache resolves within a short period. Headache is often no more than a physiological response to circumstances, but it can lead to anxiety, both for sufferers and for those who aim to unravel its cause. There are two major problems in attempting to discover the origin of a headache. First, there are some potentially very serious diagnoses, which, although rare, may be in the minds of both parties; and secondly, it can be a notoriously difficult condition to explain. There are few definitive signs or tests available to GPs or pharmacists that will confirm the diagnosis, yet headache is a common complaint that will bring many people to the pharmacy to purchase analgesics.

Fortunately, in most cases the headache will disappear spontaneously or respond to simple analgesics, proving – albeit retrospectively – to be no more than one of the transient self-limiting episodes to which most people are susceptible at some time or another. However, to distinguish the minority of cases in which serious pathology may be a possibility, it is helpful to understand the mechanisms by which headaches occur, and to arrive at some guidelines to differentiate those types that may relate to an underlying problem from those that are of no

lasting significance and can be treated symptomatically with non-prescription medicines.

### Types of headache

Headaches are usually classified as either primary (not associated with any underlying pathology) or secondary (attributed to an underlying pathological condition). Primary headache disorders are more common and include migraine, tension-type and cluster headache, which can usually be managed as minor illnesses. Secondary headaches include any head pain of infectious, neoplastic, vascular or drug-induced origin and will require referral.

Migraine is the most common severe primary headache disorder. It is characterised by unilateral (on one side), moderate to severe, pulsating or throbbing pain that builds up over minutes to hours. It can be associated with nausea and vomiting and with sensitivity to light and sound. Migraines are generally quite disabling and will limit daily activity. They can also be triggered by physical activity. The headache of migraine may be related to dilatation of blood vessels within or around the skull. Migraines can occur either with or without aura. An aura usually includes visual symptoms such as of visual loss, blurred vision, blind spots (scotomas), flashing lights and zigzagging. Sensory and speech disturbances may also occur. The symptoms of aura usually disappear within an hour and are followed by severe headache that will last between 4 and 72 hours.

Tension-type headache is the most common primary headache. It can be caused by various emotional stresses, such as tension, anxiety or fatigue. Classically it is thought to result from muscle spasm in the neck and scalp (Figure 4.1) and is often described as a tight band around the head, often spreading over the top of the head. Pain may be due in part to the tension in the muscles as well as a resulting constriction of capillaries within them, reducing their blood supply and causing a lack of oxygen. It is usually bilateral and may be described by the sufferer as a generalised ache or pain, with no specific focus, felt all over the cranium. Tension headaches can be episodic or chronic. Table 4.1 provides a useful differentiation between migraine and tension headache.

Cluster headaches cause severe, unilateral pain within and above the eye and in the temporal region. They can last for 15 minutes to 3 hours and can occur

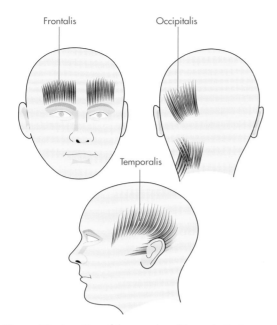

Frontalis

Occipitalis

Temporalis

**Figure 4.1** Location of the muscles of the scalp that are involved in muscular spasm in tension headache.

from once every other day to 8 times a day often with a circadian rhythm; attacks can occur at the same time of day and clusters at the same time each year. Cluster headaches are associated with autonomic features such as lacrimation, rhinitis, and forehead and facial sweating occurring at the same side as the pain and a sense of restlessness or agitation. An individual presenting with symptoms of cluster headache should be referred for medical assessment.

Chronic daily headache is defined as headache on 15 or more days per month. The pain appears to be there from morning until night and never seems to go away. It can vary in nature from an ache to a dull throb. Referral is advised for further investigation

to rule out more rare types of chronic headache, although in many cases the pain will be idiopathic (i.e. of no specific known cause).

Medication overuse headache is the most common cause of chronic daily headache and is considered to be a secondary headache. Analgesic overuse is thought to cause an increase in the number of pain receptors that are switched on, first by the pain itself and then by increased sensitisation of the receptors when analgesics are used that are not sufficient to remove the pain. Instead, there is an exaggerated response of the receptors that more frequent or more potent analgesia fails to stop, and a vicious cycle between medication and pain begins. People suffering from this type of headache will typically be taking simple or combination analgesics on more than three days a week.

Other types of secondary headache are less common but may present in a pharmacy and will require referral. The brain itself has no sensory receptors within its fabric. A lesion within the substance of the brain will therefore not produce pain until it impinges upon adjacent structures; although if the lesion is severe enough to interfere with cerebral function it may cause other symptoms, such as vomiting, confusion, drowsiness, or disturbances of balance or of intellectual function. Thus, even a lesion as severe as a stroke will not usually be accompanied by headache.

Traction headaches are caused by inflammation (e.g. meningitis), tumours or haematomas (haemorrhages). They are classified as traction headaches because the underlying pathology causes irritation and stretching of the meninges (the protective membranes that envelop the brain and spinal cord). These membranes are richly endowed with sensory

| Table 4.1 Differentiation between migraine and tension headache | |
| --- | --- |
| **Migraine** | **Tension-type headache** |
| Moderate to severe pain | Mild to moderate pain |
| Usually unilateral | Bilateral |
| Pulsating | Non-pulsating |
| Aggravated by normal activities, such that the sufferer has to stop | Not aggravated by normal activities |
| Often accompanied by sensitivity to light, nausea and/or vomiting | These symptoms are not usually present |

pain receptors which, when stimulated, will cause headache.

Tumours and cerebral abscesses are examples of space-occupying lesions, which cause headaches by compressing normal brain tissue against the skull, resulting in a raised intracranial pressure. Head injury can cause a haematoma, leading to a raised intracranial pressure. Infection and inflammation of the membranes surrounding the brain and lining the skull (e.g. meningitis) will cause headache, as will inflammation of the brain tissue itself (e.g. encephalitis) when other structures are involved or the intracranial pressure rises.

Headache can be caused by spasm or fatigue of the ciliary and periorbital muscles of the eye, as in eye strain, astigmatism and other refractive disorders. Glaucoma can cause headache. Pain may be referred from the jaw in dental pain, and from the sinuses in sinusitis.

Muscle strain or pulled ligaments in the neck or upper back are a common cause of headache. Shingles affecting the scalp or eyes can cause pain in the face and head. Temporal arteritis is a rare, but severe inflammation of the temporal artery and may occur in the elderly, producing pain and tenderness.

Hypertension rarely causes headache (although it is often believed to do so by people with high blood pressure), except very rarely in severe or so-called malignant hypertension. More serious cases of headache can be caused by rupture of a blood vessel, as in subarachnoid and subdural haemorrhages.

### Features of headache

#### Location and radiation of the pain

Often headache cannot be described as pertaining to one part of the head, but it is important to remember to ask about the exact location and any radiation of the pain, as transformation to a generalised headache might obscure the original pattern and location. The pointers given in Table 4.2 are useful.

#### Onset, duration and intensity

If a headache is recent in onset but has gradually become worse over a few days, inquiry should be made about recent head trauma, as bleeding may occur slowly, giving progressive worsening of symptoms.

A headache that has lasted only a few minutes can be regarded as minor unless it has occurred suddenly and is described as devastating and the worst pain the person has ever had. Such a headache might indicate bleeding from a ruptured blood vessel under the membrane covering the brain (subarachnoid haemorrhage), and is a medical emergency. Often under such circumstances the person collapses and becomes unconscious. A migrainous headache can occur reasonably rapidly, but usually develops over a longer period than a subarachnoid haemorrhage,

| Table 4.2 | Location of pain |
| --- | --- |
| **Location of pain** | **Description** |
| Frontal | Pain at the front of the head may indicate idiopathic headache, sinusitis or nasal congestion. |
| Occipital (back of head) | Pain at the back of the head and may suggest tension or anxiety, especially if the pain radiates over the top and sides of the head (bilateral pain). |
| Hemicranial (unilateral) | Headache on one side of the head; this is typical of migraine or sinusitis. It may spread to both sides later. The pain of shingles (herpes zoster) usually starts as a severe localised pain felt in the skin on one side of the scalp, either a day or so before the rash appears or at the same time as the rash develops. Pain on one side of the face may indicate trigeminal neuralgia. |
| Orbital | Pain behind or around the eyes and is often described in sinusitis, migraine or shingles. Pain from within the eye itself may be due to glaucoma or other serious eye diseases. |
| Temporal | Pain in the temple area at the sides of the head and may indicate temporal arteritis in people over the age of 50 years, especially if there is sensitivity to touch in this area of the scalp. Temporal pain may also be accompanied by jaw pain. This requires urgent referral to avoid more general inflammation of the arteries, which could lead to blindness if the blood supply to the optic nerve is compromised. |

which may be described as being like a blow to the back of the head.

Sufferers can often sense when a migraine is imminent, known as the prodromal phase, but this is different from symptoms of aura. If sufferers experience aura with migraine, it occurs after the prodromal phase.

It is helpful to know whether the person has suffered similar episodes before, as a new pain of some severity should be taken more seriously than recurrence of a headache that has been successfully dealt with in the past.

If a headache has become progressively more severe over a period of days (or in the case of a child, a few hours) and is not responding to treatment, referral should be considered. In the absence of any other significant factors, a headache that is becoming less painful can reasonably be treated with simple analgesics.

The frequency as well as the duration of recurrent headaches should be noted, and may reveal particular patterns. Migraine attacks classically last only a few hours, but in some people they can persist for 72 hours. Migraine usually occurs every few weeks and rarely more than once a week, whereas cluster headaches occur for 1 or 2 hours at the same time of day, every day, for several weeks.

Headache that is present on awakening can represent a serious cause, such as a space-occupying lesion, but migraines often awaken people, and people can wake up with tension headaches or chronic daily headache. Further history is therefore needed to distinguish between the causes.

Generally, a headache that does not disappear or improve over 1–2 weeks should be considered for referral to a GP, with one or two exceptions, such as tension headache (which may occur every day for several weeks in some cases).

It is useful to assess the intensity of the pain by asking the sufferer how severe the pain is and then probing the answer further by asking if it is mild and annoying or severe and debilitating. Another guide to severity is whether the person is able to carry on with their daily routine. Other useful questions are whether this is the worst pain the person has ever had or whether the pain 'stopped them in their tracks'. If the answer to either of these is yes, they should be referred to their GP or serious consideration should be given to whether referral to an Accident and Emergency department would be appropriate.

### Character of the pain

A description of the pain can give valuable pointers to a possible cause of the headache as described in Table 4.3.

### Factors that aggravate or relieve headache

Establishing a pattern to the onset of headaches, especially recurrent episodes, can help not only in seeking a possible cause but also in removing trigger factors. When appropriate, inquiries based on the list shown in Table 4.4 will be helpful.

The avoidance of trigger factors can help in diagnosing the cause of a headache as well as in relieving it. Migraine headaches are classically relieved by sleep or by vomiting. Premenstrual syndrome, which may present with a headache and other symptoms (see Chapter 6), classically improves or disappears when menstrual bleeding starts.

## Nausea and vomiting

Nausea and vomiting are associated with many disorders. For example, they may be gastrointestinal in

| Table 4.3 Character of pain | |
|---|---|
| A sudden pain | Pain that feels like a blow to the head or an explosion in the head and that stops the person in their tracks with no warning whatsoever suggests a haemorrhage (see text) and requires immediate referral, to a hospital if necessary, if the person is in obvious distress. |
| A throbbing or pounding pain | Such pain indicates a vascular cause, e.g. the vasodilatation caused by fever or migraine. |
| A constant or nagging pain | Such pain is most probably due to a tension-type headache, but if it progressively worsens, the possibility of something more serious should be borne in mind. |
| Moderate to severe pain | This is more likely to be migraine than tension-type headache, but the most easily discriminating factors are the duration and the other associations, such as nausea, vomiting or visual disturbances. |

**Table 4.4    Trigger factors for headache**

| Trigger factors or onset pattern | Possible underlying cause |
|---|---|
| Food, e.g. cheese, chocolate, caffeine, specific alcoholic drinks | Migraine |
| Exercise | Migraine; space-occupying lesion |
| Light | Migraine; meningitis |
| Hunger | Migraine |
| Neck movement | Tension; neck injury; meningitis; arthritis or fibrositis of the neck; vascular pathology |
| Cyclical pattern in women | Side effect of oral contraceptive; premenstrual tension; migraine; depression; tension |
| Present on awakening or wakes the sufferer at night | Tension; neck muscle spasm; sinusitis; space-occupying lesion causing increased intracranial pressure |
| Bending down | Space-occupying lesion; sinusitis |
| Straining, coughing, sneezing | Space-occupying lesion |
| Sudden and severe with rapid onset | Subarachnoid haemorrhage |
| Travel | Tension; migraine |
| Drugs | Various, including oral contraceptives, indometacin, vasodilators (e.g. nitrates, calcium antagonists). Check *BNF* monographs for individual drugs. |
| Ice cream, cold food | Usually no organic cause. |

origin (viral or bacterial infections such as gastroenteritis, overindulgence in either food or alcohol, or appendicitis); CNS in origin (with anxiety or severe pain); associated with ear and vestibular disorders (labyrinthitis or ear infections), often called vertigo; as a result of movement in motion sickness and high altitude in 'mountain' sickness; or associated with pregnancy ('morning sickness').

Stimulation of a complex reflex coordinated by the vomiting centre in the brain stem results in nausea and vomiting. It receives input from the vestibular system, cerebral cortex and receptor cells in the gut and visceral surfaces and the chemoreceptor trigger zone (CTZ), which is sensitive to circulating chemical abnormalities in the body such as emetic drugs, pyretics or hormones. The sufferer will experience an unpleasant sensation, which may be followed by forceful expulsion of the contents of the stomach. In vertigo the nausea is usually associated with a sensation that surroundings are moving or spinning, light-headedness and loss of balance. In motion sickness, autonomic symptoms predominate so the nausea will often be accompanied by pallor,

sweating, increased salivation, yawning, malaise and hyperventilation.

Nausea, with or without vomiting, is present alongside a number of causes of headache: migraine, glaucoma, space-occupying lesions and meningitis. Migraine sufferers often find that vomiting occurs towards the end of an attack, and is seen as a relief and a sign that the pain is about to subside. However, effortless vomiting in the morning, associated with a headache, could suggest a potentially serious problem.

Commons causes of nausea and vomiting in children are gastroenteritis, fever or ear infections and will usually be self-limiting. As with diarrhoea in children, especially younger children, dehydration is the biggest concern (see Chapter 2). In babies, differentiating between regurgitation of feed and vomiting is important. Vomiting in children under 1 year requires referral.

## Accompanying symptoms

Inquiries about concurrent symptoms can help in differentiating between types of headache and other symptoms, such as insomnia, which may present along with or independently of a headache.

### Fever

A fever in adults with headache, especially with aching muscles (myalgia), aching joints and/or general malaise, is common in viral infections, sometimes accompanied by other symptoms of upper respiratory tract infection. Fever may also accompany the headache of sinusitis, along with nasal congestion or recent symptoms of the common cold and tenderness of the sinus areas to light finger pressure (see Chapter 3). Fever may occasionally accompany the pain at the side of the head associated with temporal arteritis. In children, fever is one of the distinguishing factors in meningitis.

### Nasal congestion and rhinitis

Nasal congestion accompanies the headache of sinusitis and is also seen in some people with cluster headaches, together with rhinitis and facial flushing.

### Tender temples

Older people can develop temporal arteritis, a condition in which either one or both of the temporal arteries is inflamed and may be seen as a red, congested vessel in the temple area, running vertically up the side of the head just in front of the ear. The sufferer will find that pressure applied to the skin over the artery is very painful. Although rare, they may also have pain or an ache in the jaw, particularly after eating. This is due to obstruction of the blood supply from the cranial artery. If temporal arteritis is suspected, the sufferer requires same-day referral for a medical opinion, as vision can sometimes be affected.

### Insomnia

Insomnia is a subjective issue, with sufferers describing poor sleep, either in terms of duration or quality, and sometimes sleep that does not refresh. Insomnia is very common and may have physical, psychological or drug-related causes (Table 4.5). Temporary insomnia is often associated with stress, personal problems, painful physical illness, depression, anxiety, and excessive alcohol or caffeine intake. Normal sleep requirements vary widely, from just 3–4 hours per night, so history taking is important. Sufferers may complain of daytime fatigue, but sleepiness during the day is more likely to be associated with

| Table 4.5 Possible causes of insomnia and sleep disturbance | |
|---|---|
| **Causes** | **Examples** |
| Physical | Musculoskeletal disorders (restless legs syndrome, leg cramps)<br>Respiratory disorders (sleep apnoea, dyspnoea, cough)<br>Pain (arthritis, headaches)<br>Nocturia (benign prostatic hyperplasia, diabetes mellitus, diuretics)<br>Endocrine disorders (hyperthyroidism – sweats)<br>Perimenopausal symptoms<br>Skin disorders (pruritus) |
| Physiological | Poor sleep hygiene (caffeine, daytime naps)<br>Sleeping environment (noise, light)<br>Disturbed sleep pattern (shift work, jetlag, intellectual or physical activity immediately prior to going to bed)<br>Psychological (worry, bereavement; excessive worrying about not sleeping; nightmares, night terrors, sleepwalking)<br>Psychiatric (depression, dementia, anxiety) |
| Pharmacological | Drug withdrawal (hypnotics, alcohol – reduces time to onset of sleep, but disrupts sleep later in the night)<br>Chronic benzodiazepine misuse<br>Some antidepressants especially SSRIs and MAOIs<br>Sympathomimetics<br>Corticosteroids – agitation<br>Beta blockers |

a sleep disorder such as obstructive sleep apnoea, which should be referred for investigation.

If a headache is severe enough to interfere with sleep then a medical opinion should be sought, but more commonly sufferers will complain of early-morning wakening or an inability to fall asleep on retiring, unrelated to the headache, and this may indicate depression and anxiety, respectively. Symptoms of tiredness, poor appetite and mood changes will point to the possibility of a tension headache.

Insomnia that lasts for more than 3 weeks should be referred to a GP for further investigation.

### Visual disturbances

Failing vision requires medical referral, but visual phenomena are a common feature of migraine with aura, and constitute part of the aura that precedes the headache. Restriction of the visual field, or the appearance of haloes around lights, especially in one eye only, suggest glaucoma or the optic neuritis of multiple sclerosis, and same-day referral is required. Visual loss or double vision may occur in temporal arteritis. Any disturbance of vision, unless attributable to migraine, requires urgent referral if possible to an Accident and Emergency department.

Only around 10–20% of migraine sufferers have an aura of any description, and therefore other causes of visual disturbance resembling the descriptions associated with migraine should be borne in mind and medical referral made if there is any uncertainty, or if the duration is longer than 1 hour. Such causes may be acute vascular or neurological deficits such as stroke, retinal occlusion or other intraocular pathology.

### Neck stiffness

Neck stiffness in an adult with headache may be related to a neck strain or injury, but it could be a sign of a traction headache. Difficulty in placing the chin on the chest is a signal to refer as an emergency, particularly in children and young adults, as it raises the possibility of meningitis.

### Central nervous system symptoms

People reporting signs and symptoms of central nervous system involvement require special consideration for medical referral. Symptoms may reflect general disturbances, such as loss of coordination and balance, drowsiness, irritability, personality changes and even fits. Sometimes the symptoms will reflect more localised lesions, for example slurred speech, muscle weakness in a limb, and disturbances of the senses of smell and hearing. Such problems may accompany the headache of space-occupying lesions, such as tumours, and also subarachnoid haemorrhage and subdural haemorrhage (as in head injuries). Paraesthesia (pins and needles or numbness), usually in the arm, may occur as part of the aura of classic migraine, but this should disappear within a short time.

Any persistent unusual sensations require further investigation, as they may be a sign of a space-occupying lesion.

All of these conditions, with the exception of migraine, are rare, particularly in terms of presentation in the pharmacy. Nevertheless, they are potentially devastating diagnoses and must constantly be borne in mind.

### Rash

In children or young adults with headache, the appearance of a rash anywhere on the body is a reason to refer immediately for a medical opinion to exclude meningitis. The meningococcal rash is classically purpuric, that is it is formed by haemorrhages from small blood vessels and leaves purple marks on the skin that do not blanch when pressed (Figure 4.2). However, in the early stages the presentation can be confusing.

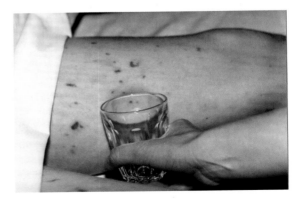

**Figure 4.2** Meningococcal rash and the glass test.
(Reproduced with permission of the Meningitis Trust.)

### Weight loss

Although the presentation in the pharmacy of weight loss (over a period of weeks or months) associated with headache will be unusual, it should always be regarded as a potentially serious sign requiring referral. It may occur in cranial arteritis and systemic disease, as well as in people with malignancy.

### Dental pain

Toothache and gingival pain are discussed in Chapter 7 but may present along with headache. Individuals may also request pain relief following dental treatment, for example a tooth extraction. In babies and toddlers, teething is a common cause of pain and usually presents along with red flushed cheek or face and dribbling more than usual. It may also be associated with slight fever. Teething occurs when the baby teeth come through the gums and is a normal part of development that usually starts around 6 months of age (but sometimes as early as 4 months) and is complete by 2–3 years of age.

### Special considerations in children

As with all illnesses it is difficult to obtain an exact history from a child, and young children who feel ill may well describe their malaise as a headache without head pain being a feature at all. Special attention should be paid to the possibility of a head injury, as young children are prone to knocks and falls.

Neck stiffness, which could be a sign of meningitis, should be considered an alarm symptom resulting in the immediate referral of the sufferer for medical investigation, although this symptom may be hard to elicit in young children. Meningitis is often notoriously difficult to diagnose, even by doctors, and it is essential that time is taken to find out whether a child looks ill or behaves oddly, appears drowsy or irritable, or is vomiting or failing to feed.

The popular conception of meningitis is that of a sudden severe illness that is fatal if not immediately treated. This is true of the rare epidemic meningococcal forms. Rash is a danger signal, but the symptoms do not all develop together and the 'warning' signs often occur relatively late on. The time from the first appearance of symptoms to a stage when the chance of survival is severely compromised can be as short as a few hours. However, viral meningitis often has a more insidious onset and could easily present – particularly in its early stages – in the pharmacy. Great caution is therefore advised in children with headaches. Where any doubts exists, same-day or more urgent referral (depending on the duration and severity) is mandatory.

Children can suffer from migraine, which can start below the age of 10 years, but its onset is more common between the ages of 11 and 15, often around the time of puberty. The symptoms are similar to those experienced by adults, but are usually shorter lasting. Abdominal pain tends to be more prevalent than in adults, and an aura is often present.

## Management options

### Pain and headache

Pain is a subjective, emotional symptom and the treatment of headache should be holistic rather than restricted to the symptom itself. A sympathetic ear and reassuring counsel will often help to alleviate the anxiety felt by some people.

Once referral has been ruled out, management of any type of pain involves removal of any causative factors and then consideration of analgesics. The choice depends on the underlying cause, severity and type of pain.

In headache, immediate referral may be required for individuals presenting with headache likely to be of secondary origin. Symptoms such as unilateral motor weakness, clumsiness or seizure-like movements, visual disturbances (other than with migraine), reduced level of consciousness, rash, headache following recent injury or a marked increase in either frequency or severity of headache require urgent referral.

Once serious pathology has been eliminated, consideration should be given to removing any possible predisposing factors or triggers. It should be emphasised that exercise-induced headache, such as migraine, should be alleviated not by avoiding exercise but by carefully increasing personal fitness so that the exercise threshold that causes the headache can be raised.

In situations where newly prescribed drugs are suspected of causing the headache, individuals should be encouraged to persist for a week or so as often an adjustment period is necessary, but this will depend on the severity of the headache. In most cases, alternative drugs will be available.

The treatment of chronic or repeated headaches, such as tension headache and migraine, lends itself to many types of non-drug therapy, such as massage, acupuncture, osteopathy and hypnotherapy. Topical application of levomenthol (available as a proprietary headache soothing stick) or lavender or peppermint oil to the forehead or temples can sometimes relieve headache without the need for analgesics.

It is easier to prevent a headache or reduce its duration by acting early, rather than trying to treat one that has already developed. This is particularly true for migraine.

Tension headaches should be treated with simple analgesics for a limited period of about 14 days before considering referral.

Anyone suspected of having medication overuse headache should be encouraged to stop taking analgesics even when they are suffering the pain to allow washout of the analgesic from the body. Simple analgesics or triptans may be stopped abruptly, but opioids should be withdrawn gradually. Structured advice and referral for professional support are advisable.

The response of individuals to simple analgesics is variable for both pharmacological and psychological reasons. Soluble and effervescent formulations of analgesics, especially aspirin, will reduce the likelihood of gastrointestinal adverse effects. No clear correlation exists between the rapid attainment of so-called therapeutic blood levels and the onset of pain relief after the ingestion of soluble tablet formulations, but the powerful placebo effect of effervescent tablets should not be ignored. They are also a rational choice in people who suffer migraine, as the reduced gut motility associated with this condition is thought to reduce and delay the absorption of drug from standard tablet formulations.

## Nausea and vomiting

Nausea may be managed with antiemetics. Choice of antiemetic type depends on the aetiology of the nausea, but the options available as GSL (general sales list) or P (pharmacy-only) medicines are limited by licensed indications.

The nausea associated with the first trimester of pregnancy is usually mild and self-limiting, but women can be advised of strategies to limit their symptoms. Rest, drinking small amounts frequently, taking small, cold, frequent, carbohydrate-rich meals, eating biscuits to boost blood sugar levels, and avoidance of caffeine, alcohol or any foods or smells that trigger nausea may help. A pregnant woman with moderate to severe morning sickness should be referred to her GP.

It is better to prevent motion sickness from occurring than trying to treat it once nausea has started. Sufferers can be advised to prevent motion sickness by use of a number of strategies: keeping motion to a minimum, for example by sitting in the front of a car; not reading or watching a film; looking at a fixed place ahead on the horizon; closing eyes or sleeping; and breathing fresh air if possible. Sufferers can also be advised to avoid heavy meals or alcohol before, and during, travelling. It may also be worth avoiding spicy or fatty foods. Antiemetics are more effective in motion sickness if given prophylactically to prevent nausea and vomiting developing and should be taken prior to travel (in some cases the night before). They can be used as treatment once it occurs, but as gastric motility is inhibited they are less likely to be effective.

Acupressure on the wrists (using proprietary pressure bands) has been found by some to be helpful for morning or motion sickness, although this is not supported by strong clinical evidence.

In children, antipyretics will help nausea associated with fever and oral rehydration therapy will prevent dehydration. Oral rehydration products may also be useful in adults suffering vomiting for several hours, for example in gastroenteritis. Unexplained nausea and vomiting at any age should be referred for medical investigation.

## Insomnia

Management of insomnia involves exploring and removing any underlying cause. Advice can be given on relaxation techniques, good sleep hygiene and a restful sleep environment. Use of a sleep diary can be helpful in determining causes and patterns of insomnia. Insomnia associated with worry or stress can be quite distressing and sufferers should be advised to discuss this with their GP if it is prolonged. There are a number of effective psychological techniques for managing insomnia that can be taught by trained professionals, but simple self-help strategies, preferably supported by written information, can be offered to the sufferer. Current guidance is that hypnotics should be avoided or limited to short courses in acutely distressed individuals.

### Non-opioid analgesics (BNF section 4.7.1)

Paracetamol has analgesic and antipyretic properties, making it an effective analgesic for many types of headache including migraine. It also has a role in providing symptomatic relief from the pain of soft tissue inflammation and joint disorders. The combination of its analgesic and antipyretic properties provides some benefit to those suffering from the symptom complexes of the common cold and flu-like illnesses, providing some relief from the generalised discomfort experienced in these conditions.

Paracetamol is safe in therapeutic doses and does not interact with other drugs. It is contained in many proprietary preparations and combination products, including cold and flu remedies, so individuals should be advised not to take different products together so as to avoid exceeding the maximum daily dose of 4 g. Paediatric liquid formulations of paracetamol are recommended for children and can be given to relieve the pain of teething or reduce fever and pyrexia.

Non-steroidal anti-inflammatory drugs (NSAIDs) have analgesic and anti-inflammatory properties and are effective in most types of headache, but as always care should be taken to inquire about any relative contraindications to NSAIDs such as history of peptic ulcer disease or cautions such as asthma. NSAIDs and aspirin should also be avoided following tooth extraction because of the increased risk of bleeding. NSAIDs are considered more fully later in this chapter in relation to soft tissue inflammation and joint disorders.

### Opioid analgesics (BNF section 4.7.2)

Both codeine and dihydrocodeine are available as P medicines combined with aspirin, paracetamol or ibuprofen as combination products. These products can be seen as a second-line approach for use when single-agent products fail to alleviate symptoms. There is limited evidence for increased clinical analgesia with these drug combinations, particularly with codeine at a dose of 8 mg, and adverse effects such as constipation are common. There is a tendency, however, for both the public and health professionals to consider them as more powerful than single agents.

Combination analgesics containing codeine are often associated with medication-overuse headache and should therefore be avoided for the management of headache wherever possible.

In 2009 the Medicines and Healthcare products Regulatory Agency (MHRA) updated its guidance on supply of products containing codeine and dihydrocodeine. It advises that these products should only be used for acute, moderate pain not relieved by paracetamol, aspirin or ibuprofen alone and should not be taken for longer than 3 days because of their addiction potential.

### Caffeine

Caffeine is often present in analgesic combinations and is claimed to potentiate the activity and the absorption of analgesics. The data to support the clinical significance of these actions are equivocal and, theoretically, caffeine can be harmful, as it can stimulate the secretion of gastric acid (enhancing the irritant effect of aspirin) and cause central excitation (counteracting the desire to obtain relief of headache by rest or sleep in some sufferers, particularly in migraine). Either an excess of (or withdrawal from) caffeine can also cause headache.

### Antimigraine drugs (BNF section 4.7.4)

Several migraine-specific combination analgesic products are available as P medicines. All contain paracetamol, usually in combination with codeine. Sedating antihistamines can be included for nausea (see below) and one product contains isometheptene, an indirect-acting sympathomimetic, which is included for its vasoconstrictor effect.

Sumatriptan is a 5HT1 receptor agonist that can be supplied as a P medicine for the treatment of acute migraine attacks in people aged 18–65 years where there is a clear diagnosis of migraine. It is recommended for individuals with an established pattern of migraine (a history of five or more attacks, with the first occurring more than 12 months ago) when simple analgesics (with antiemetic if required)

**Box 4.2  Sumatriptan should not be supplied as a pharmacy medicine in the following circumstances**

- When the person is under the age of 18 years or over the age of 65.
- When the person is aged 50 years or over and experiencing migraine attacks for the first time. (Can be considered for supply of sumatriptan as a P medicine if a doctor confirms a diagnosis of migraine.)
- For someone who had their first migraine attack within the previous 12 months or has had fewer than five migraine attacks in the past.
- For someone who experiences four or more attacks per month or if migraine headache lasts for longer than 24 hours. (Could potentially be suitable for supply of sumatriptan as a P medicine but should be referred to a doctor for assessment.)
- For individuals who do not respond to treatment.
- For people who have a headache (of any type) on 10 or more days per month.
- Women with migraine taking the combined oral contraceptive pill have an increased risk of stroke and so should be referred if the onset of migraine is within the previous 3 months, if attacks are worsening or if they have a migraine with aura.
- When the person does not recover fully between attacks.
- Pregnant or breastfeeding migraine sufferers.
- For people with three or more cardiovascular risk factors: men aged over 40 years, postmenopausal women, hypercholesterolaemia, regular smoker (10 or more daily), obesity – body mass index more than 30 kg/m², diabetes, family history of early heart disease.
- For people with contraindications to sumatriptan (see *BNF* monograph).

have failed. Box 4.2 details circumstances in which sumatriptan should not be supplied as a P medicine.

### Antiemetics (BNF section 4.6)

Antiemetics work by blocking the neurotransmitters and receptors involved at various points in the nausea pathways described above. Domperidone, a dopamine antagonist that acts on the chemoreceptor trigger zone (CTZ) and increases intestinal motility, is available as a P medicine for short-term treatment of nausea and vomiting (of less than 48 hours' duration) in adults over 16 years. It is also licensed for the gastric symptoms of over-indulgence (see Chapter 2), and as it acts on the CTZ it is unlikely to be effective in motion sickness or vertigo.

Prochlorperazine is also a dopamine antagonist and is available as a P medicine as a buccal tablet licensed for the nausea associated with migraine.

Hyoscine hydrobromide is an antimuscarinic that has central and peripheral actions and is effective in the prevention and treatment of motion sickness. The antimuscarinic adverse effects make it less tolerated than the slightly less effective sedating antihistamines.

### Sedating antihistamines (BNF section 3.4.1)

The sedating antihistamines cinnarizine and promethazine are licensed for the management of motion sickness. They are of similar efficacy but have different onset and duration of action and differ in the extent of adverse effects such as drowsiness.

Buclizine is included (along with paracetamol and codeine) in a combination analgesic for migraine associated with nausea.

Doxylamine succinate is included in combination analgesic products (along with paracetamol, codeine and caffeine) marketed specifically for tension-type headache, and it may help relax tension through its sedating effect.

The sedating antihistamines diphenhydramine and promethazine are also licensed as P medicines for the short-term management of temporary sleep disturbance. They may be useful in re-establishing a broken sleep pattern (for example in shift workers) but will not deal with the underlying cause of insomnia. Anyone who presents with insomnia with signs of anxiety or stress (for example with a tension headache) is worth referring for medical assessment and support.

## Dietary and herbal supplements

Feverfew is a herbal remedy that has had variable success in the prophylaxis of migraine in clinical trials. A Cochrane review found conflicting evidence but concluded that that feverfew is more effective than placebo.

Herbal medicines are sometimes used for relief of stress that may be a trigger for headaches. Valerian, hops and gentian as well as St John's Wort are marketed as calming herbal remedies. Valerian is also used along with passiflora in herbal products for temporary relief of sleep disturbances.

Ginger has been suggested to have antiemetic actions and some people have found it helpful in relieving the symptoms of morning sickness or motion sickness. Research evidence to support its use is insufficient to allow firm conclusions to be drawn on effectiveness.

Table 4.6 describes some interactions between analgesics available as P or GSL medicines and some prescribed drugs.

**Table 4.6   Interactions between analgesics available as a P or GSL medicines and some prescribed drugs**

| Analgesic | Interacting drug | Consequence |
|---|---|---|
| Aspirin | Methotrexate | Renal excretion of methotrexate reduced |
| Aspirin | Anticoagulants, e.g. warfarin | Extended clotting time, potential haemorrhages |
| NSAIDs (ibuprofen, diclofenac, naproxen) | | |
| Aspirin | Antidepressants, e.g. SSRIs and venlafaxine | Increased risk of bleeding |
| NSAIDs | | |
| NSAIDs | Lithium | Renal excretion of lithium reduced |
| NSAIDs | Diuretics | Increased risk of NSAID induced nephrotoxicity |
| Opioids (codeine, dihydrocodeine) | Sedating antihistamines | Increased sedation |
| Aspirin | Prescribed drugs and combination products containing the same individual components, e.g. co-codamol | Additive toxicity |

 **Re-consider the case**

Before reading further, re-consider the following questions and your initial thoughts on this case.

**Trigger questions**

- What additional information would you need before considering the appropriate management options in this case?
- What issues concern you about this case?
- Are any alarm symptoms being exhibited that require more urgent treatment or referral?

**Case study**

A woman in her mid-40s reports 'tension headaches'. She has had them before, often premenstrually when she feels stressed. Recently they have become bad enough to need treatment. The headache is usually left sided and builds up over about an hour, and she senses when one is imminent. She often feels nauseated and has tried paracetamol without effect.

Pharmacist opinion

From the symptoms described (prodromal period, unilateral pain developing over an hour with nausea), this headache sounds like migraine. It may be that the migraine is being triggered by hormones during the premenstrual period. It would be worth exploring more what the woman means by 'feeling stressed' premenstrually.

Because there appears to have been a change in severity recently it would be wise to refer to her GP for further assessment. A combination product that includes paracetamol, codeine and buclazine could be supplied until she is able to consult her GP. This codeine-containing product is suitable as paracetamol alone has been unsuccessful and the sedating antihistamine will help with the nausea.

We do not know enough about the pattern of this woman's migraine to assess her suitability for a supply of sumatriptan as a P medicine. A person suffering from migraine does not have to have had it diagnosed by a GP before supply can be made providing their symptoms and pattern of attacks indicate established migraine, i.e. five or more attacks with the first occurring more than a year ago. However, in this case, because of the changing pattern of severity, a medical assessment and evaluation would be advisable before considering supply, especially given the cyclical nature of her attacks.

 GP opinion

Headaches are an extremely common symptom with a variety of causes. Migraines are a specific type of headache that may be precipitated by stress, alcohol, fatigue, types of food, etc. Some drugs can also increase frequency of migraines, e.g. the combined oral contraceptive pill. In this case, it appears that the headache frequently occurs premenstrually owing to the reduction in oestrogen level leading up to menstruation.

A diagnosis of migraine is made on history alone; a clear history is therefore essential. There are diagnostic criteria to follow. Features supportive of migraine here are its being unilateral, severe enough to require treatment, and nausea. Migraines last over 4 hours. The feeling that a headache is imminent is common, but this is different from aura which involves either visual and/or sensory symptoms prior to the headache.

The main differential diagnosis is tension-type headache; this has less-specific features and often arises from the neck. Migraine and tension-type headache can occur together.

Symptoms suggesting more serious causes would be sudden and much more severe headache, associated confusion or unsteadiness, and persistent headaches lasting days.

Treatment of migraine is to relieve the acute symptoms, identify trigger factors and prevent future attacks. Simple analgesia with or without antiemetics is often adequate treatment. Triptans are a specific anti-migraine drugs effective in those with moderate to severe symptoms.

Treatment of premenstrual migraine would be to manipulate hormone levels. A simple option would be to use oestrogen patches several days before menstruation. Migraine sufferers can also be offered drugs to prevent migraines, e.g. beta-blockers, amitriptyline and some anticonvulsants.

**Summary of key points**

| Condition | Management |
|---|---|
| Tension-type headache characterised by bilateral pain described by the sufferer as a generalised ache or pain, with no specific focus, felt all over the cranium or as a tight band around the head, spreading over the top of the head. | Removal of possible predisposing factors or triggers. Simple analgesics. Combination analgesics if single agents have failed. Advice on relaxation and non-analgesic management such as aromatherapy oils or levomenthol. |
| Migraine characterised by unilateral, moderate to severe, pulsating or throbbing pain that builds up over minutes to hours. It may occur with or without aura and can be associated with nausea and vomiting and sensitivity to light and sound. | Avoidance of trigger factors. Simple analgesics or NSAIDs with an antiemetic if required. Sumatriptan in an established pattern of migraine when simple analgesics (with antiemetic if required) have failed. |
| Nausea and vomiting characterised by an unpleasant sensation that may be followed by forceful expulsion of the contents of the stomach. | Antiemetics (choice dependent on cause). Domperidone, especially if gastric cause. Prochlorperazine or buclizine if associated with migraine. Hyoscine hydrobromide or sedating antihistamines for motion sickness. Prevention of dehydration by maintenance of fluid intake or rehydration products. Advice on helpful strategies for pregnancy morning sickness. |
| Insomnia characterised by poor sleep, either in terms of duration or quality, and sometimes sleep that does not refresh. | Identification and removal of possible cause. Sedating antihistamines or herbal alternatives may be considered for short-term use to re-establish a broken sleep pattern. |

 **When to refer***

- Headache of sudden onset and described as explosive and the sufferer being 'stopped in their tracks'
- Headache occurring some time after a head injury
- Headache that is obviously severe, i.e. one with severe/sudden onset, that is disabling, such that the sufferer cannot move, that interferes with daily routine (and the sufferer has not experienced this before), when the sufferer appears ill
- Headache where pain is progressively worsening over weeks
- Headache that occurs 15 or more days in a month
- Headache of short duration but worsening over days
- Headache that is worse on awakening
- Cluster headache
- Suspected secondary headache with symptoms indicating underlying pathology:
  — Pain in temporal area
  — Neurological signs, e.g. paraesthesia, mood change, drowsiness, slurred speech, loss of balance, irritability and poor coordination
  — Visual disturbance (if migraine has been excluded)
  — Pupils unequal in size or not responding to light
  — Loss of consciousness
  — Jaw pain
  — Neck stiffness
  — Rash

**When to refer\*** (*continued*)

- Unexplained nausea and vomiting
- Nausea and vomiting with severe abdominal pain
- Vomiting in children under 1 year
- Nausea and vomiting where symptoms do not resolve following treatment
- Insomnia associated with anxiety or other symptoms of depression
- Unexplained insomnia
- Insomnia lasting longer than 3 weeks

\*Urgency of referral is a matter of judgement, depending on the signs and symptoms.

## Soft tissue inflammation and joint disorders

Before reading further, consider the following case and note your initial thoughts.

**Case study**

A man in his 30s is a semi-regular visitor to your pharmacy and has requested a small supply of a topical anti-inflammatory preparation and some ibuprofen tablets. This man is employed in a strenuous manual job and regards his frequent episodes of back and shoulder pain as nothing more than an occupational hazard.

**Trigger questions**

- What additional information would you need before considering the appropriate management options in this case?
- What issues concern you about this case?
- Are any alarm symptoms being exhibited that require more urgent treatment or referral?

### Assessing symptoms

The musculoskeletal system consists of the bony skeleton and associated soft tissues comprising ligaments, skeletal muscles and tendons. Ligaments are bands of tissue that connect bones, usually at a joint, and impart strength and stability to the joint, thereby limiting abnormal movement. The skeletal muscles shorten and lengthen to create movement; they are attached to bones by tendons and function together as a unit. Bursae (small fluid-filled sacs) reduce friction and serve a protective function between a bone and a tendon, between two tendons, or between a bone or tendon and the overlying skin.

Disorders of the musculoskeletal system are the result of wear, strain, overuse or trauma, resulting in inflammation or swelling and pain. It is important to consider this when choosing the management options to ensure that the appropriate approach is adopted for the cause of the injury. In managing these conditions it is important to differentiate acute injuries associated with falls or sporting activities from the symptoms of chronic conditions such as rheumatoid arthritis and backache. As the presentation of symptom complexes varies depending on the location of the injury causing the disorder, this section will consider the different areas of the musculoskeletal system from head to toe and how different conditions will present in these areas.

## The neck

Pain in the neck can be caused by strain on the ligaments and muscles resulting from unaccustomed movements or positions, including lifting heavy weights or even sitting at a desk. It may be felt in arthritis (in middle-aged to older age groups) or when a disc prolapses (in both young and older age groups). Wry neck (acute torticollis) is a condition in which the neck is bent or twisted because of muscle spasm; it is often caused by unaccustomed or repeated movement, or after exposure to cold. It is a painful condition and the neck will be tender and tense due to spasm in one or more muscles in the neck. Pain is often felt on one side of the neck and, if the powerful trapezius muscle is affected, down as far as the upper border of the scapula, close to the shoulder. The trapezius is a triangular muscle with its base running along the spine between the occiput at the base of the skull and a point just below the scapula, converging to a point at the shoulder. The condition often arises after sleeping in an awkward posture. It may also be traced to diving, heading a soccer ball or similar movements and there is usually no previous history of neck pain.

Palpation of the tender area on the affected side results in spasm of the muscles. In wry neck, the neck vertebrae are not tender. In contrast, in cervical spondylosis, which is a degeneration of the cervical spine, similar to osteoarthritis, the vertebrae are often – but not always – tender to the touch. In wry neck there will be free movement of the head away from the affected side, but there will be difficulty and pain in turning towards the affected side. This is particularly the case if the sternomastoid muscles, which lie at the side and towards the front of the neck, are affected. In arthritis or spondylosis, movement is usually equally painful to both sides but can be worse in one direction. If there is nerve root pain, movement brings a sharp pain down the shoulder and arm in the distribution of the affected nerve. Viewed from the side, the normal cervical spine has a mild forward curve. In advanced degeneration or conditions of poor posture, this curve is exaggerated so that the head appears to have slipped forwards on the neck. This can be very painful.

## The shoulders

The most common disorder affecting the shoulder joint, apart from trauma, is capsulitis (rotator cuff syndrome). Capsulitis is inflammation of the fibrous supporting tissue surrounding the shoulder joint. This may be caused by overuse or unaccustomed movement resulting in inflammation in the ring of tendons attached to the shoulder muscles. Movement is restricted in one or all directions.

A common variant is the supraspinatus syndrome. The supraspinatus muscle, which lies on the upper border of the spine of the scapula, is responsible for abduction (raising) of the arm at the shoulder joint. In this syndrome the shoulder is particularly painful when the arm is raised laterally from the body. Palpation at the outermost point of the shoulder, just behind the lateral tip of the clavicle, will reveal an acutely tender supraspinatus tendon, confirming the diagnosis. In the more widespread rotator cuff syndrome the tenderness is slightly lower, around the neck of the humerus, and extends further.

After a painful disorder of the shoulder has apparently healed, it may become apparent some time afterwards that the arm cannot be raised above the head or behind the back. This is often due to scarring or fibrosis of the muscles, tendons and ligaments around the shoulder joint, which can occur to such an extent that the syndrome known as frozen shoulder develops, often with some degree of irreversibility.

## The back

The back can be viewed in two parts; the upper back comprising the cervical and thoracic curves (including intercostal muscles) and the lower back comprising the lumbar curve, sacrum and coccyx.

Thoracic spinal pain is uncommon and should be referred unless some obvious trivial cause can be found. Pain arising in the intercostal muscles (between the ribs) may be due to a muscle strain, but it must be distinguished from the pain of a myocardial infarction, pulmonary embolus or pleurisy. Pain arising after straining, while lifting a heavy object or coughing, may be due to a muscle strain or tear, or to a prolapsed (slipped) disc, which will cause a ligament to be stretched and muscles to go into spasm. Such musculoskeletal damage must be differentiated from other serious causes of pain. Chest pain due to angina will usually disappear after resting or after the administration of glyceryl trinitrate. The pain of myocardial infarction lasts longer than 30 minutes and the sufferer will often be anxious, cyanosed and sweating, and in most cases will be obviously ill. A muscle strain or tear will cause a sharp pain in a small, defined area that will be exacerbated by coughing or deep inspiration. This is also the case with pleurisy or a pulmonary embolus, although in severe cases of these disorders the pain may be present continuously, with abnormal breathing.

Pain in the lumbar spine can be due to lumbago and can be classified as mild or severe and is most common in the third and fourth decades. In both types there will often be a strain of the spinal muscles and ligaments (soft tissue lumbago) or more seriously disorders of the vertebrae, intervertebral discs and their associated joints. Acute soft tissue lumbago can often be related to an event such as lifting or twisting. The pain may be experienced diffusely across both sides of the back at the level of the sacrum, or linearly and to one side in the vertically running spinal muscles, but there is often no pain at rest or on slow movement.

If the intervertebral discs are squeezed outwards and prolapse (slipped disc), there will be sudden severe backache. A prolapsed disc (Figure 4.3) will often impinge on the roots of nerves originating from the spinal cord. In such cases the pressure on the nerve root will cause pain in the area supplied by the nerve. Sufferers will hold themselves rigid to avoid movement because movement exacerbates the constant pain associated with a prolapsed disc. Their gait will be stiff and awkward and they will find sitting down painful and difficult. The sciatic nerve is most commonly affected by prolapsed discs, usually resulting in an intense and burning pain that radiates from the back to the buttock and the back of the leg and sometimes to the front of the thigh and is referred to as sciatica. It may also spread to below the knee and sufferers will find it difficult to flex the hip very far, making climbing stairs or sitting down uncomfortable.

Back pain that is worse after rest and improves with exercise may be due to ankylosing spondylitis, an inflammatory arthritis of the lumbar spine and sacroiliac joints that has a genetic disposition. Ankylosing spondylitis starts in young adult life and is more common in males than in females; it is characterised by pain and stiffness, especially in the morning after rest. There is a notable restriction of flexion of the spine and the sacroiliac joints are often tender.

Coccygitis produces a pain in the coccyx (tailbone) and is often caused by a fall on to a hard surface. The coccyx will be tender to the touch and painful, especially when sitting down and will take a few weeks to heal. Injury to the small spur of the vertebrae at the tip of the spine (coccyx), as in a fall, causes a painful coccydynia and inflammation of the ligaments attached to the coccyx. The pain may last for several months and the best treatment is with analgesics, but the long duration of the symptoms should be borne in mind.

It should always be borne in mind that diseases of various organs can cause backache. Inquiry should be made to exclude discomfort on micturition or colicky abdominal pain, which may indicate a urinary tract infection or renal colic. In women, any cyclical low back pain should be viewed with caution, particularly if it occurs in the middle or second half of the menstrual cycle, as this warrants consideration of a non-musculoskeletal cause. Inquiry about any menstrual irregularity or abdominal pain should be made, but even in the absence of these symptoms recurrent cyclical pain requires referral for medical investigation.

Any change in bowel habit or any weight loss should be viewed with suspicion as it may reflect a disorder in the large bowel, which lies close to the sacral area of the lower back. Persistent unexplained lumbar pain in middle age and beyond could indicate a malignant secondary tumour and must be investigated.

### The elbow

The lower end of the humerus broadens into two bony protrusions (epicondyles). One is located on the outer (lateral) side of the elbow and one on the inner (medial) side. The epicondyles are the points of insertion of the forearm muscles that move the

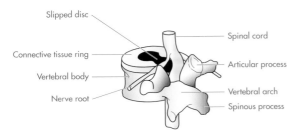

**Figure 4.3** Diagram showing prolapsed intervertebral disc causing pressure on a nerve root.

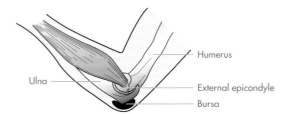

**Figure 4.4**   Diagram showing elbow-joint showing attachment of forearm muscle tendons to external epicondyle, and bursa.

fingers and wrist. The muscles are joined to the epicondyles by narrow tendons. Considerable force to, and vibration in, the muscles, as in some sports or some occupations, can cause disruption of the tendons from the epicondyles.

Pain and tenderness to the touch around the small bony protuberance on the outer side of the elbow is characteristic of tennis elbow (Figure 4.4). Tennis elbow (lateral epicondylitis) is caused by excessive force acting on the insertion of the tendons of the forearm muscles at the outer (lateral) epicondyle. This is common in racquet sports and also in activities involving repetitive twisting movements, such as turning a screwdriver. Similarly, pain and tenderness around the bony protuberance on the inner side of the elbow is known as golfer's elbow (medial epicondylitis).

Tennis elbow and golfer's elbow can be traced to overuse or unaccustomed movement, such as curling of the wrist as in powerful gripping and pulling actions, which strains the tendons of the forearm muscles attached to the outer (tennis) or the inner (golfer's) epicondyles at the elbow. The resulting stress on the elbow produces pain in both the elbow and the forearm muscles and a weakness of the wrist. Flexing the hand downwards at the wrist joint will cause pain in golfer's elbow and pain may spread to the inner aspects of the forearm. In tennis elbow the symptoms are similar to those of golfer's elbow, but pain is felt in the outer part of the forearm and may spread to the upper arm. The pain is worse when the hand is clenched or is bent backwards at the wrist.

Pain and tenderness over the tip of the elbow (the olecranon) is popularly known as student's elbow. Student's elbow can be caused either by inflammation of, or bleeding into, a bursa at the tip of the elbow. It is fairly easy to diagnose without inquiry about its onset, although there may be a classic history of

a blow to, or fall on to, the elbow, repeated flexing of the elbow, or persistent leaning on the elbow in such recreational pursuits as drinking or rifle shooting. Pain will be felt at rest and on movement of the elbow, and there may be swelling and redness. The swelling can extend to the forearm.

Despite their popular names, it is not only golfers, tennis players and students who suffer these symptoms. The symptoms of any of these syndromes will last a varying amount of time, depending on the severity of the problem. Symptoms that persist for more than 1 or 2 weeks should be referred for a medical opinion if they are particularly troublesome.

### The forearm, wrist and hand

Pain in the forearm, wrist and hand can be caused by entrapment of nerves. The most common presentations of this type of disorder are tenosynovitis and carpal tunnel syndrome. Both can produce pain and tenderness over the flexor surface of the forearm. If the pain is also felt in the palm of the hand, fingers and wrist, it suggests carpal tunnel involvement. The carpal tunnel is a narrow tunnel where the tendons that control the movements of the hands and fingers are channelled through lubricating sheaths that cross the wrist. Inflammation of the tendon sheaths at that point will reduce the space in the tunnel and compress the median nerve, which passes through it. Pain, and sometimes numbness, is felt in the forearm and the symptoms are often worse at night.

### The upper leg

Pain in the upper leg, apart from sciatica (see above), will probably be caused either by a strain or rupture of the thigh muscles or by cramp-like stiffness after unaccustomed exercise. A sudden stabbing pain in the anterior thigh after a rapid contraction of the muscles, e.g. when an athlete or sports player makes a forceful sudden movement, will most likely be due to a rupture of the quadriceps muscle. Pain at the back of the thigh will be caused by similar damage to the hamstring muscle. There will be tenderness, and often bruising and swelling.

### The knee

In young people, traumatic injuries to the knee are relatively common, whereas in older people a painful

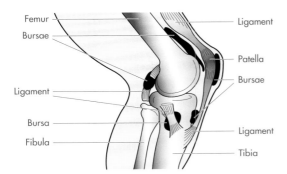

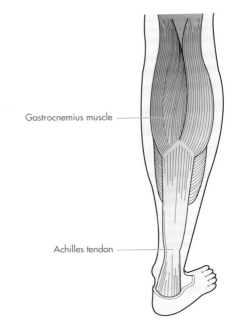

**Figure 4.5** Diagram showing location of bursae in knee joint.

knee is often caused by osteoarthritis. A swelling or lump on the back of the knee is likely to be due to a distended bursa, a condition known as Baker's cyst. The swelling is usually at least the size of a golf ball and is caused by leakage from an inflamed knee joint into the bursa at the back of the knee (Figure 4.5). Pain over the knee with swelling of the joint may be caused by prepatellar bursitis, popularly known as housemaid's knee.

Certain events, usually in sport, such as twisting, turning, or a lateral impact as in soccer, when two players kick the ball at the same time with the inside of their feet, may precipitate injuries to the joint capsule or its associated ligaments and the cartilages inside the joint itself. Pain in the knee joint that is noticed for the first time when walking up and down hills or stairs (and is worse when walking down) may be due to chondromalacia patellae. This condition involves thickening of the cartilage lining the kneecap, and is caused by overuse. A similar condition in young people causing pain and inflammation just below the kneecap, particularly on exercise, is called Osgood–Schlatter disease.

### The lower leg

Pain in the front middle part of the shin bone can be caused by an overuse injury. Other problems in the lower leg include sprained ankle, ruptured Achilles tendon (Figure 4.6) and cramp in the calf. Ruptures of muscles in the calf and of the Achilles tendon are common in sporting injuries, but can also occur in non-sporting day-to-day situations. A sudden pain in the calf, as though hit on the back of the leg, with

**Figure 4.6** Diagram of Achilles tendon.

tenderness and difficulty in contracting the muscles, may be due to rupture of the calf muscles (the gastrocnemius and soleus).

A rupture of the Achilles tendon is relatively common in many sports and it often occurs in athletes who resume training after a period out of training. At the time of rupture an intense pain is felt in the Achilles tendon, which lies above the heel and below the calf muscles. There is often a classic history of a blow or a kick on the back of the leg, and the tendon can sometimes be heard to snap. The rupture can be partial or complete, and where the tendon is totally ruptured the sufferer will not be able to walk on the affected foot. Indentation may be noted in the tendon at the site of injury as well as swelling or bruising over the lower leg and foot.

In milder cases, such as partial rupture or tendinitis (inflammation of the tendon), there will be difficulty in standing on tiptoe. Inflammation of the Achilles tendon (tendinitis) may be a result of prolonged repeated loading and is common in athletes. It is provoked by cold weather or a change in ground surface, shoes or technique. Pain and swelling occur over the tendon. Even mild cases, where the injury to the tendon is slight, must be referred for proper examination and advice. The condition could otherwise result in scarring of the tendon, which is liable to become chronically inflamed.

Cramps are common in the calf muscles, not only during strenuous exercise but also at rest. They are experienced particularly by the elderly.

### The ankle

An ankle sprain is the most common soft tissue limb injury and commonly presents with a history of excessive movement of the joint. The lateral ligament attaches the fibula (the thinner, outer bone in the lower leg) to the heel and foot bones on the outer side of the ankle joint (Figure 4.7). The lateral ligament is weaker than the broader medial ligament, which attaches the tibia to the heel bone on the inner aspect of the ankle. Sprains are caused by an inversion injury to the lateral ligament. Swelling over the lateral ligament below the ankle is less significant than swelling over the lateral ankle joint. There is usually swelling and tenderness around the front and side of the ankle. It is sometimes difficult to distinguish between a fracture and a ligament injury (sprain), and if there is any doubt then an x-ray should be taken.

### The foot

Pain at the back of the heel may be due to inflammation of a deep bursa lying between the heel bone and the attachment of the Achilles tendon or a superficial tendon located under the skin (Figure 4.8). There may be redness and swelling and it may become difficult to wear normal shoes.

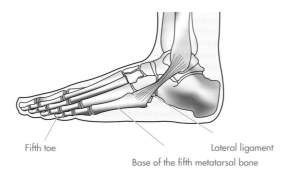

**Figure 4.7** Diagram of lateral view of the foot, showing lateral ligament.

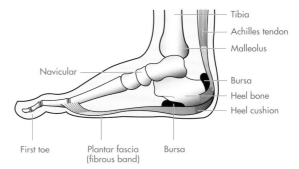

**Figure 4.8** Diagram of medial view of the foot, showing plantar fascia and bursae.

In children up to the age of 18 years fragmentation of the Achilles tendon attachment to the heel bone can occur, causing pain at the back of the heel during and for some time after walking or running.

Pain under the heel may be due to rupture of connective tissue below the heel. In such cases the heel bone becomes less firmly held and squeezes the cushion of fat normally beneath it to the side. This causes pressure on the skin, resulting in pain. There is also a bursa between the heel bone and the fat cushion, which may become inflamed.

Pain under the heel, often with pain in the sole, is commonly due to plantar fasciitis. This occurs when the arch ligaments (running under the foot from the toes to the heel) are stretched or damaged. The pain is relieved on rest, and is worse when on tiptoe or walking on the heels. There may be stiffness, particularly in the mornings.

## Management options

The treatment of soft tissue inflammation and joint disorders is generally similar and therefore in some situations a definitive diagnosis is not important as the same measures should be followed.

Treatment of acute soft tissue injury where there may be bleeding, for example in sports injuries and acute bursitis, should be immediate. The aim is to stop the bleeding, swelling, pain and tenderness. Bleeding can also delay healing, make infection more likely and distort scar tissue formation, producing a cosmetically poor result and possibly interfering with function. The well-known mnemonic

RICE comes into play here. This represents Rest, Ice, Compression, and Elevation, and may be combined with the use of NSAIDs as NICER.

### Rest and elevation

Rest allows immobilisation, which enhances healing and reduces blood flow to the affected tissue. Rest should ideally be for 24–48 hours, but this is often difficult to achieve. Elevation of the affected part also reduces blood flow and leakage of fluid into the extracellular spaces. Many disorders of the musculoskeletal system will respond to rest and therefore it is sensible advice to give anyone who complains of such a disorder. It is helpful to give an idea of the likely duration of the impairment of function caused by the condition. For example, the time taken to recover from a sprained ankle varies from person to person, but as a guide most are noticeably better after 5–7 days and fully healed at 4–6 weeks. Where rest does not bring any relief from the condition, the sufferer should be referred for medical investigation.

### Cooling

Ice packs are used to reduce blood flow to injured tissue and thus reduce bleeding and swelling. Cooling also has an analgesic effect. Ice packs should be separated from the skin by a thin towel or a handkerchief to prevent skin damage. To be effective, cooling should be continued for at least 30 minutes in, for example, a knee or ankle injury, and longer if the injury is particularly severe or when deep large muscles are involved, as in the thigh. One disadvantage of cooling is that it may encourage someone to begin exercising the affected part of the body too soon after an injury, thus causing more bleeding and delaying healing. Cooling aerosol sprays can exert an analgesic effect if a bone that lies close to the skin, such as the ankle or shin, has been knocked.

Sprays only penetrate into the skin layer. They can, however, cause injury to the skin if they are not used carefully, and should not be applied to broken skin. Their brief and superficial action means that when cooling has ceased, the blood flow increases and any beneficial effect may be lost.

### Compression

Compression of an acute injury allows haemostasis to occur and thereby reduces swelling. A supportive bandage, such as a crepe bandage or an elastocrepe, can be applied. Elasticated sports supports designed for specific areas are available.

### Heat

Heat or massage will have the opposite effect to that of cooling on blood flow. It should therefore not be used until about 48 hours after an acute injury, i.e. when the risk of bleeding has disappeared. Heat offers relief from pain arising from inflammation or overuse. As well as being of value in trauma, heat is also effective in chronic joint pain, such as rheumatoid arthritis and osteoarthritis, wry neck, backache and deep muscle pain. Heat reduces joint stiffness and relieves muscle spasm. It increases the elasticity and plasticity of collagen fibres in tissues such as tendons, preventing them from becoming stiff, and also aids gentle exercise in the rehabilitation phase. Heat is useful in preventing injury, which explains the importance of warm-up exercises, especially in cold weather.

Heat may be generated in the form of topical medication (see below), infrared lamps, heating pads, and hot baths or by ultrasound treatment, which is used by physiotherapists. Heat retainers commonly worn by sportsmen are supports made of synthetic materials that generate and retain heat as well as giving useful support and improving the mobility of joints and limbs.

### Non-steroidal anti-inflammatory drugs (BNF section 10.1.1)

The anti-inflammatory property of non-steroidal anti-inflammatory drugs (NSAIDs) makes them a suitable choice for any pain associated with inflammation. NSAIDs such as ibuprofen can give effective relief of musculoskeletal pain when used either alone or in conjunction with other treatments, and they should be recommended as first-line treatment. Ibuprofen is particularly effective for symptomatic relief in musculoskeletal conditions. These drugs may be helpful in acute injury as well as more chronic conditions such as torticollis, sternocostal joint strain, frozen shoulder, carpal tunnel syndrome, back pain and coccygitis.

Ibuprofen is widely available as a GSL and P medicine for use by adults and children, with some newer products being formulated with ibuprofen lysine, a much more highly soluble salt which manufacturers claim is absorbed faster. Diclofenac is also available as a P medicine for short-term relief of pain in people over 14 years of age and naproxen is licensed for period pain in women over 15 years (see Chapter 6). Care should be taken to inquire about any relative contraindications to NSAIDs, such as a history of peptic ulcer or upper gastrointestinal disorders and asthma.

Aspirin is one of the oldest drugs available as a GSL and P medicine and can provide adequate analgesia in most situations but it is contraindicated in children under the age of 16 years because of its association with Reye syndrome. Five per cent of people with asthma are hypersensitive to aspirin, and in its most severe form this allergy can manifest as a life-threatening asthmatic attack. Therefore, care needs to be taken when considering NSAID use in people with asthma.

NSAIDs cause gastric irritation; they should be taken with food and should not be recommended for anyone with a history of peptic ulcer or dyspepsia or in women who are pregnant. Owing to the potential risk of increased bleeding, NSAIDs should not be recommended for individuals who are taking anticoagulants, nor for those already taking aspirin (such as for cardiovascular secondary prevention). In situations where NSAIDs are cautioned or contraindicated, paracetamol would normally be considered to be a suitable alternative.

### Glucosamine (BNF section 10.1.5)

Glucosamine is a natural substance that it is suggested has some beneficial effects in osteoarthritis. It is believed to be localised in cartilage after oral ingestion and there is some evidence of a modest symptomatic effect in osteoarthritis. Therefore, it is reasonable to recommend it for chronic joint conditions, although it must be noted that the Scottish Medicines Consortium has advised that this product should not be used within the NHS in Scotland for the symptomatic relief of mild to moderate osteoarthritis of the knee.

### Rubefacients and other topical antirheumatics (BNF section 10.3.2)

Topical medication applied to aches and pains is a traditional remedy and is generally effective. Most preparations containing rubefacients cause vasodilatation and produce a sensation of warmth. They encourage healing and also provide analgesia. They are useful as a preventative and rehabilitative measure, but should not be used in the acute stage of injury, when there is a risk of bleeding.

The traditional constituent of embrocations and liniments is methyl salicylate, present in many proprietary balms, liniments and balsams. The concentration varies between different products, and the resultant differences in potencies between products should be borne in mind because of this. Branded products also often include turpentine oil and a variety of salicylates and nicotinates. The efficacy of most topical medications is enhanced by massage during application, which will itself induce vasodilatation.

Topical preparations of the NSAIDs include ibuprofen, diclofenac and piroxicam, which are useful analgesic and anti-inflammatory agents. There has been considerable controversy about the efficacy of topical NSAIDs, but there is anecdotal evidence that they do provide symptomatic relief in some people and can be used for muscular aches, sprains and strains, and rheumatoid symptoms and can be used immediately after acute injury.

### Cod liver oil

Fish oils, particularly cod liver oil, taken orally are perceived to be helpful in the symptomatic relief of chronic joint pain such as arthritis.

### Arnica

Arnica is an old herbal remedy. Topical arnica preparations have a traditional use for sprains and bruises. Arnica contains some terpenoids, which have pharmacological activity in animal models, but there is a paucity of clinical evidence.

### Re-consider the case

Before reading further, re-consider the following questions and your initial thoughts on this case.

**Trigger questions**

- What additional information would you need before considering the appropriate management options in this case?
- What issues concern you about this case?
- Are any alarm symptoms being exhibited that require more urgent treatment or referral?

**Case study**

A man in his 30s is a semi-regular visitor to your pharmacy and has requested a small supply of a topical anti-inflammatory preparation and some ibuprofen tablets. This man is employed in a strenuous manual job and regards his frequent episodes of back and shoulder pain as nothing more than an occupational hazard.

### Pharmacist opinion

In assessing the symptoms in this case it would be important to establish whether the pain that this man is experiencing is acute or chronic in nature. In general terms acute pain of a musculoskeletal nature can safely be managed using the mnemonic RICE (Rest, Ice, Compression and Elevation). However, chronic pain or stiffness should be referred for medical assessment as it may not respond to RICE or the use of analgesia that can be supplied without a prescription. In some cases it may be necessary to consider local steroid injections into the joint to manage the condition.

In differentiating between acute and chronic pain in this case, it would be necessary to establish whether the frequent episodes described are actually a series of acute attacks of back and shoulder pain triggered by the repetition of a specific activity as part of his job. If this is the case then measures can be taken to avoid this activity or undertake it in a way that does not trigger the pain. However, referral for any pain that persists or recurs should be considered to rule out or monitor for the occurrence of a chronic condition such as osteoarthritis. In a man of this age, ankylosing spondylitis would be a risk that should be ruled out.

The use of NSAIDs on a longer-term basis also poses a risk for this man developing gastrointestinal side effects and therefore the man should be advised that the use of NSAIDs supplied without a prescription is a short-term measure and they should not be used on a long-term basis.

Although no alarm symptoms are described in this case and the use of NSAIDs, either topical or oral, appears appropriate in this case, referral to a physiotherapist may also be a useful course of action for this man to consider given that he has described a series of episodes of back and shoulder pain. A physiotherapist would be able to provide advice on a specific course of exercises that would improve this man's symptoms but also prevent long-term problems associated with fibrosis and scarring of the muscles, e.g. in capsulitis.

### GP opinion

It would be helpful to know the natural course of these episodes of pain, how long do they last? How severe is the pain? Is he able to continue everyday tasks and stay at work? Does he gain complete relief of symptoms between episodes or has it become a chronic problem?

### GP opinion (*continued*)

Occupational hazards are an important issue to address. Has this man had an occupational health assessment? Has he needed to take time off work? Is he reluctant to address these issues with his seniors at work? Or is he self-employed?

Self-management of these types of problems is entirely reasonable. He should be made aware of possible side effects of NSAIDs. He should also be made aware of symptoms that warrant immediate medical assessment, e.g. perineal numbness, incontinence and muscle weakness.

In someone who is persistently troubled by musculoskeletal problems, an assessment from a physio-therapist would be helpful. This would identify specific injuries or defects, and in this case may confirm areas of his work which are specifically causing problems. A physiotherapist could also recommend specific exercises or treatments to address on-going problems.

### Summary of key points

| Condition | Management |
| --- | --- |
| Acute torticollis is characterised by a muscle spasm causing pain, discomfort and a possible twisted neck. | General advice using the RICE mnemonic where appropriate. Immobilisation of the neck as far as practical and application of heat may provide some relief. NSAIDs can provide symptomatic relief from the pain and reduce any associated inflammation. |
| Capsulitis or rotator cuff syndrome is characterised by pain and tenderness in the tendons supporting the shoulder. | A programme of exercises should help restore mobility and prevent possible scarring and fibrosis of the joint. |
| Lumbago is characterised by diffuse pain across the lower back or to one side of the spine but often will not be experienced at rest or on slow movement. | General advice using the RICE mnemonic where appropriate. Rest is the main course of action in treating lumbago. Paracetamol or NSAIDs can provide symptomatic relief from the pain and reduce any associated inflammation. |
| Prolapsed or slipped disc is characterised by a constant pain with a stiff and awkward gait. | General advice using the RICE mnemonic where appropriate. Rest and application of heat may provide some relief. NSAIDs can provide symptomatic relief from the pain and reduce any associated inflammation |
| Tennis or golfer's elbow is characterised by pain and tenderness around the elbow joint. | General advice using the RICE mnemonic where appropriate. Resting the elbow and avoidance of activities that aggravate the condition. NSAIDs can provide symptomatic relief from the pain and reduce any associated inflammation. |
| Carpal tunnel syndrome is characterised by pain and tenderness over the flexor surface of the arm with pain felt in the palm of the hand. | General advice using the RICE mnemonic where appropriate. Resting and splinting of the arm is usually required. NSAIDs can provide symptomatic relief from the pain and reduce any associated inflammation. |
| Housemaid's knee is characterised by swollen knee joint due to inflammation of a bursa in the joint. | General advice using the RICE mnemonic where appropriate. Resting and elevating the knee where appropriate. NSAIDs can provide symptomatic relief from the pain and reduce any associated inflammation. |
| Ruptured Achilles tendon is characterised by an intense pain, perhaps with a sound if the tendon has snapped. | In the acute phase rest and cooling, and later heat. Ruptured Achilles tendons require medical treatment. |

### When to refer

- There have been substantial impact forces and a fracture cannot be ruled out
- If there is pain at rest or the pain is severe
- Pain is not relieved by simple analgesia
- Improvement in function of the affected limb is not obvious in 5–7 days
- Sufferer is elderly or a child
- There is a bony abnormality or tenderness (by observation or touch)
- Cannot weight bear for four steps
- There is obvious deformity
- Suspected prolapsed disc
- Achilles tendon problems
- Tenderness of the bony protuberance of the ankle (malleolus)
- Tenderness of the fifth metatarsal bone on the outer edge of the foot (Figure 4.7)
- Tenderness of the navicular bone in the foot just below the ankle joint on the instep (Figure 4.8)
- History of a sporting, traffic or industrial injury, previous slipped disc or arthritis in individuals with chronic lumbago
- Lower back pain with disturbance in bowel or bladder function

## Obesity

Since 1980 worldwide obesity has more than doubled. The World Health Organization (WHO, 2011) has reported that overweight and obesity are the fifth leading risk for global death and that 44% of diabetes and 23% of ischaemic heart disease burden are attributable to overweight and obesity.

Overweight and obesity are terms used to describe an excess accumulation of body fat. Although not strictly minor illnesses or major diseases in themselves, these conditions can be considered as warning signs that the risk of disease may increase, having a major impact on the health of the population; they are therefore included here as a pro-active measure to prevent the mortality and morbidity associated with obesity.

The reclassification of orlistat as a P medicine provides access through pharmacies to an effective weight loss aid for people who are overweight or obese.

Before reading further, consider the following case and note your initial thoughts.

### Case study

A 39-year-old woman comes into the pharmacy on a cold winter day and asks about appetite suppressants or other drugs that she can take to help her lose weight. She recently spoke with a friend who reported losing almost 20 kg in weight over a period of 3 months with the aid of herbal diet pills. She is uncertain where to obtain these but thinks that the pharmacist would be the best information source. The woman states that she hopes 'to lose weight in time for a family wedding in six weeks'.

**Trigger questions**

- What additional information would you need before considering the appropriate management options in this case?
- What issues concern you about this case?
- What health promotion issues affect this case?

## Assessing suitability for supply

### Body mass index (BMI)

In order to supply pharmacological agents for weight reduction to anyone it is necessary to make an assessment of body fatness. Precise measurement of fat in adipose tissue is very difficult, so a calculation of relative weight for height, known as the body mass index, is often used:

$$BMI = \frac{weight(kg)}{height\ squared(m^2)}$$

The WHO classification of obesity in adults in terms of BMI is shown in Table 4.7.

It should be noted, however, that 'overweight' does not always mean 'over-fat' as in the example of some athletes with a greater proportion of muscle contributing to their body weight. Additionally, BMI does not reflect distribution of fat within the body. Waist circumference is a simple measure of fat distribution and can be used to predict risk of other diseases; for example, it is the most accurate predictor of risk of type II diabetes mellitus. Table 4.8 provides cut-off values for disease risk. Waist-to-hip ratio may be the most accurate predictor of risk of myocardial infarction (NICE 2006).

Accurate measurement of waist and hip circumference, following agreed protocols, is essential. The International Society for the Advancement of Kinanthropometry advises that waist circumference should be measured at the narrowest point of the abdomen, as the person is viewed from the front. The tape should be passed around the waist and the measurement taken at the end of a normal expiration. Hip circumference should be measured with the feet together; the tape is passed around the buttocks and measurement taken at the level of the greatest protuberance of the buttocks when viewed from the side. A flexible steel tape is the instrument of choice as elastic tapes commonly available are prone to stretching.

Evidence suggests that ethnic differences exist in the relationship between waist circumference and cardiovascular disease risk factors; South Asians have higher cardiovascular risk factors at lower waist circumferences compared with Western populations. Since, then, the effects of obesity may be seen at different threshold levels, it is difficult to set specific cut-off values for ethnic populations. However, cut-offs for those of Asian origin with increased risk have been recommended as a waist circumference of ≥90 cm for men and ≥80 cm for women.

In a simplistic explanation, obesity arises due to an imbalance between energy intake and energy expenditure over a long period of time. However the aetiology is, in fact, much more complex and multifactorial in nature. A very small proportion of individuals develop obesity as a consequence of genetic or endocrine abnormalities, for example Prader–Willi syndrome and hypothyroidism respectively. In other cases of obesity, genetic predisposition, metabolic, behavioural and environmental factors are all likely to be involved.

It is estimated that approximately 20–30% of those presenting for treatment of obesity may have binge eating disorder (BED), a term used to describe individuals who binge eat in the absence of compensatory behaviours, such as purging. Although it is not classified officially as an eating disorder, and therefore not considered a psychiatric condition, a set of research criteria has been developed to provide guidance to healthcare professionals.

**Table 4.7　WHO classification of obesity**

| Category | BMI (kg/m²) |
|---|---|
| Underweight | <18.5 |
| Healthy weight | 18.5–24.9 |
| Pre-obese (overweight) | 25–29.9 |
| Obese Class I (moderately obese) | 30–34.9 |
| Obese Class II (severely obese) | 35–39.9 |
| Obese Class III (morbidly obese) | >40 |

**Table 4.8　Waist circumference cut-off values for disease risk**

| Risk | Male | Female |
|---|---|---|
| Low risk | <94 cm | <80 cm |
| Increased risk | 94–102 cm | 80–88 cm |
| High risk | >102 cm | >88 cm |

The research criteria for binge eating disorder (American Psychiatric Association 1994) are:

- Recurrent episodes of binge eating. An episode of binge eating is characterised by both of the following:
  — Eating, in a discrete period of time (e.g. within any 2-hour period), an amount of food that is definitely larger than most people would eat in a similar period of time under similar circumstances
  — A sense of lack of control over eating during the episodes (e.g. a feeling that one cannot stop eating or control what or how much one is eating).
- The binge-eating episodes are associated with three (or more) of the following:
  — Eating much more rapidly than usual
  — Eating until feeling uncomfortably full
  — Eating large amounts of food when not feeling physically hungry
  — Eating alone because of being embarrassed by how much one is eating
  — Feeling disgusted with oneself, depressed, or very guilty after overeating.
- Marked distress regarding binge eating is present.
- Binge eating occurs, on average, at least 2 days a week for 6 months.
- The binge eating is not associated with regular use of inappropriate compensatory behaviours (e.g. purging, fasting, excessive exercise) and does not occur exclusively during the course of anorexia nervosa or bulimia nervosa.

It is essential that individuals seeking obesity treatment have BED identified – or excluded – as those with BED are likely to require prior, or concurrent, interventions such as cognitive behavioural therapy to address the binge eating behaviour.

## Management options

### Diet

The main energy-yielding nutrients in the human diet are carbohydrates, fats, proteins and alcohol. The available energy content varies between these macronutrients and Table 4.9 shows the energy provision per gram.

**Table 4.9  Energy content of macronutrients**

| Macronutrient | Energy provision (kJ/g [kcal/g]) |
|---|---|
| Carbohydrate | 16 (3.75) |
| Fat | 37 (9) |
| Protein | 17 (4) |
| Alcohol | 29 (7) |

However, humans consume a complex mix of nutrients in the form of foods, rather than individual nutrients, so estimation of energy intake can be difficult without the support of food composition tables or a good understanding of food labelling.

The Department of Health has calculated standardised estimated requirements for the macronutrients and various micronutrients for the general UK population based upon epidemiological and research evidence identifying levels for 'good health', toxicity or deficiency.

As a more prescriptive tool to support balanced energy contribution of the macronutrients, individuals are advised to consume approximately 50–55% total daily energy from carbohydrate, 30–35% energy from fat, and 15% energy from protein. This concept can be difficult for some individuals to understand, as it first requires a calculation of total energy requirements, often based on prediction equations incorporating basal metabolic rate and physical activity factors specific to the individual.

So, to aid individuals in selecting a balanced diet of both macro- and micronutrients, the UK Food Standards Agency designed the Eatwell Plate (Figure 4.9), which visually describes the approximate contribution that the main food groups should make to our diets. However, this health promotion tool does not indicate portion size of foods and therefore is insufficient alone in educating and supporting obese individuals to achieve weight loss.

### Dietary interventions

A number of dietary approaches to weight reduction and management have been proposed over the years, with varying levels of scientific evidence or success. Skipping meals has been one of the most commonly used methods in the belief that less total energy is consumed. However, it is now understood that this

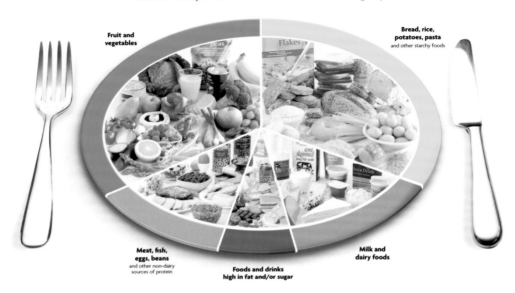

**Figure 4.9** UK Food Standards Agency Eatwell plate.

(Crown copyright: Department of Health in association with the Welsh Assembly Government, the Scottish Government and the Food Standards Agency in Northern Ireland).

approach is likely to disrupt appetite regulation, resulting in increased hunger and lapses in dietary control.

To achieve the suggested weight loss of approximately 0.5-1 kg per week, individuals are encouraged to restrict their food intake by a modest amount (approximately 2500 kJ (600 kcal)) below their maintenance energy requirements. Alternatively, an individual may choose to increase their exercise levels, or indeed undertake a combination of these measures. Evidence suggests that those who include exercise as part of their weight loss programme have a greater likelihood of sustaining their new body weight.

The traditional approaches to managing weight have relied on providing persuasive, expert dietary guidance linked to associated risk reduction in the belief that these are sufficient for individuals to instigate and sustain change. Evidence now, however, suggests that few people respond to this method

without concurrent motivational and behavioural approaches by skilled practitioners.

### Drugs used in the treatment of obesity (BNF section 4.5)

Various pharmacological agents have been used to support weight loss over the years, involving a variety of modes of actions. Owing to the withdrawal of many of them as a result of identified health risks, the only drug currently licensed specifically for the management of obesity is orlistat.

Orlistat is a specific and long-acting gastrointestinal lipase inhibitor causing malabsorption of approximately 30% of dietary fat when taken at a dose of 120 mg. The resulting increase in faecal fat causes an energy deficit, which should support weight loss. However, individuals considering taking orlistat need to understand that it is only an aid to weight loss, and must also be used in conjunction with a reduced-energy and reduced-fat diet to maximise weight loss and prevent unpleasant side effects of steatorrhoea (excessive excretion of fat in stools) and associated symptoms.

The remaining fat absorbed allows for sufficient absorption of fat-soluble vitamins, but it may be necessary for some individuals to take additional vitamin supplements containing fat-soluble vitamins to avert any deficiencies (particularly vitamin D) (see Chapter 8).

Orlistat was reclassified in 2009 as a P medicine and therefore can be supplied to members of the public from a pharmacy without prescription. Its status as a P medicine permits its use for weight loss in adults (age 18 years or older) who are overweight (BMI $\geq$ 28 kg/m$^2$) when used in conjunction with a mildly hypocaloric, lower-fat diet. Its status as a P medicine also requires it to be prescribed at a lower recommended dose of one 60 mg capsule three times daily during or within one hour of a main meal. It is important that the dose is omitted if a meal is missed or contains no fat.

Prior to commencing treatment with orlistat, individuals should be advised to start a lower-fat diet and increase their levels of activity. Treatment with orlistat should not exceed 6 months and if after 12 weeks an individual has been unable to lose weight then their treatment needs to be reviewed. If it is

clear that the individual has implemented the necessary lifestyle changes but is still not losing weight then they should be advised to seek advice from their doctor. People who get no benefit from taking orlistat should not continue to take it.

The diet-related side effects that occur with orlistat are the most common side effects and are largely manageable. These include wind with or without oil spotting, sudden bowel motions, and fatty or oily stools or soft stools. These are largely within the control of the individual, their presence being an indication of excessive fat in the diet. The chances of experiencing these effects can be minimised by reducing the fat content of the diet.

There are some situations in which orlistat should not be used or where individuals should talk with their doctor first before commencing treatment. Orlistat is contraindicated in breastfeeding, chronic malabsorption syndrome and cholestasis (a blockage of bile flow from the liver). Orlistat also has the potential to interact with different groups of drugs and therefore care should be taken to assess concurrent drug therapy for potential interactions. Orlistat is contraindicated in anyone taking ciclosporin or warfarin and care should also be taken with anyone who is taking medication for diabetes mellitus because improved metabolic control may accompany any weight loss and their drug treatment may need to be adjusted to compensate.

### Re-consider the case

Before reading further, re-consider the following questions and your initial thoughts on this case.

**Trigger questions**

- What additional information would you need before considering the appropriate management options in this case?
- What issues concern you about this case?
- What health promotion issues affect this case?

**Case study**

A 39-year-old woman comes in to the pharmacy on a cold winter day and asks about appetite suppressants or other drugs that she can take to help her lose weight. She recently spoke with a friend who reported losing almost 20 kg in weight over a period of 3 months with the aid of herbal diet pills. She is uncertain where to obtain these but thinks that the pharmacist would be the best information source. The woman states that she hopes 'to lose weight in time for a family wedding in six weeks'.

Pharmacist opinion

Assuming that this woman's weight and height measurement reveal a BMI >28 kg/m², she would be suitable to be supplied with orlistat. There is no indication that she has any medical history that would make the supply inappropriate or that she is taking any drugs that could interact with the orlistat. Considering her age, it would be sensible to confirm whether she is taking an oral contraceptive.

There is no evidence that there is a specific drug interaction between orlistat and oral contraceptives. However, there is potential for an indirect reduction in the availability of oral contraceptives resulting in an unplanned pregnancy. Therefore, additional contraceptive methods are recommended to prevent possible failure of oral contraception in the case of severe diarrhoea.

One of the most important aspects in supplying orlistat is managing the expectations of the individual concerned. It is important that they understand that orlistat is not a 'quick fix' and that they cannot continue to eat what they want while taking orlistat. This woman's comment that she wants 'to lose weight before a family wedding in six weeks' suggests that she may view orlistat as a 'quick fix' and therefore some time needs to be spent explaining to her the various aspects of this particular drug and establishing that she is committed to making the necessary lifestyle changes.

If she is committed to making the necessary lifestyle changes then it would be appropriate to supply orlistat as part of a programme of weight loss, i.e. lowering dietary fat and increasing physical activity. It is important to set realistic weight loss targets for the use of orlistat, not only as a means of maintaining motivation but also as an important monitoring parameter. Individuals who despite implementing lifestyle changes do not lose weight after 12 weeks should not continue treatment with orlistat and should be referred to their GP. It is also important to monitor weight loss because once an individual's BMI falls below 28 kg/m² then they are no longer eligible to be supplied with orlistat and will need to continue their weight loss via dietary control and increased physical activity. This underlines the importance of the commitment to make lifestyle changes prior to using orlistat as a time will come when weight loss needs to be maintained without it.

 Dietitian opinion

It is important not to make assumptions about this individual at first presentation. First, you must establish whether she does need to lose weight. On the day in question, a cold winter's day, she may have many layers of clothes on, giving the impression of excess body weight. In some cases, a person's body image perception may be incorrect and it is important to establish a baseline of measurements to correctly identify overweight or obesity and, in part, to determine suitability for various treatment options.

The woman in this case is requesting medication to facilitate management of a nutritional disorder. It should be established whether she has made any dietary changes to support weight management. This aids in determining her motivation for change and likelihood of adhering to the appropriate dietary guidance while using obesity management medications. If prior weight loss attempts have failed to achieve or maintain clinically significant or successful weight loss, defined as 5–10% reduction from original body weight, this woman may be suitable for a supply of orlistat as a P medicine.

It is important to support this woman to develop a realistic view of her food consumption habits. Research has shown that overweight and obese individuals have a tendency to under-report their food

Dietitian opinion (*continued*)

energy intake by approximately 30–50%, compared with 20% under-reporting in non-obese subjects. This is rarely through a deliberate attempt to misguide health professionals, but rather due to a lack of awareness of energy consumption, which partly explains their weight gain.

Basic dietary advice should be given, or reference to supporting resources for orlistat to ensure that this woman achieves the hypocaloric diet required in conjunction with the use of orlistat. This should include recommending following the Eatwell Plate model, restrictions of portion sizes and fat intake, and regular meals. Detailed dietary and lifestyle advice is best given by a healthcare professional who has received additional training to support individuals in these areas.

The weight loss expectations of an individual are a key factor. Expectations may be based purely on a set weight loss, which may or may not be achievable in the identified timescale. However, some individuals associate other personal or social expectations with weight loss, which cannot be guaranteed e.g. 'I'm not married because I am overweight. If I lose this weight, I will find a suitable partner.' It is particularly relevant to establish and sensitively discuss motivating factors with individuals, since failing to achieve these may drive them, in the longer term, into weight regain and weight cycling.

## Smoking cessation

Since the 1970s smoking rates in the United Kingdom have declined because of the association between cigarette smoking and serious illness. Nevertheless, there are still large numbers of adults who smoke. The prevalence of smoking in the UK as reported by the General Lifestyle Survey in 2008 was 21% (males 22% and females 21%) with an estimated 114 000 deaths per year in the UK attributable to smoking.

The provision of smoking cessation services from community pharmacies is now commonplace, whether that be the sale of nicotine replacement products to smokers who visit the pharmacy or through NHS-run smoking cessation services. During 2009 an estimated 6.5% of smokers in Scotland made a quit attempt with an NHS smoking cessation service; 56% of quit attempts were made through pharmacy services.

Before reading further, consider the following case and note your initial thoughts.

**Case study**

Mr Smith has decided that he wants to give up smoking and has visited your pharmacy to enrol in a smoking cessation scheme. He has agreed a time to visit your pharmacy each week. He seems determined to succeed after smoking about 30 cigarettes a day for 15 years. Although he is confident about not smoking while at work, he is concerned about when he is socialising with friends who smoke.

**Trigger questions**

- What additional information would you need before considering the appropriate management options in this case?
- What issues concern you about this case?
- What health promotion issues affect this case?

## Assessing suitability for supply

Healthcare professionals should take any opportunity to discuss with smokers their smoking habit and whether they have ever considered quitting smoking. This should be undertaken in a manner that does not leave the individual feeling pressurised and the approach should be one of assessing the willingness of the smoker to quit and offering them help to do so. The first milestone in the process may just be to achieve a state of mind in which the smoker will at least consider quitting. This can be achieved by offering to work with the smoker and monitor their progress ('support' may be a wrong choice of words and appear patronising, whereas 'working together' may sound better).

If it has not already been done, it is pertinent at this stage to discuss the risks and benefits of quitting smoking. If the individual does not accept the reasons for giving up then they will not quit.

The second milestone is to agree a timeframe and a date to quit. Some means of reinforcement may be helpful here. For example, the smoker could be provided with a diary, which might also contain a table of benefits for the smoker to refer to (Table 4.10),

and at this stage an action plan can be drawn up and summarised in the diary, with an outline of the time intervals for monitoring the number of cigarettes smoked during the treatment period.

The process should be taken one step at a time, both at this stage and later when monitoring or reviewing progress. A timescale can be worked out for each step of the monitoring plan, which must be agreed by both parties and be realistic.

### Assessment of the smoker's motivation

There is no doubt that the success of a smoking cessation programme depends largely on the individual's motivation to give up. Motivation varies with time, and smokers may not always be honest about their real feelings. Surveys indicate that about 70% of smokers want to quit, and motivation can be judged by asking a number of questions:

- Has the individual made an attempt to stop smoking on a previous occasion?
- Do they want to stop smoking for good?
- Do they want to start the smoking cessation programme very soon?

| Table 4.10 Timetable of the benefits of quitting smoking | |
| --- | --- |
| **Timeline** | **Benefit** |
| 20 minutes after quitting | Blood pressure and pulse return to normal. |
| 8 hours after quitting | Oxygen concentration in the blood increases to normal. Nicotine and carbon monoxide concentrations in the blood are reduced by 50%. |
| 24 hours after quitting | Carbon monoxide has been eliminated from the body. Lungs begin to clear mucus and debris. Risk of myocardial infarction decreases. |
| 48 hours after quitting | Nicotine has been eliminated from the body. Sense of taste and smell improve. |
| 72 hours after quitting | Breathing is easier and bronchi begin to relax. Energy levels begin to increase. |
| 2–12 weeks after quitting | Circulation improves, making physical activity easier. |
| 3–9 months after quitting | Lung function has increased by 10%. Cilia in airways regrow. Coughing, shortness of breath and wheeziness improve. |
| 5 years after quitting | Risk of myocardial infarction falls to half that of a smoker. Risk of cancer of the mouth, throat and oesophagus is half that of a smoker. |
| 10 years after quitting | Risk of lung cancer is half that of a smoker. |
| 15 years after quitting | Risk of myocardial infarction falls to the same as someone who has never smoked. |

- Would they like someone to work with them as an adviser during the treatment period?

However, even a high degree of motivation at this stage does not predict the success of the attempt. Success in quitting also depends on the degree of dependence on nicotine. Dependence can be judged by the degree of difficulty a smoker has in refusing a cigarette at times when they would normally smoke, for example on awakening or on social occasions.

A commonly used measure of dependence is the Fagerström test (Table 4.11), which is useful for assessing the smoker's level of nicotine dependence; a high score (greater than 9) suggests a high level of dependence. This may be useful in illustrating to a smoker how addicted they are to nicotine and therefore may be a powerful tool in encouraging someone who has previously not considered quitting to at least re-evaluate their smoking habit.

## Management options

### Starting the programme

The choice of products to be used in the cessation plan should be agreed and a start date suggested within the following 2 weeks unless the plan is to reduce first then quit later. At this stage the smoker should be reminded that it may be necessary to make some changes in lifestyle or habits, even temporarily, such as not attending social gatherings in places where others may be smoking. The next step is to agree follow-ups, and the need to maintain the effort should be stressed to the smoker. It may not be appropriate to put negative thoughts into the individual's mind, but it should be remembered that relapse is not uncommon, and that although 4-week quit rates may be 50% this can decline to less than 20% over a longer period. Weekly support reviews for the first fortnight, followed by every 2 weeks, and then monthly, would be a suitable programme. If a person following the programme does not attend for a follow-up interview they should be contacted by telephone and several attempts should be made before they are designated as 'lost to follow-up'.

### Nicotine (BNF section 4.10)

It is thought that nicotine stimulates dopaminergic pathways in the brain, which results in the stimulation of the mesolimbic system that gives rise to feelings of pleasure. The absorption of nicotine from the

**Table 4.11   The Fagerström test for nicotine dependence**

| Questions | Answers | Points |
|---|---|---|
| 1. How soon after waking do you smoke your first cigarette? | (a) Within 5 minutes<br>(b) 6–30 minutes<br>(c) 31–60 minutes<br>(d) After 60 minutes | (a) 3<br>(b) 2<br>(c) 1<br>(d) 0 |
| 2. Do you find it difficult to refrain from smoking in places where it is forbidden (e.g. cinemas, restaurants)? | (a) Yes<br>(b) No | (a) 1<br>(b) 0 |
| 3. Which cigarette would you hate most to give up? | (a) The first in the morning<br>(b) Any other | (a) 1<br>(b) 0 |
| 4. How many cigarettes per day do you smoke? | (a) 31 or more<br>(b) 21–30<br>(c) 11–20<br>(d) 10 or fewer | (a) 3<br>(b) 2<br>(c) 1<br>(d) 0 |
| 5. Do you smoke more frequently during the first few hours after waking than during the rest of the day? | (a) Yes<br>(b) No | (a) 1<br>(b) 0 |
| 6. Do you smoke if you are so ill that you are in bed most of the day? | (a) Yes<br>(b) No | (a) 1<br>(b) 0 |

A score of 9 or above indicates high dependence.
A score of 4–8 indicates medium dependence.
A score of 3 or less indicates low dependence.

| Box 4.3 Some of the chemicals found in tobacco smoke |
|---|
| ● Acetone |
| ● Ammonia |
| ● Arsenic |
| ● Benzene |
| ● Cadmium |
| ● Carbon monoxide |
| ● Cyanide |
| ● Formaldehyde |
| ● Shellac |
| ● Tar |

| Box 4.4 Outline of behavioural support for smoking cessation |
|---|
| ● Give support both during the time the smoker expresses an interest to give up as well as during the treatment period. |
| ● Give advice on the choice of method/ formulation, in keeping with the person's lifestyle. |
| ● Monitor progress using diary cards, regular follow-ups, telephone calls. |
| ● Provide feedback using carbon monoxide monitors. |
| ● Maintain motivation, e.g. calculate the financial savings of smoking cessation to the individual on a weekly basis and record in the diary card. |
| ● If a course of NRT fails, then encourage the individual to try again. |
| ● Encourage quitting with a friend to provide motivation and encouragement. |
| ● Plan ahead, especially in the initial stages, but take a practical day-to-day approach. |

smoke in the lungs is rapid and gives rise to high concentrations of nicotine in the brain within a few seconds. Nicotine replacement therapy (NRT) aims to replace the nicotine absorbed from cigarette smoking, thereby avoiding the withdrawal effects of nicotine dependence such as change in mood and performance which are normally reduced or eliminated by the next cigarette. This then permits the smoker to gradually reduce their nicotine intake over a prolonged period, avoiding these withdrawal effects.

Nicotine replacement therapy is safer than smoking because there is no exposure to harmful smoke and the chemicals it contains (Box 4.3). It can be used in those with cardiovascular disease because, although nicotine is a vasoconstrictor, the lower levels of concentration produced by NRT, together with the lack of smoke, mean that the individual should come to less harm than if they were smoking. The use of NRT is cautioned in severe or unstable cardiovascular disease, for example following a recent myocardial infarction or a stroke, and it would be prudent in this situation for NRT to be initiated under medical supervision.

Nicotine replacement therapy doubles the cessation rates achieved by any other non-pharmacological method of intervention and maximum effect is gained when it is part of a programme that includes behavioural support (see Box 4.4). Nicotine replacement products can be provided without a prescription or via a patient group direction (PGD), whereby local arrangements allow NHS funding to pay for the cost of the products.

Nicotine replacement therapy is a broad term that encompasses a range of different types of formulation that deliver controlled amounts of nicotine to the body thereby eliminating the need for someone addicted to nicotine to smoke a cigarette. The choice of formulation to a certain degree is one of personal choice but should take account of the smoker's lifestyle. Table 4.12 summarises the different types of nicotine replacement products that are available.

Smokers may ask if they will become addicted to NRT and can be assured that this is extremely rare, because the blood concentrations of nicotine that occur with NRT are much lower than with cigarette smoking.

In pregnancy NRT is again safer than cigarettes, and 20% of women who smoke in the UK continue to do so throughout pregnancy. Carbon monoxide binds to haemoglobin and reduces the availability of oxygen to the fetus. Smoking causes fetal growth retardation. However, concentrations of cotinine in the blood of pregnant women who are being treated

**Table 4.12  Summary of nicotine replacement products**

| Type of formulation | Comment |
| --- | --- |
| 24-Hour transdermal patch | • Convenient to use as it is applied each day and left on for 24 hours.<br>• Simple, discrete and requires least effort.<br>• Available in different strengths and delivers a controlled amount of nicotine to the body over 24 hours.<br>• Initial strength of the patch is decided by the number of cigarettes smoked per day. Decreasing patch strengths are used over 10–12 weeks to reduce the physical dependence on nicotine.<br>• Patches left on for 24 hours can cause sleep disturbance in some people. In this situation, removal of the patch before retiring is preferable.<br>• Useful for those who crave a cigarette immediately on waking. |
| 16-Hour transdermal patch | • Similar to the 24-hour transdermal patch but delivers nicotine over 16 hours. This patch is removed at night before going to bed. |
| Chewing gum | • Chewing gum is used whenever an urge to smoke is felt.<br>• The gum is chewed slowly until its taste changes, it is then rested.<br>• Once taste fades, the gum should then be chewed again.<br>• Chewing releases nicotine from the gum.<br>• This is known as the 'chew–rest–chew' technique.<br>• Onset of action is 10 minutes, and for optimal effect the average usage would be about 15 pieces of gum per day.<br>• The gum is provided in two strengths, depending on the number of cigarettes smoked per day. |
| Lozenges | • These are sucked when there is a craving to smoke.<br>• The lozenge is sucked on a 'suck–rest–suck' regime, like that for gum.<br>• Treatment can be continued for 3 months and then reduced, with a maximum period of treatment of 6 months.<br>• Maximum dosage should not exceed 15 lozenges per day.<br>• No food or drink should be taken while the lozenge is in the mouth; some drinks may decrease the absorption of nicotine and are best avoided for 15 minutes before sucking a lozenge. |
| Sublingual microtab | • These are allowed to dissolve under the tongue for about 30 minutes.<br>• One or two tablets per hour can be used as required.<br>• Use may be continued for up to 6 months, reducing the dosage after 12 weeks to one or two tablets per day. |
| Nasal spray | • This is used to spray nicotine directly into the nostrils, where it is absorbed rapidly.<br>• Peak blood concentrations of nicotine are produced between 5 and 10 minutes after inhalation.<br>• Provides rapid relieve of cravings.<br>• The nasal spray may cause some local irritant effects, such as a sore throat, but these usually resolve within a few days. |
| Inhalator | • This device is designed to be held like a cigarette and contains a replaceable nicotine cartridge.<br>• Provides a source of nicotine in a format that simulates the behavioural habit of the hand-to-mouth action of the smoker.<br>• Users draw on it like a cigarette, releasing nicotine which is absorbed through the buccal lining with an onset of action of around 15 minutes. |

with NRT are lower than those in pregnant women who smoke.

### Bupropion (BNF section 4.10.2)

The mode of action of bupropion in smoking cessation is unknown, but it is thought to have an effect on noradrenaline and dopamine neurotransmission. In the UK it is a prescription-only medicine, although in some locations there may be local arrangements for it to be supplied via a patient group direction.

If the latter arrangement does not exist but it is felt that this drug may be the best option for a smoker, they should be referred to their GP. However, similarly to NRT, bupropion is most effective as an aid to smoking cessation when combined with behavioural support.

Adverse effects of bupropion include weight gain and rarely seizures, and therefore it is contraindicated in anyone with a low threshold for seizures, such as those with diabetes, eating disorders, head trauma, or alcohol misuse. Bupropion is also contraindicated in pregnancy and breastfeeding and must be administered with extreme caution to anyone already taking other drugs known to lower seizure threshold.

### Varenicline (BNF Section 4.10.2)

Varenicline is a selective nicotine receptor partial agonist used as an aid to smoking cessation; however, in the UK it is a prescription-only medicine. It is mentioned here for completeness but if it is required then referral to a GP is necessary for its supply. As with NRT and bupropion, it should only be prescribed as part of a programme of behavioural support.

### Re-consider the case

Before reading further, re-consider the following questions and your initial thoughts on this case.

**Trigger questions**

- What additional information would you need before considering the appropriate management options in this case?
- What issues concern you about this case?
- What health promotion issues affect this case?

**Case study**

Mr Smith has decided that he wants to give up smoking and has visited your pharmacy to enrol in a smoking cessation scheme. He has agreed a time to visit your pharmacy each week. He seems determined to succeed after smoking about 30 cigarettes a day for 15 years. Although he is confident about not smoking while at work, he is concerned about when he is socialising with friends who smoke.

### Pharmacist opinion

Mr Smith's decision to seek support to quit smoking should be seen as a positive sign that he is committed to giving up smoking. It might be useful to explore this further with Mr Smith to confirm that he is truly committed and understands what is involved with quitting. It might prove beneficial to complete the Fagerström test with Mr Smith to assess his level of dependence on nicotine; however, regardless of the result it is still a positive choice that Mr Smith has made to seek support in his attempt to quit smoking.

The various nicotine replacement products should be outlined to Mr Smith and a shared decision made as to what product(s) he wishes to use. In this case there are no contraindications to the use of any product so it would be entirely appropriate to commence with a nicotine replacement product, only considering the likes of bupropion or varenicline if NRT proves unsuccessful. However, Mr Smith would need to see his GP to have these products prescribed.

An exploration of Mr Smith's concern about smoking while socialising with his friends should be undertaken. Situations where this is likely to occur should be identified so that they can be avoided, thus minimising the chance of Mr Smith having a cigarette with his friends. However, it should be made clear to Mr Smith that this does not mean he cannot quit successfully. Sharing his intention to quit smoking with his friends may help in this regard as they can be supportive of his attempt by not smoking while socialising with him.

### Summary of key points

| Condition | Management |
|---|---|
| Obesity | Dietary modification and increased physical activity.<br>Orlistat can be used in people who have a BMI ≥28 kg/m² and are aged 18–65. |
| Smoking cessation | The smoker needs to be motivated to quit smoking.<br>A quit date should be set.<br>Nicotine replacement therapy can be used without prescription. The smoker should select a product that most suits his or her preferences and lifestyle. |

# Bibliography

American Psychiatric Association (1994). *Diagnostic and Statistical Manual of Mental Disorders*, 4th edn. (DSM-IV). Washington, DC: American Psychiatric Association.

Anon (2002). Is glucosamine worth taking for osteoarthritis? *Drug Ther Bull* 40: 81–82.

ASH Scotland (2010). *Smoking and Tobacco Statistics Factsheet*. Available from: http://www.ashscotland.org.uk/media/3624/ASHS_smokingstats_factsheet.pdf (accessed 1 April 2011).

ASH Scotland (2011). *Smoking Cessation Information*. Available from: http://www.ashscotland.org.uk/information/key-topics/smoking-cessation (accessed 31 March 2011).

British Association for the Study of Headache (BASH) (2010). *Guidelines for All Healthcare Professionals in the Diagnosis and Management of Migraine, Tension-type, Cluster and Medication-Overuse Headache*. Hull: BASH.

Department of Health (1991). *Dietary Reference Values for Food Energy and Nutrients for the United Kingdom*. Reports on Public Health and Medical Subjects no. 41. London: HMSO.

Douglas G *et al.* eds (2005). *MacLeod's Clinical Examination*. Edinburgh: Churchill Livingstone.

Electronic Medicines Compendium (2009). *Summary of product characteristics for alli 60mg hard capsules*. Available from: http://www.medicines.org.uk/EMC/medicine/21670/SPC/alli+60+mg+hard+capsules (accessed 31 March 2011).

Ernst E, Pittler MH (2000). Efficacy of ginger for nausea and vomiting: a systematic review of randomized clinical trials. *Br J Anaesth* 84(3): 367-371.

International Society for the Advancement of Kinanthropometry (2006) *International Standards for Anthropometric Assessment*. Potchefstroom: ISAK.

Kumar P, Clark M, eds (2005). *Clinical Medicine*. London: Elsevier Saunders.

Lin J *et al.* (2004). Efficacy of topical non-steroidal anti-inflammatory drugs in the treatment of osteoarthritis: meta-analysis of randomised controlled trials. *Br Med J* 329: 324–326.

Mason L *et al.* (2004). Topical NSAIDs for acute pain: a meta-analysis. *Fam Pract* 5: 10–19.

Matthews A *et al.* (2010). Interventions for nausea and vomiting in early pregnancy. *Cochrane Database Syst Rev* Sep 8; (9): CD007575.

Medicines and Healthcare products Regulatory Agency, (2009). *Codeine and Dihydrocodeine-containing Medicines: Minimising the Risk of Addiction*. London: MHRA.

Moore RA *et al.* (1998). *Quantitative systematic review of topically applied non-steroidal anti-inflammatory drugs*. Br Med J. 316: 33–38.

National Institute for Health and Clinical Excellence (2006). *Clinical Guideline 43: Obesity – Guidance on the Prevention, Identification, Assessment and Management of Overweight and Obesity in Adults and Children*. Available from: http://guidance.nice.org.uk/CG43 (accessed 31 March 2011).

Office for National Statistics. *General Household Survey 2008 – Smoking and Drinking among Adults*. Available from: http://www.statistics.gov.uk/downloads/theme_compendia/GLF08/GLFSmokingandDrinkingAmongAdults2008.pdf (accessed 1 April 2010).

Pittler MH, Ernst E (2004). Feverfew for preventing migraine. *Cochrane Database Syst Rev*. (1): CD002286.

Royal Pharmaceutical Society (2011). *Practice guidance: OTC Sumatriptan*. Available from: http://www.rpharms.com/support-pdfs/otcsumatriptanguid.pdf (accessed 30 March 2011).

Scottish Intercollegiate Guidelines Network (2008). *Diagnosis and Management of Headache in Adults*. Edinburgh: Scottish Intercollegiate Guidelines Network.

Stevinson C *et al.* (2003). Homeopathic arnica for prevention of pain and bruising: randomised placebo-controlled trial in hand surgery. *J R Soc Med*. 96: 60–65.

The British Pain Society (2008). *The British Pain Society*. Available from: http://www.britishpainsociety.org/index.htm (accessed 1 April 2011).

World Health Organization (2011). *Obesity and Overweight Factsheet*. Available from: http://www.who.int/mediacentre/factsheets/fs311/en/index.html (accessed 31 March 2011).

# Self-assessment questions

The following questions are provided to test the information presented in this chapter.

*For questions 1–7 select the best answer in each case.*

1. Select which of the following is not normally a symptom of migraine:
   a. Pulsating or throbbing pain that builds up over minutes to hours
   b. Bilateral pain
   c. Nausea and vomiting
   d. Sensitivity to light and sound
   e. Visual disturbances

2. Select which of the following people could be treated with an NSAID:
   a. A 42-year-old woman with headache who takes lansoprazole 10 mg daily
   b. A 22-year-old man with toothache who uses a salbutamol inhaler four times daily
   c. A 33-year-old woman with headache who takes lithium carbonate 600 mg daily
   d. A 32-year-old man with back pain who takes carbamazepine 1 g daily for epilepsy
   e. A 67-year-old female with knee pain who takes bendroflumethiazide 2.5 mg daily

3. Select which of the following is not a feature of a wry neck:
   a. Caused by unaccustomed movement
   b. Can occur after exposure to the cold
   c. Caused by a fall on a hard surface
   d. The neck is tender and tense to the touch
   e. Pain is felt on one side of the neck

4. Select which of the following best describes the term body mass index:
   a. Is a quantitative measure of disease
   b. Is a way of comparing weight relative to height
   c. Can accurately measure body fat percentage
   d. Is determined by measuring waist circumference and weight
   e. Is rarely used in nutritional assessment of individuals

5. Select which of the following a body mass index of 28.5 kg/m² would be classified as according to the World Health Organization:
   a. Under weight
   b. Normal weight
   c. Overweight
   d. Obese Class I
   e. Obese Class IV

6. Select which of the following is viewed as a benefit of quitting smoking for 24 hours:
   a. Carbon monoxide is eliminated from the body
   b. Risk of lung cancer is half that of a smoker
   c. Cilia in airways regrow
   d. Lung function increased by 10%
   e. Coughing, shortness of breath and wheeze improve

7. Select which of the following is capable of delivering nicotine to the body over 24 hours:
   a. Nicotine gum
   b. Nicotine sublingual tablets
   c. Inhalator
   d. Nasal spray
   e. Transdermal patch

*For questions 8 and 9 select from the list below one lettered option which is most closely related to it. Each lettered option may be used once, more than once, or not at all.*
   a. tension-type headache
   b. migraine
   c. cluster headache
   d. chronic daily headache
   e. traction headache

8. Is commonly caused by overuse of analgesics.

9. Is characterised by unilateral pain around the eye often associated with lacrimation, rhinitis, forehead and facial sweating.

*For questions 10–12 select from the list below one lettered option which is most closely related to it. Each lettered option may be used once, more than once, or not at all.*
   a. acute torticollis
   b. capsulitis
   c. lumbago
   d. lateral epicondylitis
   e. ruptured Achilles tendon

10. Is characterised by pain and tenderness in the shoulder joint.

11. Is a common injury in racquet sports.

12. Is characterised by an intense pain and the sound of a snap.

*For questions 13–16. Each of the questions or incomplete statements in this section is followed by three responses. For each question one or more of the responses is/are correct. Decide which of the responses is/are correct and then choose a–e as indicated in the table below.*

| Directions summarised | | | | |
|---|---|---|---|---|
| **a** | **b** | **c** | **d** | **e** |
| If 1, 2 and 3 are correct | If 1 and 2 only are correct | If 2 and 3 only are correct | If 1 only is correct | If 3 only is correct |

13. The following medicines can be supplied from a pharmacy without a prescription to treat nausea and vomiting associated with migraine:
    1 – prochlorperazine buccal tablets
    2 – cyclizine tablets
    3 – metoclopramide capsules

14. The following measures can be used to treat someone complaining of lumbago:
    1 – rest
    2 – ibuprofen tablets
    3 – ibuprofen topical gel

15. Select in which of the following situations the use of ibuprofen tablets would be contraindicated:
    1 – pregnancy
    2 – active peptic ulceration
    3 – severe heart failure

16. Select which of the following can be supplied without a prescription from a pharmacy as an aid to smoking cessation:
    1 – nicotine replacement therapy
    2 – varenicline
    3 – bupropion

*Questions 17–20 consist of two statements linked by the word* because; *decide whether each statement is true or false. If both statements are true then decide whether the second statement is a correct explanation of the first statement. Choose a–e as your answer as indicated in the table below.*

| Directions summarised | | |
|---|---|---|
| | **First statement** | **Second statement** | |
| a | True | True | Second statement is a correct explanation of the first statement |
| b | True | True | Second statement is not a correct explanation of the first statement |
| c | True | False | |
| d | False | True | |
| e | False | False | |

17.

| Sumatriptan can be supplied as a P medicine to treat migraine in people with an established pattern of migraine | BECAUSE | Migraine does not respond well to simple analgesics |
|---|---|---|

18.

| NSAIDs should not be used in anyone taking warfarin tablets | BECAUSE | People who take warfarin tablets are at an increased risk of bleeding |
|---|---|---|

19.

| Orlistat is a drug that can be used in the pharmacological management of obesity | BECAUSE | Orlistat inhibits gastro-pancreatico-intestinal lipases |
|---|---|---|

20.

| Nicotine replacement therapy is contraindicated in anyone with cardiovascular disease | BECAUSE | People with cardiovascular disease are at an increased risk of side effects from nicotine replacement therapy. |
|---|---|---|

## Answers

1-b; 2-d; 3-c; 4-b; 5-c; 6-a; 7-e; 8-d; 9-c; 10-b; 11-d; 12-e; 13-d; 14-a; 15-a; 16-d; 17-c; 18-a; 19-a; 20-e

# 5

# Infections and Infestations

*Gwen Gray and Alyson Brown*

| This chapter will cover the following conditions: | This chapter will cover the following range of medicines: |
|---|---|
| • Threadworms<br>• Chickenpox<br>• Measles<br>• Impetigo<br>• Cold sores | • Antiviral drugs<br>• Mebendazole<br>• Piperazine |

In this chapter some common infections and infestations that are encountered in pharmacies will be considered. A range of infections affecting various body systems will present in the pharmacy and these will be covered in other chapters of this book. When dealing with infections and infestations it is important to consider differential diagnosis to determine whether a major disease, which cannot be managed by purchasing medicines from a pharmacy, is present.

## Chickenpox and measles

Before reading further, consider the following case and note your initial thoughts.

## Case study

A young mother comes into the pharmacy and asks for something to treat her 6-year-old daughter's rash. The rash is red and she describes it as blister-like in appearance. It is present mainly on the trunk although the face is also affected. She tells you that her daughter has had a fever and has generally been feeling quite tired. She is at home with her dad as she has not been well enough to attend school.

### Trigger questions

- What additional information would you need before considering the appropriate management options in this case?
- What issues concern you about this case?
- Are any alarm symptoms being exhibited that require more urgent treatment or referral?

## Assessing symptoms

### Rash on face and trunk

Rash is characteristic of many skin conditions as detailed in Chapter 9. A rash may be diagnosed and classified by observing the lesions and collecting a detailed history. Age may give some clue to the likelihood of particular diagnoses as some conditions are more common in certain age groups.

Chickenpox is now the most common infectious disease of childhood. It is most common in children under the age of 10 years, although it can occur at any age. It is caused by the varicella-zoster virus and is very infectious. It spreads readily among school and family contacts, either by droplet infection from the respiratory tract or by contact with the vesicular exudate. The incubation period is between 10 and 24 days. Chickenpox is infectious from 1–2 days before the rash appears until all the vesicles have dried or crusted over. This usually takes about 5–6 days although this may take longer in people who are immunocompromised.

The chickenpox rash appears as characteristic tiny vesicles (small blisters) surrounded by reddened areas, mainly on the trunk rather than the face and limbs (Figure 5.1); it may also appear on the scalp. The vesicles are extremely itchy. The rash develops over 2–5 days and the vesicles eventually burst and form crusts or scabs, which disappear after about 10 days. The vesicles appear in crops, and early on both forms of the rash, i.e. vesicles and scabs, will be found simultaneously in different areas of the body. The rash is more likely to be widespread in adults with chickenpox than in children.

Once the infection subsides, the virus persists in the nerve tissues of the body and years later it may be reactivated and herpes zoster (shingles) occurs. It is possible to catch chickenpox from a person with shingles, but not vice versa. Chickenpox may start with a prodromal period in adolescents and adults, where nausea, headache and myalgia may occur. Loss of appetite, fever and a feeling of general malaise may also be experienced when chickenpox occurs. Complications are rare in children but may occur in adults. The infection can be more severe in pregnancy, neonates and immunocompromised individuals; hence these people must be referred to a doctor for treatment.

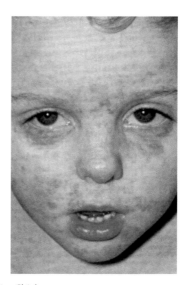

**Figure 5.1** Chickenpox.

(Reproduced with permission from Mark Clarke/Science Photo Library, SPL M130/200.)

Rash on the face and trunk is characteristic of measles. The measles virus is spread by droplet infection from the respiratory tract, and the incubation period is 7–14 days. It is a highly contagious infection and most commonly occurs in children aged 1–4 years, although anyone who has not been vaccinated may catch it. Measles has become uncommon nowadays because of widespread immunisation, although the number of cases of measles has been increasing owing to a fall in uptake of the MMR vaccine.

The condition begins with a fever and symptoms of an upper respiratory tract infection. Conjunctivitis and greyish-white specks on a red base on the buccal mucosa (known as Koplik's spots) will often be present. These spots strongly suggest that measles is present. These symptoms occur during the prodromal phase before the rash appears. After about 4–5 days the blotchy, flat rash appears, starting behind the ears and spreading onto the face and then spreading down to the trunk and limbs (Figure 5.2). It lasts about 7 days. Treatment is not normally necessary as the body fights off the infection and then develops immunity to the measles virus. Complications of measles are possible such as pneumonia and encephalitis.

Cellulitis is a bacterial infection of the skin and subcutaneous tissue caused by either streptococci or staphylococci, and sometimes both together. The infection may arise at the site of trauma, but it can also affect previously healthy skin. If the skin is damaged this creates a point of entry for bacteria, which then attack the skin. It is important that skin wounds are cleaned thoroughly as this helps to minimise the risk of infection developing. A similar condition caused by streptococci is called erysipelas when the infection is superficial; however, it is sometimes difficult to determine the depth of tissue involved and distinguish between the two conditions. The rash is red, painful and often hot and oedematous, and blister formation is possible (Figure 5.3).

Cellulitis is commonly seen on the legs but can also affect the face and arms. Lower limb oedema is a predisposing factor and hence cellulitis is common in older people. Those at risk of developing cellulitis include people who are obese, poorly controlled diabetics, immunocompromised individuals and intravenous drug users. There is often headache, fever, malaise, nausea and shivering present and referral to a doctor for treatment is required. In most serious cases of cellulitis hospital admission is required for treatment.

### Fever and malaise

Fever and malaise commonly occur when infection is present. Fever occurring along with rash allows for differential diagnosis of the cause of rash as most

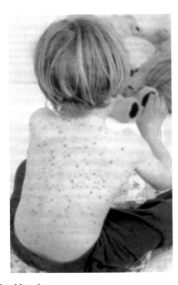

**Figure 5.2** Measles.

(Reproduced with permission from the Wellcome Trust Medical Photographic Library.)

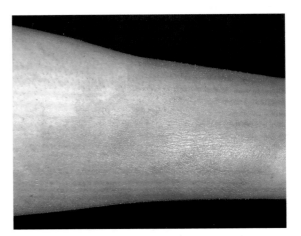

**Figure 5.3** Cellulitis.

(Reproduced with permission of Dr P. Marazzi/Science Photo Library, SPL M130/739.)

skin conditions are not accompanied by fever. Fever may occur in chickenpox, measles and cellulitis.

## Accompanying symptoms

### High temperature

If a person with chickenpox develops a high temperature and experiences pain and redness around the chickenpox lesions, this may indicate a bacterial superinfection. Referral to a doctor is necessary in such circumstances to ensure appropriate management.

### Dehydration

If signs of dehydration such as reduced urine output, lethargy and reduced skin turgor develop, referral for medical attention is required.

### Respiratory symptoms

Lung problems such as pneumonia may occur in adults with chickenpox. Smokers are at greater risk of developing lung problems. Referral is required for medical attention if respiratory symptoms occur in adults with chickenpox.

Symptoms of an upper respiratory tract infection occur at the start of measles. Pneumonia may occur as a complication of measles and referral for medical attention is required.

## Management options

People suffering with chickenpox should be persuaded not to scratch the lesions as this may cause scarring and also releases the virus from the vesicles. It is advisable to ensure that the nails are kept short to minimise damage caused by scratching. It should be advised that the most infectious period is 1–2 days before the rash appears but also that the chickenpox sufferer will remain infectious until all the lesions have crusted over and that contact with other people should be avoided. During this time children should be excluded from school or nursery and return only when the rash is dry and crusted and no vesicles are present. Contact with people who are immunocompromised, pregnant women and neonates should be avoided. Adequate fluid intake should be encouraged to avoid dehydration and smooth, cotton fabrics should be worn to minimise irritation to the skin.

Paracetamol may be used to provide relief of fever associated with chickenpox. It may also be used in measles to relieve aches, pains and fever. Adequate fluid intake is also advisable to avoid dehydration in measles. As measles is highly infectious, contact with other people should be avoided for at least 5 days after the rash has appeared.

If cellulitis is suspected, referral to a doctor for appropriate antibiotic treatment is required, but paracetamol can be recommended for symptomatic relief of fever and pain. It is also advisable to elevate the leg affected by cellulitis and ensure adequate fluid intake to avoid dehydration.

### Antipruritics (BNF section 13.3)

Topical calamine lotion may be used to relieve the itch of chickenpox.

### Antihistamines (BNF section 3.4.1)

Oral antihistamines are useful for pruritis. Chlorphenamine is commonly used to provide symptomatic relief of chickenpox itch. It can be used from age 1 year.

 **Re-consider the case**

Before reading further, re-consider the following questions and your initial thoughts on this case.

**Trigger questions**

- What additional information would you need before considering the appropriate management options in this case?
- What issues concern you about this case?
- Are any alarm symptoms being exhibited that require more urgent treatment or referral?

## Case study

A young mother comes into the pharmacy and asks for something to treat her 6-year-old daughter's rash. The rash is red and she describes it as blister-like in appearance. It is present mainly on the trunk although the face is also affected. She tells you that her daughter has had a fever and has generally been feeling quite tired. She is at home with her dad as she has not been well enough to attend school.

 Pharmacist opinion

The child has a rash accompanied with fever and malaise, which suggests that it is unlikely to be a simple skin condition. The appearance and presentation would suggest that this child is suffering from chickenpox as it commonly affects the trunk, although the face may be affected, and the rash appears as small vesicles as is the case in this child. It would be worthwhile checking with the mother whether she was aware of an outbreak of chickenpox at school as this would also help to establish whether chickenpox was likely. The presence of fever and malaise in this child also suggests that infection is likely and in chickenpox the infection is caused by varicella-zoster virus. The mother should be advised that providing symptomatic relief is the only management option for chickenpox. Paracetamol can be recommended for fever and calamine lotion may be used for itch. The possibility of using an oral antihistamine to relieve itch would also be considered and if appropriate chlorphenamine would be recommended. Further discussion with the mother would also be required to establish whether contact with anyone with a low immune system, pregnant women or babies under 4 weeks of age had occurred. If so it would be important that those persons were assessed by a doctor as a matter of urgency. The child has not been attending school and it would be important to advise the mother that school absence should continue until all the vesicles have crusted over as chickenpox is very infectious and spreads easily.

 General practitioner opinion

This child almost certainly has chickenpox caused by the varicella-zoster virus. It is likely that the mother would know of other children in contact with her daughter who have been affected. The virus is transmitted via the upper respiratory system. The time between initial contact with the virus and development of lesion is usually 10–14 days, but can be as long as 21 days. The lesions are recognised by their classic blister appearance, which turns into crusty lesions. Initially lesions appear on the trunk and head and then may seem to spread to the limbs. Sometimes lesions can be found in the mouth and on the genitalia. Lesions are classically itchy, but less so in younger children. A fever usually precedes the outbreak of lesions for 2–3 days.

Treatment would be supportive with fluids, antipyretics and, if needed, antihistamines. Calamine lotion may be of some help to treat an itch. Symptoms generally last less than a week. A child with prolonged symptoms would need further investigations. This 6-year-old girl should avoid contact with pregnant women, neonates and immunocompromised individuals. Her mother may well be at risk of pregnancy and should be given appropriate advice. Complications of chickenpox are rare but can be very serious. Secondary bacterial infection of lesions may require antibiotics. Viral pneumonia presents with wheeze, chest pain and difficulty breathing. Viral encephalitis presents with confusion, irritability, drowsiness and vomiting.

Summary of key points

| Condition | Management |
|---|---|
| Chickenpox is characterised by a rash that presents as small itchy vesicles, which then crust over. It mainly affects the trunk and may be accompanied by other symptoms such as fever and malaise. | Symptomatic relief with paracetamol, calamine lotion and oral antihistamines. |
| Measles is characterised by a blotchy rash that starts on the face and spreads to the trunk and limbs. Fever and upper respiratory tract symptoms precede the rash. | Symptomatic relief with paracetamol. |

 When to refer

- Erythematous rash or ulceration on the lower leg or ankles in an elderly person
- Chickenpox in special cases such as in pregnancy or in a mother less than 4 weeks after childbirth, or if the sufferer is prescribed steroids, is immunocompromised or is unwell
- Suspected bacterial superinfection of chickenpox
- Signs of dehydration in sufferers of chickenpox or measles
- Respiratory symptoms such as pneumonia in adults with chickenpox or measles (see Chapter 3)
- Refer anyone with diabetes who shows signs or symptoms of skin infection, especially if recurrent, such as boils or cellulitis

## Impetigo and cold sores

Before reading further, consider the following case and note your initial thoughts.

 Case study

A young father comes into the pharmacy and asks for advice on the rash that his 8-year-old son has on his face. The area around his mouth and nose has a crusty rash, although he explains that it started as small blisters that were weeping. He has never had a rash like this before.

**Trigger questions**

- What additional information would you need before considering the appropriate management options in this case?
- What issues concern you about this case?
- Are any alarm symptoms being exhibited that require more urgent treatment or referral?

### Assessing symptoms

#### Crusty rash on face

The rash of impetigo begins with vesicles that rupture and weep, with the affected skin beneath becoming very red. The exudate then dries to form yellowish-brown crusted lesions (Figure 5.4). The skin is sore, and scratching the lesions can cause the infection to spread.

Impetigo is caused by a staphylococcal or streptococcal infection of the skin. The rash occurs most commonly on the face, chiefly around the nose and

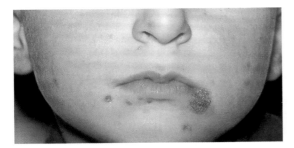

**Figure 5.4** Impetigo.
(Reproduced with permission from the Wellcome Trust Medical Photographic Library.)

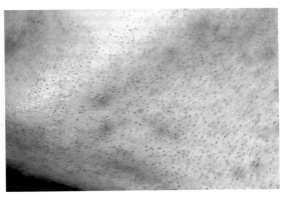

**Figure 5.5** Sycosis barbae.
(Reproduced with permission from the Science Photo Library, SPL M160/014.)

mouth, but sometimes also affects the limbs. This occurs most commonly in children during the early school years. The condition is contagious and children should be kept from school until the lesions have dried up (usually only a few days). It may be difficult to differentiate from infective eczema in some cases, although the crusts of impetigo are very characteristic. In either case, referral to a doctor is necessary for topical or systemic antibiotic therapy. Impetigo may cause psychological distress to the individual, but complications of impetigo such as cellulitis are very rare.

Lesions on the lips may be caused by infection with the herpes simplex virus, which causes cold sores. Cold sores start with a tingling or pricking sensation on the skin of the lips. Blisters then develop, which burst and eventually dry up to form a yellow crust. Although cold sores occur on the lips, they may also appear on the nose or round the mouth. Cold sores last from 7 to 10 days and are often self-diagnosed; they may be triggered by sunlight or cold weather. Attacks are common in individuals who are ill or feeling run down.

Crusting may be present in infection of the beard area of the face. The presence of red papules or pustules in the beard area is characteristic of a staphylococcal infection of the hair follicles called sycosis barbae. It may sometimes be caused by a tinea (ringworm) infection. Sycosis barbae and tinea barbae are characterised by a crusted, raised, pustular folliculitis in the beard area (Figure 5.5). It is most commonly seen in middle-aged men and is exacerbated by shaving. Mild cases may resolve if shaving is stopped for a few days, but failure to resolve requires referral for medical attention.

## Accompanying symptoms

### Atopic eczema

Sufferers of atopic eczema who come into contact with the herpes simplex virus are at risk of developing herpetiform eczema. This is a widespread herpes simplex infection that occurs in atopic eczema. It is rare but can be life threatening. Referral for medical attention is required in such circumstances.

### Fever and malaise

The presence of fever and malaise indicates infection, and referral to a doctor for treatment is required. Cellulitis may occur on the face.

Fever and malaise can occur before the rash of shingles develops. Shingles may occur on the face. Referral to a doctor is required for appropriate treatment.

## Management options

Anyone suffering from impetigo should be reassured that the condition usually heals completely without scarring and it is rare that serious complications occur. They should be advised of the importance of hygiene measures to aid healing and to stop the infection spreading to other areas of the body and to other people. The affected areas should be washed with soapy water and hands should be washed thoroughly after touching affected areas and after applying antibiotic creams. Fingernails should be kept short and clean and scratching should be avoided. Towels, flannels and clothing should not be shared.

The importance of staying away from school until the lesions have dried up should be reinforced.

Sufferers of cold sores should be reassured that the condition is self-limiting and that the lesions will heal without scarring. Advice should be given to try to minimise the spread of the virus. The lesions should not be touched other than when treatment is being applied to the area. Hands should be thoroughly washed after touching the lesions and care should be taken to avoid contact with the eyes. Items that come into contact with the lesion such as eating utensils or lipsticks should not be shared, and kissing should be avoided until the lesions have healed. The bursting of blisters should be avoided. Children who have cold sores can attend school as normal.

### Antiviral preparations (BNF section 13.10.3)

Antiviral creams such as aciclovir or penciclovir can be used to treat cold sores as they stop the virus from multiplying and thus shorten the duration of the attack. These should be applied to the lesion as early as possible, at the time when a tingling sensation is felt. Aciclovir should be applied 5 times a day for at least 4 days but may be continued for up to 10 days if healing has not occurred. Anyone using aciclovir should be warned that it may cause initial stinging when applied. Penciclovir should be applied every 2 hours during awake hours (approximately 8 times a day) and treatment should be continued for 4 days. It is not recommended for children under 12 years of age.

**Re-consider the case**

Before reading further, re-consider the following questions and your initial thoughts on this case.

**Trigger questions**

- What additional information would you need before considering the appropriate management options in this case?
- What issues concern you about this case?
- Are any alarm symptoms being exhibited that require more urgent treatment or referral?

**Case study**

A young father comes into the pharmacy and asks for advice on the rash that his 8-year-old son has on his face. The area around his mouth and nose has a crusty rash, although he explains that it started as small blisters that were weeping. He has never had a rash like this before.

Pharmacist opinion

The child has a crusty rash around his mouth and nose, which started as small blisters. This presentation suggests that he may either have cold sores or impetigo. Both conditions appear initially as blisters that then crust over. Although cold sores commonly occur on the lips, the area around the mouth and nose may be affected. The child has never had this before so this may suggest that it is more likely to be impetigo, particularly since the lips are not affected. By visually observing the lesions it would be possible to determine the cause as the crusts of impetigo are very characteristic.

If impetigo was suspected the child would be referred to a doctor for appropriate treatment with antibiotics. General advice on hygiene measures to minimise the spread of infection would also be given. If cold sores were suspected then an antiviral cream such as aciclovir would be recommended and advice given on how to use the cream. It would also be important to give advice regarding measures to take to minimise the spread of the virus such as avoiding sharing eating utensils and kissing.

General practitioner opinion

This is a classic description of impetigo, a very contagious superficial skin infection. This requires treatment, which may be topical or oral. Care must be taken to avoid touching the lesions and to wash hands thoroughly if this is unavoidable. If using topical treatment, the skin should be cleaned with warm water to allow removal of crusty skin. The antibacterial will then be more easily absorbed through the skin.

There may be an underlying predisposing factor, e.g. a pre-existing skin condition or poor hygiene. These issues must be addressed in order to prevent further infection. Recurrent infection may be due to nasal colonisation and this can also be addressed by eradication with topical antibiotics.

Summary of key points

| Condition | Management |
| --- | --- |
| Impetigo is characterised by a weeping, vesicular rash that then forms yellowish-brown crusted lesions. It mostly affects the face of school-aged children. | Referral is required for antibiotic therapy. |
| Cold sores start with a tingling sensation, followed by blisters that then form a yellowish crust. They commonly occur on the lips of the face. | Antiviral creams such as aciclovir. |

When to refer

- Papular rash, with or without vesicles and crusting, in the beard area of men
- Rash around the mouth or nose of children that changes to weeping vesicles, eventually forming yellow crusts
- Anyone who suffers from atopic eczema who has come into contact with an active cold sore
- Skin lesions accompanied by fever and malaise

# Threadworm

Before reading further, consider the following case and note your initial thoughts.

Case study

A mother comes into the pharmacy and asks for her advice regarding her two children, aged 2 and 7 years. She has noticed that her youngest daughter has been itching around the anus for the last few days and her older daughter is now complaining about discomfort as well as itching. She has noticed what she describes as 'white threads' in her youngest daughter's nappy that morning.

**Case study** (*continued*)

**Trigger questions**

- What additional information would you need before considering the appropriate management options in this case?
- What issues concern you about this case?
- Are any alarm symptoms being exhibited that require more urgent treatment or referral?

## Assessing symptoms

### Perianal itch

This is a common symptom in someone who has a threadworm infection and is caused primarily by the worms laying their eggs around the anal area. The eggs are often laid at night when the conditions favour worm activity as it is usually warm and there is little movement. Through itching, it is then easy for the eggs to be transferred as they become stuck under the fingernails and can be easily ingested or passed on to others.

### White threads in nappy

These white threads are the worms themselves, which can be 2–13 mm in length. They will often be apparent in young children's nappies, although in older children and adults they can be difficult to spot. They will also appear on clothing and bedclothes and so care must be taken to ensure good hygiene and washing practices.

## Accompanying symptoms

Other than the itch and the visible presence of worms, there are usually no other symptoms that commonly occur with an infestation of threadworm. Symptoms that would suggest referral to a doctor would include presence of a fever, accompanied by bedwetting or pain when urinating, and vaginal discharge in young girls as the worms can move to the vaginal area and lay eggs there which can cause further complications. Similar to the gastrointestinal illnesses referral criteria, vomiting, diarrhoea and unexplained weight loss would also be referred to a doctor for further investigation.

## Management options

Treatment is not always necessary as adult worms only live for around 6 weeks, although this management option would require strict hygiene measures as mentioned below.

Pharmacological treatments include mebendazole and piperazine, both of which are available for supply to the public as non-prescription medicines. The purpose of this treatment is to kill the worms, but good hygiene practices must also be undertaken to ensure the eggs are removed from the anal area and to prevent further infection. If a pregnant woman (or her family) present with worms, then no medication can be given if she is in the first trimester, although general hygiene measures may be enough (Box 5.1).

### Drugs for threadworms (BNF section 5.5.1)

Mebendazole is available for supply as a non-prescription medicine as 100 mg tablets. Treatment can be given to children over 2 years of age. All household members should be treated at the same time and if symptoms persist a repeat dose should be given after 14 days. Mebendazole is not licensed for use during pregnancy or breastfeeding.

Piperazine is available for supply as a non-prescription medicine as a sachet and can be given to anyone over 3 months old. Again the whole household should be treated at the same time and a second dose is required after 14 days. Piperazine should not be supplied to anyone with epilepsy, but mebendazole could be offered as an alternative in this case.

## Box 5.1 Hygiene measures with threadworm

**At the same time as treatment**

- Wash all bed linen, sleepwear, towels and any toys that children have in bed with them.
- Thoroughly clean the house and ensure the cloth is thrown out after use.
- Ensure that the bathroom is cleaned and all towels and flannels are washed.

**For the following two weeks**

- Wear loose fitting clothes in bed and change in the morning.
- If particularly itchy at night, consider wearing gloves.
- Ensure that children and adults are fully bathed in the morning.

**General hygiene advice**

- Ensure that nails are kept short and washed regularly.
- Always wash hands after using the bathroom.
- Do not bite nails and avoid putting hands in the mouth.
- Avoid sharing towels and flannels.

### Re-consider the case

Before reading further, re-consider the following questions and your initial thoughts on this case.

**Trigger questions**

- What additional information would you need before considering the appropriate management options in this case?
- What issues concern you about this case?
- Are any alarm symptoms being exhibited that require more urgent treatment or referral?

**Case study**

A mother comes into the pharmacy and asks for her advice regarding her two children, aged 2 and 7 years. She has noticed that her youngest daughter has been itching around the anus for the last few days and her older daughter is now complaining about discomfort as well as itching. She has noticed what she describes as 'white threads' in her youngest daughter's nappy that morning.

Pharmacist opinion

The symptoms that the children have are suggestive of threadworm. The perianal itch is one of the most common symptoms, caused by irritation of the area by the eggs that are laid. The presence of 'white threads' is usually the deciding factor in making a diagnosis of threadworm. These are commonly seen in the faeces or around the anal area. Threadworms are usually not harmful and can easily be treated with non-prescription medicines, although all family members should be treated, even those who are not displaying symptoms. Treatment is usually mebendazole or piperazine. Hygiene advice is

**Pharmacist opinion** (*continued*)

also important as the worms are spread by itching and then getting onto the fingers and beneath the fingernails. Threadworms can also live away from the body for up to 2 weeks and so it is also important to advise washing of bedding and clothes as well as the initial treatment, and then the continuation of good hygiene practice. This will also help in preventing re-infection.

**General practitioner opinion**

This is a clear history of threadworms and there is enough evidence here to make a diagnosis. Anal itching in children is usually caused by threadworms and presence of 'white threads', which are often moving, is diagnostic. Skin conditions can present with itching in the anal and genital area so it is worth keeping that it mind.

Threadworms lay their eggs around the anus and must be ingested in order to mature in the small intestine. The eggs are transferred to the child's fingernails during scratching and then ingested whilst biting nails or eating with fingers, etc. Hence, prevention of threadworms is to improve personal hygiene with washing of hands regularly and avoiding scratching.

Treatment is not mandatory as adult threadworms only live for 6 weeks. If there is no opportunity for eggs to mature, the adult threadworms will die and the infestation ends. This route of management requires diligent care for hand washing, cleaning clothes and bedding and keeping nails short and well-scrubbed.

Most families will want definitive treatment. All family members should be treated at the same time as asymptomatic infestation is common. Treatment should coincide with cleaning of all bedclothes. Mebendazole can be used in children over the age of 2 years and kills worms. It is given as a single dose and is best repeated after 2–3 weeks in case of re-infection. Piperazine can be used in younger children from 3 months; it paralyses the worms and is combined with senna to expel them from the bowel. Treatment with piperazine is repeated after 14 days.

**Summary of key points**

| Condition | Management |
|---|---|
| Threadworm is characterised by a perianal itch and the presence of worms, which are similar in appearance to 'white threads'. | General hygiene measures are important during infestation and to prevent recurrence. Pharmacological treatment is not always necessary as adult worms only live for around 6 weeks; however, good hygiene is important during this time. Mebendazole and piperazine are available to treat threadworms, and the whole household should be treated at the same time. |

**When to refer**

- Vaginal discharge
- Bedwetting
- Problems passing urine
- Loss of appetite
- Weight loss

# Bibliography

Douglas G *et al.*, eds (2005). *MacLeod's Clinical Examination*. Edinburgh: Churchill Livingstone.

Kumar P, Clark M, eds (2005). *Clinical Medicine*. London: Elsevier Saunders.

## Self-assessment questions

The following questions are provided to test the information presented in this chapter.

*For questions 1–4 select the best answer in each case.*

1.  Select which of the following is not a symptom associated with chickenpox:
    a.  Fever
    b.  Malaise
    c.  Myalgia
    d.  Conjunctivitis
    e.  Itch

2.  Select from the following infectious skin conditions those for which exclusion from school or work is not necessary:
    a.  Shingles
    b.  Impetigo
    c.  Cold sores
    d.  Chickenpox
    e.  Measles

3.  Select which of the following is not a risk factor for developing cellulitis:
    a.  Hypertension
    b.  Obesity
    c.  Intravenous drug use
    d.  Poorly controlled diabetes
    e.  Immunosuppression

4.  Select which of the following is not a symptom associated with cellulitis:
    a.  Nausea
    b.  Diarrhoea
    c.  Shivering
    d.  Fever
    e.  Headache

*For questions 5–7 select from the list below one lettered option that is most closely related to it. Each lettered option may be used once, more than once, or not at all.*

    a.  small itchy vesicles that crust over
    b.  yellowish brown crusted lesions
    c.  Koplik's spots
    d.  red, painful, hot rash
    e.  red papules or pustules

5.  Characteristic of sycosis barbae.

6.  Characteristic of measles.

7.  Characteristic of cold sores.

*Questions 8–11: Each of the questions or incomplete statements in this section is followed by three responses. For each question one or more of the responses is/are correct. Decide which of the responses is/are correct and then choose a–e as indicated in the table below.*

| Directions summarised | | | | |
|---|---|---|---|---|
| **a** | **b** | **c** | **d** | **e** |
| If 1, 2 and 3 are correct | If 1 and 2 only are correct | If 2 and 3 only are correct | If 1 only is correct | If 3 only is correct |

8.  Select which of the following groups of people should be referred to their doctor for treatment if contact with a person who has chickenpox has occurred:
    1 – pregnant ladies
    2 – neonates
    3 – people taking oral corticosteroids

9.  Select which of the following items of advice should be given to anyone who has impetigo:
    1 – keep affected areas clean
    2 – avoid sharing towels
    3 – the condition is not contagious

10.  Select which of the following may be used to relieve the itch associated with chickenpox in a 10-month-old child:
    1 – chlorphenamine liquid
    2 – crotamiton cream
    3 – calamine lotion

11.  Select which of the following people can be treated with mebendazole supplied as a P medicine:
    1 – a 3-year-old child with symptoms of perianal itching and 'white threads' visible on the underwear
    2 – a woman who is 8 weeks pregnant and whose daughter has threadworms
    3 – a 6-year-old child who has symptoms of perianal itch and has been bedwetting for the past 3 weeks

*Questions 12–14 consist of two statements linked by the word* because; *decide whether each statement is true or false. If both statements are true then decide whether the second statement is a correct explanation of the first statement. Choose a–e as your answer as indicated in the table below.*

## Directions summarised

|   | First statement | Second statement |   |
|---|---|---|---|
| a. | True | True | Second statement is a correct explanation of the first statement |
| b. | True | True | Second statement is not a correct explanation of the first statement |
| c. | True | False |   |
| d. | False | True |   |
| e. | False | False |   |

**12.**

| Aciclovir cream may be sold as a P medicine to treat cold sores | BECAUSE | Topical antivirals are used to treat herpes zoster infection |
|---|---|---|

**13.**

| Anyone with measles who has severe respiratory symptoms must be referred to their general practitioner for management | BECAUSE | Pneumonia is a possible complication of measles |
|---|---|---|

**14.**

| Perianal itch is a common symptom of threadworm | BECAUSE | Threadworms lay their eggs around the anal area, which causes irritation |
|---|---|---|

## Answers

1-d; 2-c; 3-a; 4-b; 5-e; 6-c; 7-a; 8-a; 9-b; 10-e; 11-d; 12-c; 13-a; 14-a

# 6

## Obstetrics, Gynaecology and Urinary System

*Ruth Edwards*

| This chapter will cover the following conditions: | This chapter will cover the following groups of medicines: |
|---|---|
| • Urinary tract infections (UTIs) (cystitis)<br>• Benign prostatic hyperplasia (BPH)<br>• Vaginal infections (vaginal candidiasis, bacterial vaginosis and trichomoniasis)<br>• Sexually transmitted infections (STIs)<br>• Menstrual disorders (dysmenorrhoea, menorrhagia and premenstrual syndrome (PMS))<br>• Emergency contraception<br>• Pregnancy and ovulation testing | • Sodium bicarbonate<br>• Potassium citrate<br>• Sodium citrate<br>• Tamsulosin<br>• Preparations for vaginal and vulval candidiasis<br>• Antibacterials (azithromycin)<br>• NSAIDs and analgesics<br>• Tranexamic acid<br>• Dietary and herbal supplements<br>• Emergency hormonal contraception<br>• Folic acid |

Pharmacists commonly encounter people with conditions relating to the urinary and reproductive systems. In addition, promoting good sexual health is an important aspect of the pharmacist's health promotion role. In this chapter we will consider the symptoms of common minor illnesses of the urinary tract and the reproductive system that are encountered in pharmacies and the major diseases that these need to be differentiated from. This chapter will also consider general approaches to dealing with these conditions and with sexual health issues and the specific groups of drugs that can be used to treat and manage these conditions. In addition we will consider the supply of emergency hormonal contraception and

specific issues encountered in pharmacies around pregnancy testing and preconception care.

The reproductive system comprises the reproductive organs and is responsible for sexual reproduction. In the male, the organs include the testes, accessory ducts, accessory glands, prostate gland and penis. In the female, the organs include the uterus, uterine tubes, ovaries, vagina and vulva. Control of the female menstrual cycle involves a complex interaction of physiological processes, which are illustrated in Figure 6.1. The majority of conditions that can be dealt with as minor illness relate to the female reproductive system and most conditions that occur in men require medical referral.

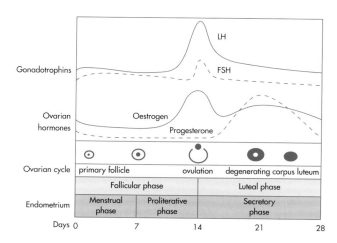

**Figure 6.1** Hormone levels, follicular development and endometrial changes in the normal menstrual cycle.

(Reproduced from Period Problems: disorders of menstruation in adolescents, Peacock, A, Alvi, NS, Mushtaq, T, *Archives of Disease in Childhood*, Jun 24 2010 with permission of BMJ Publishing Group Ltd.)

Contraception involves preventing conception from occurring, and this can be achieved by either hormonal or non-hormonal methods. In order to fully understand the mode of action of contraceptives it is important to know how the female reproductive cycle is controlled and how conception occurs. This is outside the scope of this text and we refer you to a physiology text for a deeper understanding of this process. A male hormonal contraceptive has been under development for some years, but at present most forms of hormonal contraception interfere with the control of the female menstrual cycle in some way.

The urinary and renal systems are responsible for excretion of waste and homeostasis or maintaining fluid and electrolyte balance. The urinary system is made up of the kidneys, the ureters, which connect the kidneys to the bladder, and the urethra, which opens to allow urine to be passed out of the body. The kidneys and ureters are usually referred to as the upper urinary tract and the bladder and urethra as the lower urinary tract. In men, the prostate gland, which is part of the reproductive system, is located at the bottom of the bladder and surrounds the urethra.

## Sexual health services in pharmacy

Public health activity and sexual health services are well-established pharmacy roles, especially in community pharmacy where there is convenient access without the need to make an appointment. Specialist clinical pharmacists also contribute to delivery of HIV and genitourinary medicine (GUM) services. A growing range of non-prescription medicines and products for use in this area has allowed this contribution to broaden over the past decade.

Emergency hormonal contraception (EHC) has been available over the counter in pharmacies in the United Kingdom since 2001. Often referred to as 'the morning-after pill', EHC allows community pharmacists to play a significant role in contraception services, through which they can contribute generally to the public health agenda and specifically to meeting national sexual health agenda objectives.

Unwanted pregnancies and subsequent abortions are a significant public health issue in the UK. EHC is an effective means of preventing accidental pregnancy and the related anxiety it causes when unprotected sex has occurred. Pharmacists should be able to offer a non-judgemental and sensitive service in a private area (preferably a consulting room) in the pharmacy.

Since EHC became available as a non-prescription medicine in 2001, about a third of all users have bought it from a pharmacy. Studies have shown that a significantly higher number of patients who access EHC from a pharmacy were able to do so within 24 hours of unprotected sex compared with other routes of supply. At least a half of EHC supplied through community pharmacies is accessed out of hours or over a weekend.

Prevention and treatment of sexually transmitted infections (STIs) is another area where pharmacists can contribute to promoting good sexual health. STIs commonly affect both the reproductive and urinary systems and pharmacists have traditionally had a role in prevention of STIs by the supply of condoms and advice on safe sex. The reclassification of azithromycin for treatment of asymptomatic *Chlamydia trachomatis* establishes another aspect of the pharmacists' role in managing sexual health.

## Consultation and behavioural skills for sexual health consultations

Before considering the conditions in this chapter, it is important to reflect on the consultation skills needed to conduct a consultation around sexual health or any other intimate issue. Discussing sexual health issues or conditions in intimate body areas can be embarrassing for individuals and for healthcare professionals and it is important that the person is put at ease.

Professionals need to be aware of their own attitudes towards sex and the existence of different sexual cultures and orientations, and to treat everyone with respect and in a non-judgemental way. Sensitivity towards sexual orientation is important; for example, not making assumptions about the gender of sexual partners and using neutral language (e.g. the use of 'their' or 'his/her' can be helpful here). When discussing personal and sexual issues, privacy is extremely important and wherever possible the consultation should take place in a private area where it cannot be overheard. The language used in these types of consultations is also worth reflecting on; professionals should explore the language they use around sexual functions and body parts but must also be able to respond to the use of colloquialisms without being drawn into using phraseology they are uncomfortable with. Child protection is another issue of which healthcare professionals need to have an awareness, especially when dealing with consultations with individuals under the age of 16 years. All UK NHS Trusts have guidance available for health professionals on child protection issues and information on how to seek help locally if concerns arise.

## Urinary tract disorders

Before reading further, consider the following case and note your initial thoughts.

**Case study**

A regular customer comes into the pharmacy and asks for something to ease their symptoms of pain and discomfort when passing urine as they do not want to bother their doctor.

**Trigger questions**

- What additional information would you need before considering the appropriate management options in this case?
- What issues concern you about this case?
- Are any alarm symptoms being exhibited that require more urgent treatment or referral?

### Assessing symptoms

#### Dysuria

Dysuria is difficulty and pain when passing urine, which is often described as a stinging, burning sensation and is frequently accompanied by urinary urgency and frequency. This cluster of symptoms is often called cystitis. Dysuria in women is commonly due to inflammation of the urethra, which can be caused by bacterial infection, irritation by perfumed soaps, antiseptics or spermicides, sexual intercourse, or sexually transmitted infections, and can also occur with vaginal infections. In women, organisms from the bowel, such as *Escherichia coli*, staphylococci and enterococci, may be carried from the perianal area to the urethra, which is relatively short in women, thereby facilitating the passage of bacteria to the bladder. In men, due to the longer urethra and the antibacterial properties of the prostatic fluid, cystitis is less common and men presenting with symptoms should be referred to exclude conditions such as enlarged prostate, prostate infection or sexually transmitted infections.

It is important to consider symptom onset; bacterial infections are likely to be acute in onset. It is worth asking about any likely triggers including recent sexual activity. If sexual intercourse with a new partner has occurred, particularly unprotected, it is important to consider an STI.

Duration of symptoms will influence whether the condition can be managed as a minor illness. If the symptoms have been present for longer than 5–7 days, there may be a risk that the infection has moved from the lower urinary tract to the kidneys and may have developed into pyelonephritis. Dysuria in men over 45 presenting as hesitancy, weak stream and urgency of several months' duration may be indicative of benign prostatic hyperplasia (BPH). Symptoms of prostate enlargement are caused by the enlarged prostate placing pressure on the bladder and urethra. This can cause 'functional' lower urinary tract symptoms such as difficulty when starting urinating, urinating for longer or more frequently, needing to do so again within a short period of time, and needing to get up to urinate several times at night. Urinary frequency is also a presenting feature of diabetes. If this symptom has lasted for more than a few days, is marked at night, and is accompanied by thirst and weight loss, the individual should be referred.

Frequent recurrence of symptoms may also suggest that the individual has some predisposing condition, such as diabetes, or an anatomical or physiological abnormality in the urinary tract and they should be referred for assessment.

The age of the person experiencing the symptoms is relevant; cystitis is common in women of reproductive age. About one in two women will be treated for a symptomatic urinary tract infection (UTI) during their lifetime. At the menopause, changes in the urethral and vaginal epithelium may increase the likelihood of infection in some women. In elderly women, cystitis may also be indicative of underlying pathology such as diabetes. Elderly women are also much more prone to complications such as pyelonephritis and so should be referred to their doctor for assessment. Cystitis can occur in children, particularly female children, but should be referred to a doctor for assessment. Any concerns about child abuse or sexual intercourse under the age of consent should be handled sensitively and any health professional with concerns should take local advice from child protection support workers. Cystitis is rare in young men. It may be a manifestation of a renal stone, causing damage and infection in the renal tract. In such cases, the sufferer will complain of episodes of severe colicky loin pain spreading, over days or longer, downwards to the groin and the testicles, and this requires medical appraisal. Cystitis is more common in older men, but referral is needed for exclusion of prostatic disease and bladder neoplasms.

Pregnant women often present with the symptoms of cystitis. These may result from the mechanical effects of pressure from an enlarging uterus and will often resolve spontaneously in a few days. However, if symptoms are either persistent or recurrent, the woman should be referred.

Drugs such as cytotoxics or tiaprofenic acid can precipitate cystitis.

## Accompanying symptoms

Dysuria can be accompanied by other symptoms and it is important to take a full history and consider any accompanying symptoms to determine the likely cause.

### Pain, fever, nausea and vomiting

In an upper UTI, dysuria is often accompanied by pain in the lower abdomen, sometimes described as loin pain, or pain in the lower back indicating that the infection may have moved up the urinary tract to the kidneys and therefore anyone reporting these symptoms should be referred. Signs of a kidney infection also include high fever with shaking chills, nausea and vomiting.

### Appearance of the urine

The urine may appear cloudy and may smell strong or 'fishy'. Presence of blood in the urine may indicate a more severe infection or inflammation and again would require referral.

### Discharge

A discharge from the urethra, often accompanied by redness around the opening of the urethra in a man, may indicate presence of an STI such as chlamydia or gonorrhoea. Dysuria can accompany abnormal vaginal discharge in women and this will be discussed later in this chapter.

### Visual abnormalities

Presence of any visual abnormalities in the genital area in either women or men requires referral. In genital herpes a vesicular rash affects the tip or shaft of the penis or the labia and vulva and there is local pain, which is aggravated by sexual intercourse. Genital warts are not usually associated with dysuria but appear either as a frond-like growth, which is almost certainly sexually transmitted, or a flat, common skin wart, which is not. They may be found around the anus, particularly in homosexual men, and are not serious but are difficult to treat and often recur.

### Suspected sexually transmitted infection

Dysuria, frequency, vaginitis, discharge, urethritis and rashes in the genital region are all possible symptoms of an STI and may occur within a few days of sexual intercourse with an infected partner. STIs will not present frequently to pharmacists, but because incidence of STIs in the UK is increasing (especially of chlamydia, syphilis, genital herpes and warts) it is important to be aware of symptoms associated with such a timescale, especially in young adults, those with a new sexual partner, those returning from holiday, or whose job involves a lot of travel, and individuals (or their partners) who have been treated previously for STIs. Where an STI is suspected the individual should be referred for appropriate testing. They may express concerns about the possibility of HIV infection, when no symptoms will be evident. These concerns should be handled sensitively, explaining the low probability among heterosexuals, the need for safe sex, and that the antibody blood test will not be accurate until 3 months after exposure. Referral for counselling is recommended.

## Management options

Assuming the individual does not have any referable or 'alarm' symptoms, symptomatic relief can be offered. Mild cases of cystitis usually resolve spontaneously within a few days and symptomatic relief from cystitis is commonly achieved by drinking plenty of fluids. Symptoms that persist beyond 3 days require referral so that antibiotic treatment can be considered.

Simple analgesics such as paracetamol can be offered for pain relief providing this does not prevent the individual from seeking appropriate medical advice.

Counselling can include advice to empty the bladder as completely as possible after urinating, and to avoid delay in emptying the bladder. Perianal hygiene is important, and people should be encouraged to wash the area with water and unperfumed soap after a bowel movement, and to wipe from front to back to prevent re-infection.

Sufferers should be advised to try to avoid known triggers such as spermicides or perfumed soaps. If symptoms are related to sexual intercourse, the perianal skin should be washed beforehand and the bladder should be emptied before and after intercourse. A lubricant should be used to prevent trauma and soreness. Care should be taken to avoid tight underwear made of synthetic material. Detergents should be thoroughly rinsed out after washing underwear.

If an STI is suspected, then the individual should be referred to their GP or to local sexual health services for testing and follow-up. They may also choose to buy a chlamydia test kit providing they are over 16 years of age and asymptomatic. This involves posting a urine sample to a testing laboratory which will test for *Chlamydia trachomatis* but not for other sexually transmitted bacteria such as *Neisseria gonorrhoeae* (gonorrhoea), *Treponema pallidum* (syphilis) or viruses such as herpes simplex virus (HSV), human papillomavirus (HPV) or human immunodeficiency virus (HIV). Advice should also be provided on safe sex and condom use.

### Alkalinising agents (BNF section 7.4)

The alkalinising action of sodium bicarbonate, sodium citrate or potassium citrate on the urine can relieve the symptoms of cystitis. Potassium citrate is available as a mixture that needs to be mixed with water, and a number of proprietary products, formulated as sachets of powder to be dissolved in water, are available as non-prescription medicines. Robust clinical trials have not been conducted into the use of alkalinising agents for symptoms of UTIs, but women who use them report symptomatic relief. Cautions regarding the use of alkalinising agents are outlined in Table 6.1.

### Cranberry juice

Cranberry juice has been found to contain substances that prevent bacteria (particularly *E. coli*) from adhering to the uroepithelial cells on the walls of the bladder and urethra. No evidence has been found of efficacy in treating UTIs, but there does

**Table 6.1 Contraindications and need for care in the use of potassium and sodium containing preparations**

| Contraindication | Need for care |
|---|---|
| Renal disease | There may be impaired ability to excrete potassium in potassium citrate |
| Pregnancy, hypertension | Caution over extra sodium intake with sodium bicarbonate and citrate |
| Taking ACE inhibitors or potassium-sparing diuretics | Potassium citrate may cause hyperkalaemia |
| Taking nitrofurantoin | Nitrofurantoin is inactivated in alkaline urine |
| Taking lithium | Sodium salts can reduce plasma lithium levels |

appear to be evidence for benefit in preventing infections. It is not clear what is the optimum dosage or method of administration, for example juice, tablets or capsules, and large numbers of dropouts in studies indicate that cranberry juice may not be acceptable over long periods. High-strength cranberry capsules (containing at least 200 mg of cranberry extract) may be used in prevention of recurrence and may be more acceptable than juice. Although there is no evidence for benefit in treating UTIs, sufferers of cystitis may choose to take cranberry juice as part of their increased fluid intake, possibly along with other treatments. This is safe to do unless they take drugs that interact with cranberry such as anticoagulants.

## Tamsulosin (BNF section 7.4)

Tamsulosin is licensed as a P medicine for treatment of the symptoms of benign prostatic hyperplasia (BPH) in men aged 45 to 75 years who meet certain criteria. Tamsulosin is an alpha$_1$-blocker that works by relaxing smooth muscle in BPH, producing an increase in urine flow rate and an improvement in obstructive symptoms.

Symptoms of BPH are described in Assessing symptoms above. To be eligible for supply of tamsulosin from a pharmacy, the individual should be within the age range above, have had the symptoms of BPH for a minimum of 3 months, not meet any of the referral criteria listed in Box 6.1 and not have been prescribed any other BPH treatment. The manufacturer of tamsulosin advises use of a symptom check questionnaire (which incorporates the International Prostate Symptom Score) to determine the severity of symptoms and impact on quality of life.

A pharmacist can make a 2-week initial supply of tamsulosin as a P medicine and a further 4 weeks' supply if there has been an improvement in symptoms. If there has been no improvement in symptoms after the initial 2 weeks or if symptoms get worse, the man should be referred to his GP. Men who are supplied with tamsulosin must be advised to see their GP within 6 weeks of starting treatment for assessment and confirmation that they can continue treatment. The pharmacist can make a further supply after 6 weeks if they ensure (by asking the individual) that this clinical assessment has taken place, and the man should be reviewed by his GP every 12 months.

## Antibacterials (BNF section 5.1)

Although not available as non-prescription medicines for UTIs, in some areas of the UK antibacterials may be supplied for uncomplicated UTIs in women by accredited pharmacists under Patient Group Directions (PGDs). Trimethoprim and cephalosporins are the main agents used and strict inclusion and exclusion criteria usually apply such as previous diagnosis

---

**Box 6.1   Referral criteria for tamsulosin as a P medicine**

*Tamsulosin should not be supplied and men should be referred to their general practitioner when:*

- There is pain on urination, bloody or cloudy urine, or fever that may indicate a urinary tract infection.
- There is blood in the urine, which can be a sign associated with bladder cancer.
- There is incontinence or leaking of urine, as this may indicate chronic urinary retention.
- There is unstable or potentially undiagnosed diabetes, for example characterised by excessive thirst and tiredness as this may result in damage to the autonomic nervous system.
- There are liver, kidney or heart problems.
- There are reports of fainting, dizziness or weakness when standing (postural hypotension) as alpha-blockers can reduce blood pressure.
- Cataract surgery is planned or there is recent blurred or cloudy vision that has not been examined by a general practitioner or optician (as cataracts may be indicated) owing to the risk of intraoperative floppy iris syndrome (IFIS) during cataract surgery in some men taking tamsulosin.
- The man has had prostate surgery.
- There is allergy or hypersensitivity to tamsulosin.

by a GP, fewer than three episodes per year, and absence of alarm symptoms.

In the UK, public consultations have been held by the Medicines and Healthcare products Regulatory Agency (MHRA) on behalf of manufacturers making applications for the reclassification of trimethoprim and nitrofurantoin to P medicines for uncomplicated acute bacterial cystitis in women who had been previously diagnosed by a doctor. Neither drug has been reclassified, possibly because of concerns about the implications of wider availability of antibacterials and antibiotic resistance.

Azithromycin is licensed as a P medicine for confirmed asymptomatic genital *Chlamydia trachomatis* infection and epidemiological treatment of sexual

partners aged over 16 years. In some areas of the UK, it can also be supplied under PGD for individuals aged 13 years or over, but this depends on the inclusion criteria of the individual PGD.

The supply of azithromycin as a P medicine can only be made following positive laboratory testing for *C. trachomatis*, which the product licence requires to be confirmed by a test result letter. This will be sent to the individual receiving the positive result, known as the index patient. For sexual partners, supply can be made following production of a Partner Notification (PN) slip, which they will have been given by the index patient. The contraindications to the supply of azithromycin as a P medicine are listed in Box 6.2.

---

**Box 6.2** Circumstances when azithromycin cannot be supplied as a P medicine

*Azithromycin should not be supplied as a P medicine in the following circumstances:*

● Anyone with symptoms of chlamydia or its complications such as:

**In women**

- pain when passing urine
- bleeding between periods
- unusual vaginal discharge
- bleeding after sex
- pain when having sex
- any unexpected pain below the belly button (indicating lower abdominal pain and pelvic pain).

**In men**

- discharge from the penis
- pain when passing urine
- pain or swelling in the testicles (indicating epididymo-orchitis).

● Anyone with symptoms suggestive of other STIs (any unusual lumps, bumps, blisters, sores around genital or anal area).
● Children under the age of 16 years.
● Known hypersensitivity to azithromycin or any macrolide antibiotic or any of the excipients.
● Renal or hepatic impairment.
● Anyone with a history of cardiac disease.
● Pregnant women and anyone who is breastfeeding.
● Individuals receiving ciclosporin, digoxin, ergotamine, terfenadine, theophylline, disopyramide, rifabutin and coumarin anticoagulant therapy, such as warfarin because of the interaction with azithromycin.
● Individuals taking azithromycin for any other infection.
● Individuals who have already taken azithromycin or another treatment for chlamydia in the last 6 months (this is because the risk of serious complications increases each time a person is infected).

**Re-consider the case**

Before reading further, re-consider the following questions and your initial thoughts on this case.

**Trigger questions**

- What additional information would you need before considering the appropriate management options in this case?
- What issues concern you about this case?
- Are any alarm symptoms being exhibited that require more urgent treatment or referral?

**Case study**

A regular customer comes into the pharmacy and asks for something to ease their symptoms of pain and discomfort when passing urine as they do not want to bother their doctor.

Pharmacist opinion

In this case a lot more information needs to be obtained from the person before deciding on management options. The treatment options available in a pharmacy will only give symptomatic relief, so an important consideration is determining whether this person needs to be referred to their GP for further assessment or treatment.

The individual should be asked to describe the pain in more detail, giving specific information about location, occurrence and duration. Are they experiencing pain in their abdomen or in their lower back, which may indicate a kidney infection? It would also be important to explore what they mean by 'discomfort'. Is it a sharp and burning pain in the urethra and a feeling or urgency, which would indicate cystitis, or are they experiencing any difficulty in passing any urine? Alarm symptoms requiring referral need to be ruled out such as fever, nausea and vomiting, loin or back pain, and presence of blood in the urine. It would also be worth inquiring sensitively about recent sexual activity.

At this stage it needs to be considered whether the individual is male or female and immediate referral is required for any man who describes the symptoms of cystitis. Their age is also relevant; cystitis is quite common in women of child-bearing age but is less common and more of a concern and cause for referral in children and the elderly.

If the symptoms were of short duration (less than 3 days), indicative of cystitis, and referral has been ruled out, an alkalinising agent can be supplied. The choice would depend on the woman's personal preference and coexistence of any medical problems. Although potassium citrate mixture is cheap, it has a particularly unpleasant taste so it is worth recommending a proprietary brand of sachet as these have been formulated to mask the flavour. This needs to be explained to the woman and she should be given the choice.

As well as advice to drink plenty of fluids, they need an explanation that the treatment is only providing symptomatic relief and if the symptoms continue or worsen or if they develop any 'alarm symptoms' they should contact their GP. If the symptomatic relief is unsuccessful, it is worth encouraging the woman to inform the GP receptionist of this, allowing the surgery to assess the urgency of providing an appointment.

In a man with symptoms of benign prostatic hyperplasia, assessment could be made of suitability for supply of tamsulosin.

General practitioner opinion

Some important considerations here are duration of symptoms, age and sex of the person and previous history of urological, gynaecological or gastrointestinal problems.

Dysuria may be a symptom of simple UTI, but also of atrophic vaginitis, urethral syndrome, sexually transmitted infections and bladder irritation caused by stones or tumour. Symptoms of this nature may be accompanied by signs of systemic illness, e.g. high temperature, sweats and rigors.

A simple urinary infection in a woman in her early twenties may be resolved with no antibiotic treatment or it may develop into a serious pyelonephritis affecting the kidneys and causing significant morbidity. A urinary infection in an elderly person can be much more disabling and can cause confusion. In assessing for presence of UTI, a GP would normally use dipstick urinalysis. The diagnosis of UTI is made using a combination of clinical signs and urinalysis. A positive urinalysis for nitrites is most indicative of UTI and is extremely helpful in those with milder symptoms. Confirmation of infection would then be sought by sending a mid-stream urine sample to the microbiology laboratory for culture and sensitivity. This will not only identify presence of infection but will also identify antibiotics that the bacterium is sensitive to and resistant to.

Persistent symptoms would require further investigation and treatment tailored to the specific cause. People who 'don't want to bother their doctor' are very often those who actually need medical assessment. Some people will use that phrase to cover up fear about their symptoms; it is the task of the health professional to unravel the significance of statements like this in combination with the clinical picture.

 Summary of key points

| Condition | Management |
| --- | --- |
| Urinary tract infection (cystitis) is characterised by stinging, burning pain when passing urine accompanied by urinary urgency and frequency. | Alkalysing agents can be used for symptomatic relief. Drink plenty of fluids. Cranberry products may be useful in preventing recurrence. |
| Sexually transmitted infections (STIs) are characterised by any or all of dysuria, frequency, vaginitis, discharge, urethritis, and rashes in the genital region, particularly after unprotected sexual intercourse. | Referral for appropriate testing. Azithromycin may only be supplied if the individual is asymptomatic and has had a positive test for chlamydia or is the sexual partner of someone who has tested positive. Advice on safe sex and condom use. |
| Benign prostatic hyperplasia (BPH) is characterised by difficulty when starting urinating, urinating for longer or more frequently, needing to do so again within a short period of time, and needing to get up to urinate several times at night in men aged around 40 years or above. | Referral for appropriate medical assessment. Consideration for supply of tamsulosin if the man meets the supply eligibility. |

 When to refer

- Men with symptoms of cystitis
- Elderly women or children with cystitis

**When to refer** (*continued*)

- Presence of alarm symptoms: duration longer than 5-7 days, fever, nausea, vomiting, loin pain and tenderness, back pain, presence of blood in the urine
- Suspected STI or visual abnormalities in the genital area
- Symptoms of undiagnosed diabetes
- Drug-induced cystitis
- Recurrent episodes of cystitis (more than 3 in 12 months)
- Where symptoms do not improve within 3 days or after 2 days of treatment with a non-prescription medicine or where symptoms get worse
- Persistent or recurrent symptoms in pregnant women

# Vaginal infections

Before reading further, consider the following case and note your initial thoughts.

**Case study**

One busy afternoon a 32-year-old woman comes into the pharmacy with her two young children to buy nappies and baby milk. Once she has paid for her shopping, she says quietly 'Would it be possible to have a quick word with the pharmacist?' She explains, rather embarrassedly, that she has a vaginal discharge and some itching around the area. The discharge is white and she is not aware of any smell. She had similar symptoms when she was expecting her first child but cannot remember what her doctor prescribed at the time.

**Trigger questions**

- What additional information would you need before considering the appropriate management options in this case?
- What issues concern you about this case?
- Are any alarm symptoms being exhibited that require more urgent treatment or referral?

## Assessing symptoms

### Vaginal discharge

A slight vaginal discharge is normal in most women and provided the discharge has not changed in any way, such as amount, smell or texture, and is not irritant or blood-stained then reassurance may be all that is needed.

Abnormal discharge can be caused by infection of the vagina, most commonly with yeasts such as *Candida albicans* (candidiasis or thrush), bacteria such as *Gardnerella vaginalis* (bacterial vaginosis) or protozoa such as *Trichomonas vaginalis* (trichomoniasis).

The vagina contains lactobacilli, which produce lactic acid and make the vagina slightly acidic, which prevents other organisms from growing there. Disruption of the pH balance (for example with use of perfumed bubble baths) or a reduction in the lactobacilli (for example following a course of antibiotics) will affect the natural bacterial balance in the vagina and pre-dispose to infections.

In vaginal candidiasis there is often (but not always) a characteristic vaginal discharge, which is usually described as thick and white or creamy, curd-like (resembling cottage cheese) but odourless.

Any offensive, smelly discharge requires referral, as it may represent a trichomonal or bacterial infection. The thin, white discharge of bacterial vaginosis has a fishy odour, which is often prominent after intercourse or during the menstrual period. Bacterial vaginosis is not transmitted sexually but is more common in sexually active women. It is usually caused by disruption of the natural bacterial balance in the vagina. The discharge of trichomoniasis, which is transmitted sexually, is often profuse and frothy, and may be white, yellow or green in colour. Similarly, blood in the discharge or any bleeding not associated with menstruation should be referred to exclude a sinister cause.

Changes in the urethral and vaginal epithelium due to reducing oestrogen levels at the menopause may increase the likelihood of infection in some women. A thin, watery discharge in a postmenopausal woman may be due to candidal infection but may also be due to atrophic vaginitis or possibly carcinoma and therefore referral is required to exclude these.

It is important to ascertain duration, frequency and onset of symptoms to help determine the likely cause. Onset of symptoms in candidal infections tends to be acute, although sometimes it may be a chronic complaint and sufferers may complain of a discharge for several weeks. A long-standing discharge, however, is unlikely to be candidiasis, and is more often associated with bacterial infections (which are usually insidious in onset), pelvic inflammatory disease (PID; which is a complication of bacterial vaginosis), hormonal disturbance or other systemic illness all of which require referral. Anyone with symptoms lasting more than 7 days despite treatment should be referred. This is because the differential diagnosis can be difficult, and conditions such as STIs, bacterial infection, trichomoniasis, genital herpes and warts may present with similar (although often more severe) soreness, inflammation and oedema.

Recurrence of symptoms is also important and may determine whether a referral is required. Referral should be made if similar symptoms have been experienced on more than two previous occasions in the previous 6 months, so that any underlying predisposing condition, such as diabetes, can be identified and a differential diagnosis made to exclude other diseases. If the woman is known to have diabetes and has recurrent episodes of candidiasis, she should be questioned about the control of her diabetes and referred if appropriate, as high levels of glucose may encourage an overgrowth of *Candida*

in the vagina. If symptoms are recurrent around the time of menstruation in younger women and do not respond to non-prescription medicines, then they should be assessed by a doctor.

It is important to assess whether the symptoms have been triggered by anything. Infections of the vagina can be a complication or accompany a course of antibiotics or steroids. Antibiotics can affect the natural vaginal flora and cause an overgrowth of *Candida*. Pregnancy also predisposes to an overgrowth of *Candida* owing to hormonal changes; the use of oral contraceptives may alter the vaginal environment and cause candidiasis, but this is controversial and may not be the case with low-dose oestrogen pills. Pregnancy or suspected pregnancy requires referral.

In cases of vaginal candidiasis, women should be asked about their use of local topical applications, such as vaginal deodorants or bath additives, as these can predispose to or exacerbate the condition. Tampons and intrauterine contraceptive devices may aggravate vaginal candidiasis, as might menstruation and sexual intercourse. Tight underclothing made from synthetic material, such as nylon tights, will increase the temperature and humidity of the perianal and perivulval region, thus fostering ideal conditions for the growth of bacteria and *Candida*. A change in sexual partner is often associated with the onset of bacterial vaginosis.

### Vulvovaginitis

Vulvovaginitis or inflammation of the vaginal and vulval area is associated with pain, itching, redness and swelling of the genital area. Vaginal candidiasis usually presents as vulval soreness, itching, and a burning sensation in the vulval area. There is often redness or swelling of the vulva along with the discharge. These symptoms are not specific to thrush and can occur in each of the causes of vaginal discharge as well as with STIs.

## Accompanying symptoms

Other symptoms accompanying vulvovaginitis that should be regarded as unusual and require referral include vaginal blisters, abdominal pain, fever, vomiting and diarrhoea, which may indicate other local pathology or pelvic inflammation.

### Dysuria

Pain and discomfort when passing urine has been dealt with earlier in this chapter but can be associated with vaginal infections.

### Dyspareunia

Dyspareunia (painful intercourse) may be caused by candidiasis, but could indicate other pathology and requires referral for a full examination and assessment. Postmenopausal vaginal atrophy is accompanied by symptoms such as dryness, irritation, discomfort and painful intercourse. Bleeding after sexual intercourse is normally associated with STIs or a more serious pathology.

### Symptoms in men

Although less common in men, thrush can cause itching, burning and/or redness at the tip of the penis or under the foreskin. A burning sensation is felt on urinating. A penile discharge is best referred to exclude an STI. In men, candidal infection of the penis may be noticed after sexual intercourse.

## Management options

Vaginal candidiasis may be managed with either topical or oral azoles. Other suspected bacterial or protozoal infections require referral.

The decision to treat vaginal candidiasis rests on whether the woman has had the symptoms diagnosed before and whether it is a recurrent problem. If this is the first time the symptoms have appeared, or if the woman has had more than two recurrences in the previous 6 months, she should be referred. This is because in the first instance it is crucial that diagnoses such as bacterial vaginosis, which can cause serious complications, are excluded. Recurrent cases of candidiasis may suggest an underlying condition such as diabetes causing relapses and re-infection, or the presence of a more resistant species of *Candida*, which is resistant to short-term azole treatment.

Non-drug remedies have been advocated, such as the local application of yogurt; the lactobacilli produce lactic acid which inhibits the growth of *Candida*. Acidifying agents, such as dilute vinegar, are also sometimes used to restore the normal slightly acidic pH but non-drug remedies should be discouraged for a few days before and after the use of topical imidazoles, as the latter are less effective in an acid environment.

Over-the-counter products that are advertised for the treatment of 'embarrassing itching' and that contain local anaesthetic agents, such as benzocaine, can sensitise perianal and perivulval skin, thereby aggravating rather than relieving the condition. Women should be advised of other measures that can be taken to reduce symptoms. These include avoiding perfumed products, such as soaps and bubble baths, which may exacerbate the skin irritation. Hot baths can cause irritation, as can wearing synthetic underwear, tights and tight-fitting trousers. After defecation the anus should be wiped from front to back to prevent the transfer of infection from the bowel to the vagina.

Women taking oral contraceptives who are having recurrent candidal infections may benefit from switching to a low-dose oestrogen pill or an injectable progestogen. If the woman is pregnant, referral is necessary as although topical treatments are safe and effective, they are not licensed as a P medicine for use in pregnancy. Anyone who is immunocompromised, for example by receiving immunosuppressive drugs or having HIV infection, should be referred. Referral should also be made if the woman, or her partner, has a known history of STIs so that both can be treated and relapses prevented.

Any individual with symptoms lasting more than 7 days despite treatment should be referred. This is because the differential diagnosis can be difficult, and conditions such as STIs, bacterial infection, trichomoniasis, genital herpes and warts may present with similar (although often more severe) soreness, inflammation and oedema.

### Preparations for vaginal and vulval candidiasis (BNF section 7.2)

The most effective treatment for vulvovaginal candidiasis is one of the azole preparations. The choice is between a single-dose oral preparation (such as fluconazole) and topical preparations in the form of creams or pessaries (imidazoles such as clotrimazole). These are only recommended for use as a P medicine for uncomplicated candidiasis in women who have previously suffered from, and are able to recognise, the condition. A single-dose treatment, either orally or intravaginally may be preferable for some people. An intravaginal preparation or oral dose is necessary to treat the infection, which lies high in the vagina. Oral and intravaginal imidazoles are equally effective, so individual preference will determine the most suitable option.

Imidazole creams may be applied night and morning and can give symptomatic relief where there is extensive vulval or labial irritation. If seepage occurs from daytime use of the cream, usage can be restricted to a bedtime dose when the woman is lying flat.

Male sexual partners may be asymptomatic carriers of *Candida*, but treating them with antifungal creams is not recommended. However, symptomatic men can be treated with a single dose of oral fluconazole and an imidazole cream.

Azoles are inhibitors of the hepatic microsomal metabolism of some drugs. Caution is therefore advised in people taking warfarin, and it is suggested that the prothrombin ratio (INR, measured routinely in people taking warfarin) be checked within or at the end of a 7-day treatment period. In theory, the arrhythmogenic potential of the antihistamines known to cause arrhythmias, i.e. terfenadine and astemizole, might be enhanced by both oral and topical imidazoles. Blood concentrations of theophylline, ciclosporin, rifampicin and oral sulphonylureas may be increased by the imidazoles. Except for ciclosporin, these latter interactions are unlikely to be of any clinical significance.

Antifungals as non-prescription medicines are not licensed for use in vaginal candidiasis in girls under the age of 16 years or in women over the age of 60.

### Vaginal moisturisers (BNF section 7.2)

Menopausal women who are experiencing symptoms of vaginal atrophy may be referred for consideration whether local application of oestrogen may be helpful. Non-hormonal, acidic vaginal moisturisers are also available and may provide some relief of symptoms by rehydrating the vaginal epithelium and returning the pH to the premenopausal range.

 **Re-consider the case**

Before reading further, re-consider the following questions and your initial thoughts on this case.

**Trigger questions**

- What additional information would you need before considering the appropriate management options in this case?
- What issues concern you about this case?
- Are any alarm symptoms being exhibited that require more urgent treatment or referral?

**Case study**

One busy afternoon a 32-year-old woman comes into the pharmacy with her two young children to buy nappies and baby milk. Once she has paid for her shopping, she says quietly 'Would it be possible to have a quick word with the pharmacist?' She explains, rather embarrassedly, that she has a vaginal discharge and some itching around the area. The discharge is white and she is not aware of any smell. She had similar symptoms when she was expecting her first child but cannot remember what her doctor prescribed at the time.

Pharmacist opinion

It would be important to deal with this patient's request sensitively owing to her obvious embarrassment by taking her to one side, preferably into a consulting room. Her symptoms indicate vaginal thrush and, since she has had a previous episode diagnosed by her doctor, she meets the product licence criteria to be treated with a P medicine. After questioning to rule out any other cause of vaginal discharge, she may be offered an antifungal, either oral fluconazole or intravaginal clotrimazole depending on which route of administration she prefers. The only caution in this case is that she last had thrush while pregnant, so if, after careful questioning, there is a possibility that she may be pregnant again, she should be referred to her doctor as thrush in pregnancy is outside the product licence as a P medicine. There is no need to treat her partner unless he is experiencing symptoms. Although it appears the woman is in a stable relationship it is important not to make assumptions and it may be worth sensitively checking that she has not had a change of partner recently, to rule out the possibility of an STI. She should consult her doctor if she does not respond to treatment within 7 days, if her symptoms get worse, or if there is a recurrence.

 General practitioner opinion

It sounds like this woman has vaginal thrush, particularly if she has had successful treatment for the same symptoms in the past. Candidiasis is more prevalent in pregnancy; it might be worth suggesting a pregnancy test in this case. Other predisposing factors are diabetes mellitus, treatment with broad-spectrum antibiotics, chemotherapy, and vaginal foreign body, e.g. retained tampon.

Treatment may be topical or oral depending on individual preference, e.g. clotrimazole or fluconazole. If the vulva is particularly inflamed and swollen it may be more appropriate to use the oral route to avoid any further discomfort. General advice would include wearing loose fitting underwear, avoiding topical irritants, and good hygiene.

Occasionally recurrent symptoms occur; confirmation of the infection with swabs should be done and any predisposing factors should be identified. Longer courses of treatment may be required or cyclical courses.

Advice on preventive measures should be given.

 Summary of key points

| Condition | Management |
| --- | --- |
| Vaginal candidiasis (thrush) is characterised by vulvovaginitis with thick and white or creamy, curd-like, odourless discharge. | Oral or intravaginal azoles. Topical imidazole creams for external irritation. Avoidance of triggers such as perfumed products, synthetic underwear, tight-fitting clothing. Advice on avoiding re-infection. No need to treat the sexual partner unless they are symptomatic. |
| Bacterial vaginosis is characterised by vulvovaginitis with thin, white, smelly discharge. | Refer. |
| Trichomoniasis is characterised by vulvovaginitis with smelly profuse and frothy, white, yellow or green discharge. | Refer. |

**When to refer**

- First occurrence
- Discharge with a strong smell
- Bloodstained discharge
- Dyspareunia
- Suspected STI
- Diabetes
- Pregnant women
- Women under 16 and over 60 years
- Recurrence more than twice in last 6 months
- If symptoms do not improve after 7 days or where symptoms get worse

# Menstrual disorders (dysmenorrhoea, menorrhagia and premenstrual syndrome)

Before reading further, consider the following case and note your initial thoughts.

**Case study**

A 22-year-old woman asks for something to manage her period pain. She experiences a cramping pain in her abdomen just before her periods start each month. The first day of bleeding is pretty sore and then the pain usually eases off on the second day. She normally takes paracetamol, and when she was a student she 'curled up with a hot water bottle' all day when the pain was bad. She usually feels pretty 'low and irritable' for the few days leading up to her periods. Since graduating last month, she has started a new job and really cannot take time off each month for period pain.

**Trigger questions**

- What additional information would you need before considering the appropriate management options in this case?
- What issues concern you about this case?
- Are any alarm symptoms being exhibited that require more urgent treatment or referral?

## Assessing symptoms

### Dysmenorrhoea

Dysmenorrhoea or period pain is painful cramping in the lower abdomen or pelvic area, sometimes radiating to the back or thighs. It occurs shortly before or during menstruation, or both. Dysmenorrhoea is the most common gynaecological symptom reported by women and affects between 40% and 70% of menstruating women, compromising daily activity in 10% of women. It is caused by increased myometrial activity induced by an excessive production of prostaglandin.

In deciding whether to manage dysmenorrhoea in the pharmacy, it is important to distinguish between primary (absence of any identifiable underlying pelvic pathology) and secondary dysmenorrhoea (underlying pelvic pathology), and careful questioning about onset, duration, type and severity of pain along with associated symptoms can help differentiate between them. It is important to establish whether the onset of pain relates to the menstrual cycle; mid-cycle pain may be caused by an ovulation syndrome, whereas pain around the time of menstruation is likely to be due to dysmenorrhoea or some secondary underlying cause such as endometriosis.

Table 6.2 summarises the key features that help to differentiate between primary dysmenorrhoea, which can be managed using remedies available as non-prescription medicines and secondary dysmenorrhoea, which should be referred.

### Premenstrual syndrome

Premenstrual syndrome (PMS) is a group of symptoms that occur in women during the luteal phase of the menstrual cycle. Mild physiological symptoms occur in up to 80% of women of reproductive age, with 40% experiencing moderate symptoms that disrupt their daily lives and around 5% experiencing severe debilitating symptoms. Symptoms of PMS include fatigue, irritability and low mood, bloating, weight gain, breast pain and tenderness (mastalgia), headache and abdominal pain. In 2011, the International Society for Premenstrual

Disorders (ISPMD) published a classification for diagnosis of premenstrual disorder (Box 6.3) to aid clinicians in effective diagnosis and management of this condition.

---

**Box 6.3　Criteria for diagnosing premenstrual disorder (ISPMD classification) (O'Brien _et al._ 2011)**

- It is precipitated by ovulation.
- Symptoms are not defined, although typical symptoms exist.
- Any number of symptoms can be present.
- Physical and psychological symptoms are important.
- Symptoms recur in the luteal phase.
- Symptoms disappear by the end of menstruation.
- A symptom-free week occurs between menstruation and ovulation.
- Symptoms must be prospectively rated.
- Symptoms are not an exacerbation of an underlying psychological or physical disorder.
- Symptoms cause substantial impairment.

---

**Table 6.2　Features that help to differentiate between primary and secondary dysmenorrhoea**

| Primary dysmenorrhoea | Secondary dysmenorrhoea |
|---|---|
| Most common between the ages of 16 and 25 years | More commonly occurs in older women, aged 30–45 years |
| Starts at or shortly after (6–12 months) menstrual periods start | Tends to occur several years after menstrual periods start |
| Pain is usually described as cramping or spasmodic | Pain may be described as cramping but more usually as dull and continuous |
| Pain typically begins within 24 hours of onset of menstruation and persists for 8–72 hours | Pain may occur throughout or last for the whole of the menstrual cycle |
| Periods are usually normal or light | Periods are often heavy |
| Other gynaecological symptoms are not usually present | Other gynaecological symptoms are often present (e.g. dyspareunia, vaginal discharge, menorrhagia, intermenstrual bleeding, postcoital bleeding). The specific symptoms will be determined by the underlying pathology |
| Response to NSAIDs or COCs is usually good | There may be little or no response to NSAIDs or COCs |
| Pelvic examination is normal | Pelvic examination may be abnormal (but absence of abnormal findings does not exclude secondary dysmenorrhoea) |

## Accompanying symptoms

Primary dysmenorrhoea is often accompanied by fatigue, irritability, dizziness, headache, lower backache, and gastrointestinal symptoms such as diarrhoea or nausea and vomiting.

### Menorrhagia

Menorrhagia is described as excessive and prolonged uterine bleeding that occurs at the regular menstrual intervals. In around one-third of cases menorrhagia occurs as a result of underlying gynaecological pathology such as endometriosis, fibroids, endometrial cancer or ovarian tumours. It may also be associated with an intrauterine contraceptive device (IUD). In the majority of cases, however, no known cause can be identified and this is known as dysfunctional uterine bleeding. What is considered normal menstrual flow varies widely between women. As a guide, menstrual loss requiring pad or tampon changes every 1–2 hours with anything longer resulting in 'accidents' is considered to be excessive, especially if the periods last longer than 8 days. Women may also describe it as impacting on their physical, social or emotional quality of life, for example by preventing daily activities.

### Anaemia

Blood loss due to menorrhagia is the most common cause of iron deficiency in premenopausal women. If anaemia is suspected or if the woman is experiencing prolonged menorrhagia, it is worth referring to her doctor for a full blood count to be carried out.

### Gastrointestinal symptoms

Many women experience changes in bowel habit around the time of their menstrual period. One-third of otherwise asymptomatic women may experience gastrointestinal (GI) symptoms and women who have existing GI disorders can also experience exacerbations at the time of menstruation. The physiological basis of this is not known but appears to be related to the raised serum levels of progesterone and the resultant effects on the gut during the luteal phase of the menstrual cycle. In some cases it can also be related to pathology such as endometriosis. Careful history taking can help determine whether the GI symptoms are related to the menstrual cycle.

## Management options

Management of menstrual disorders focuses on relief of the symptoms the woman presents with. Primary dysmenorrhoea can be managed with analgesics and NSAIDs; menorrhagia with antifibrinolytics; and PMS with a variety of dietary and herbal supplements. If a woman is experiencing GI symptoms associated with menstruation, these should be managed according to Chapter 2 and any anaemia associated with menorrhagia should be managed according to Chapter 8.

Many women find heat can be helpful in reducing period pain. Hot-water bottles, heat patches and hot baths can be used. Application of topical heat has been found to be as effective as ibuprofen in reducing pain. Gentle exercise has been suggested as a non-medical approach to the management of the symptoms of dysmenorrhoea and, although not supported by strong evidence, exercise may reduce some symptoms during the menstrual phase. Drinking herbal teas such as peppermint or chamomile may also help as they are thought to have some antispasmodic action.

Dysmenorrhoea is more common and more severe in smokers, but it is not known whether stopping smoking improves symptoms. However, smoking cessation is associated with many other health benefits (see Chapter 4 for further information).

If dysmenorrhoea or menorrhagia is associated with use of an IUD, switching to a progesterone-releasing intrauterine system (IUS) may help.

### Analgesics (BNF section 4.7)

Simple analgesics such as paracetamol, either alone or in combination with an opioid analgesic, may be useful in managing the pain of dysmenorrhoea, especially if NSAIDs are contraindicated. Analgesic use, cautions and advice are covered in Chapter 4.

### Non-steroidal anti-inflammatory drugs (NSAIDs) (BNF section 10.1)

NSAID use, contraindications and advice are covered in depth in Chapter 4. In primary dysmenorrhoea, NSAIDs are likely to be effective due to inhibition of prostaglandin synthesis and the resultant reduction in uterine prostaglandin and therefore in uterine contractility. Ibuprofen is commonly used in period pain but needs to be taken at maximal licensed dose as a P medicine for best effect. Naproxen is licensed as a P medicine for treatment of primary dysmenorrhoea in women aged 15 to 50 years. Treatment with NSAIDs is most effective if started 1–2 days before the periods begin. NSAIDs have also been shown to reduce blood loss by 20–50% and are useful in women with menorrhagia associated with dysmenorrhoea. Prostaglandin levels are known to be increased in women with menorrhagia and therefore NSAIDs are a logical treatment choice; however, none of the NSAIDs available as non-prescription medicines are licensed for menorrhagia.

## Antispasmodics (BNF section 1.2)

Hyoscine butylbromide is licensed for relief of spasm of the genitourinary tract and alverine citrate is licensed for dysmenorrhoea. Both drugs act by relaxing smooth muscle and, although there is a lack of published evidence on their efficacy for this indication, some women may find them helpful, especially if NSAIDs are contraindicated.

## Combined oral contraceptives (BNF section 7.3)

Although only available as a prescription-only medicine (POM), combined oral contraceptives (COCs) are a commonly used second-line treatment for primary dysmenorrhoea. Pain is lessened directly by inhibiting endometrial growth and indirectly by inhibiting ovulation and subsequent progesterone production. If management using a P medicine has failed then it is worth referring the woman to her doctor for assessment of suitability for the COC. Dysmenorrhoea that does not respond to COC is more likely to be secondary in origin.

## Tranexamic acid (BNF section 2.11)

Tranexamic acid is an antifibrinolytic drug that is licensed as a P medicine for reduction of heavy menstrual bleeding over several cycles in women over 18 years of age with regular, 21- to 35-day cycles with no more than 3 days individual variability in cycle duration. It has been shown to reduce menstrual loss by up to 58%. Tranexamic acid can be used as long as periods remain regular and heavy, but referral to a doctor is necessary if menstrual bleeding is not reduced after three menstrual cycles. Contraindications and cautions for the use of tranexamic acid as a P medicine are listed in Table 6.3. Gastrointestinal adverse effects such as nausea, vomiting and diarrhoea are common with

**Table 6.3** Contraindications and cautions for use of tranexamic acid as a P medicine

| Contraindications | Cautions |
|---|---|
| Mild to moderate renal insufficiency (because of the higher risk of blood clots) | A doctor should be consulted if menstrual bleeding is not reduced after three menstrual cycles. |
| Hypersensitivity to tranexamic acid or any of the excipients | Women over the age of 45 years should consult their doctor before taking. |
| Active thromboembolic disease | People who are obese and diabetic should consult their doctor before taking (because of the higher risk of endometrial cancer and thromboembolic disease) |
| A previous thromboembolic event and a family history of thrombophilia | Those with polycystic ovary syndrome or a history of endometrial cancer in a first-degree relative should consult their doctor before taking. |
| Haematuria | Women receiving unopposed oestrogen should consult their doctor as they should not be having menstrual periods. |
| Irregular menstrual bleeding | Women taking tamoxifen should consult their doctor before taking (because of the increased risk of endometrial cancer). |
| Taking warfarin or other anticoagulants | Treatment should be withdrawn from anyone who experiences visual disturbance. |
| Taking oral contraceptives | |
| Pregnancy and breastfeeding | |

antifibrinolytics but can be minimised by limiting treatment to the first 3 days of menstruation or by reducing the dose.

### Dietary supplements and herbal remedies

A number of dietary supplements and herbal remedies are advocated for relief of the symptoms of PMS, but rigorous evidence of benefit is only available for a few of these. Calcium supplementation at a dose of 1000–1200 mg/day appears to substantially decrease the symptoms of PMS. Plasma calcium levels in premenstrual women have been shown to be lower than in the week following menstruation and this appears to explain why calcium may be of benefit. Vitamin $B_6$ (pyridoxine) is a co-factor in the synthesis of neurotransmitters, so would appear to have a possible role in alleviating PMS symptoms. Vitamin $B_6$ may be effective in the management of the psychological symptoms of PMS, but the evidence is of low quality and there is the potential for adverse effects such as neuropathy, at high doses (>200 mg/day).

Research into the efficacy of magnesium and evening primrose oil for PMS has produced conflicting results and *Vitex agnus castus*, ginkgo biloba and St John's Wort, although commonly marketed for PMS, do not appear to be supported by strong evidence. Many women continue to use supplements and herbal remedies for PMS despite a lack of established efficacy, possibly because of the lack of availability of conventional therapies for this condition.

If PMS is having a significant impact on quality of life, especially if psychological symptoms are severe, the women should be referred for medical assessment. Selective serotonin reuptake inhibitors (SSRIs) have been found to be of benefit in these situations.

A systematic review of the efficacy and safety of herbal and dietary therapies for dysmenorrhoea showed some evidence of effectiveness for magnesium (over placebo) with the need for additional medication being less. Other therapies such as vitamins $B_6$, $B_1$ and E, and omega-3 fatty acids were either ineffective or not supported by strong evidence.

### Re-consider the case

Before reading further, re-consider the following questions and your initial thoughts on this case.

**Trigger questions**

- What additional information would you need before considering the appropriate management options in this case?
- What issues concern you about this case?
- Are any alarm symptoms being exhibited that require more urgent treatment or referral?

**Case study**

A 22-year-old woman asks for something to manage her period pain. She experiences a cramping pain in her abdomen just before her periods start each month. The first day of bleeding is pretty sore and then the pain usually eases off on the second day. She normally takes paracetamol, and when she was a student she 'curled up with a hot water bottle' all day when the pain was bad. She usually feels pretty 'low and irritable' for the few days leading up to her periods. Since graduating last month, she has started a new job and really cannot take time off each month for period pain.

### Pharmacist opinion

The onset and character of symptoms, along with this woman's age, would indicate primary dysmenorrhoea. Providing she has no contraindications to taking NSAIDs, the best choice of management would

### Pharmacist opinion (*continued*)

be ibuprofen or possibly naproxen. She should be advised to take it with food and if possible, if she has a regular cycle, to start taking it a couple of days before her periods are due. She could also be encouraged to continue to use her hot-water bottle when she returns home from work and she may wish to consider heat patches during the day. If she wants to take something for the PMS symptoms of being 'low and irritable', she could be advised of the existence of complementary therapy options, but also that there is little evidence of benefit except with calcium. If the NSAID does not help, she should make an appointment with her GP. Even if the NSAIDs are effective, she may wish to consider discussing the combined oral contraceptive with her GP or family planning clinic.

### General practitioner opinion

In a woman with history of dysmenorrhoea it would be prudent to check for other symptoms of sexually transmitted infections also. Does she have intermenstrual bleeding, postcoital bleeding, discharge or dyspareunia? Is she using any hormonal methods of contraception? Is she indeed currently sexually active?

Painful periods often coexist with heavy periods; although it is not described here, further questioning may reveal that menorrhagia is also a problem. She also describes symptoms of psychological aspects of premenstrual syndrome. She will probably recognise these as such and may be able to cope, understanding that they are related to her menstrual cycle. Some women with underlying psychological disorders may find that their symptoms become difficult to manage just before a period, or indeed present to their doctor at that time.

There are several treatment options here and the choice warrants discussion. Dysmenorrhoea alone can be treated successfully with non-steroidal anti-inflammatories, taken a few days before a period and stopped after the first 2–3 days of bleeding. Mefenamic acid and naproxen seem to be the preferred choice. Use of the combined oral contraceptive pill is also effective in reducing pain, heavy bleeding and sometimes premenstrual symptoms. It can also be used to reduce the number of periods in a year by running three packs of pills together without a break. In a woman who needs contraception this would seem a sensible option providing there are no contraindications. Even in those who do not need contraception, it would be a reasonable option that many women would choose.

It is worth remembering that endometriosis can present with dysmenorrhoea; the treatment would be to control pain as described above. However, endometriosis can lead to fertility problems in the future, so if this woman is trying to conceive she may need further investigation.

### Summary of key points

| Condition | Management |
|---|---|
| Primary dysmenorrhoea is characterised by cramping, spasmodic pain in the lower abdomen starting within 24 hours of menstruation and persisting for 8–72 hours and is more common in younger women. | NSAIDs can be used as first line, or simple analgesics if NSAIDs are contraindicated. Antispasmodics may be helpful in some people. Topical heat application may provide relief. Referral for COC if OTC treatment is ineffective. |

## Summary of key points (*continued*)

| Condition | Management |
| --- | --- |
| Secondary dysmenorrhoea is characterised by dull continuous pain in the lower abdomen, occurring throughout the menstrual cycle, may be associated with heavy periods and is more common in older women. | Refer for medical assessment of underlying pathology. |
| Menorrhagia is characterised by excessive and prolonged uterine bleeding which occurs at the regular menstrual intervals. | Tranexamic acid if individual meets eligibility criteria or referral for medical assessment. |
| Premenstrual syndrome (PMS) is characterised by fatigue, irritability and low mood, bloating, weight gain, mastalgia, headache and abdominal pain prior to the menstrual period. | Complementary therapies such as calcium or vitamin B6 may be considered, or referral if symptoms are having a significant impact on quality of life. |

## When to refer

- Primary dysmenorrhoea that fails to respond to treatment with non-prescription medicines
- Suspected secondary dysmenorrhoea
- Severe PMS that is impacting on QOL
- Menorrhagia suspected to be due to secondary causes or in women for whom OTC treatment is contraindicated
- Menorrhagia that does not respond to OTC treatment after three menstrual cycles
- Anaemia due to prolonged menstrual bleeding

# Emergency hormonal contraception

Before reading further, consider the following case and note your initial thoughts.

## Case study

A 26-year-old woman asks for a private consultation with the pharmacist and, when comfortably seated in the consultation room, asks for the 'morning-after pill'. She and her partner had an 'incident' with a burst condom last night and she explains that it is really important for her not to get pregnant at the moment as she will be sitting her professional accountancy examinations in the next 12 months.

### Trigger questions

- What additional information would you need before considering the appropriate management options in this case?
- What issues concern you about this case?
- What health promotion issues affect this case?

## Assessing suitability for supply

A number of questions are necessary before a decision can be made about the appropriateness of emergency hormonal contraception (EHC). These can be asked by the pharmacist or, if the woman prefers, a questionnaire can be completed prior to the consultation to relieve any initial embarrassment on her part.

*Age of the woman.* Is the woman 16 years of age or older? Some Patient Group Directions may allow the supply of EHC to a woman under the age of 16; however, the licence for supply as a P medicine requires women to be over 16.

*Who is requesting supply?* Is the EHC for the woman who is requesting it? EHC should only be supplied to a third party in exceptional circumstances to ensure that the pharmacist can make an assessment of appropriateness of supply.

*How long ago was the unprotected sex?* Within the last 72 hours? The product licence for EHC requires it to be used within 72 hours of unprotected sex. EHC is most effective (85–95%) when taken within 24 hours, with effectiveness decreasing to 58% at 72 hours. If a woman presents after 72 hours, she should be referred to her GP or family planning clinic as an intrauterine device may be fitted within 5 days of unprotected sex or ulipristal (a progesterone receptor modulator), which is effective if taken within 5 days of unprotected sex, may be prescribed.

*Has she had unprotected sex previously in this cycle?* This is to determine whether there is a possibility of the woman already being pregnant. Although EHC will not harm a woman who is in the early stages of pregnancy, it will not be effective at this stage and pregnancy is a contraindication. The manufacturer of levonorgestrel states that use more than once in the cycle is not advisable because of the possibility of disturbance of the cycle, although its use is not contraindicated. In such cases women may be directed to seek advice about contraception from a family planning clinic or GP, and told that EHC can disrupt the cycle and cause intermenstrual bleeding or 'spotting', which may lead to confusion about the timing of the last menstrual bleed.

*When was her last menstrual period and was it normal?* Again this is to determine whether the woman may already be pregnant. Some women bleed slightly during the early stages of pregnancy around the time the period is due, so if her last period was much lighter than normal it may be worth carrying out a pregnancy test before taking EHC.

*Is she taking other medicines or herbal remedies?* Various drugs will interact with levonorgestrel, and these are indicated in Table 6.4. If a woman is taking a hepatic enzyme-inducing drug, she should be referred to her doctor as she can be prescribed an unlicensed dose of 3 mg levonorgestrel.

Further questions should be asked to ascertain whether levonorgestrel may be inappropriate. If the answer to any of the following questions is positive, the woman should be referred to a GP or family planning clinic.

- Does the woman have any known allergy to levonorgestrel? Some contraceptive pills contain levonorgestrel, and previous intolerance should be inquired about.

**Table 6.4   Drug interactions with EHC (levonorgestrel)**

| Interacting drug class | Examples | Consequence |
|---|---|---|
| Antibacterials | Rifabutin, rifampicin | These drugs increase the metabolism of levonorgestrel and may reduce its efficacy. Referral is necessary for consideration of an increased (unlicensed) dose or insertion of an IUD. Rifampicin and rifabutin are such potent enzyme-inducing drugs that an alternative method is always recommended. |
| Anticonvulsants | Barbiturates (e.g. phenobarbital, primodone), carbamazepine, phenytoin, topiramate) | |
| Antifungals | Griseofulvin | |
| Antivirals | Protease inhibitors (e.g. nelfinavir, ritonavir), nevirapine | |
| Other drugs | Aprepitant, modafinil, St John's Wort (Hypericum perforatum), troglitazone | |
| | Ciclosporin | Levonorgestrel inhibits the metabolism of ciclosporin and increases the risk of ciclosporin toxicity and therefore referral to a general practitioner is necessary. |

- Is there any small-bowel disease (including Crohn disease) or any liver problems? Such conditions may interfere with the absorption or metabolism of the pill.
- Are there any problems that may affect absorption of the pill, such as vomiting or severe diarrhoea?

## Management options

Emergency hormonal contraception is relatively expensive to purchase as a P medicine in the UK. However, many women do obtain it in this way. Some pharmacists participate in a scheme by which the pill is provided under a Patient Group Direction (PGD) protocol, whereby the drug is supplied on the NHS. Ideally, a supply of EHC should be accompanied by counselling regarding STIs and other methods of contraception.

Sexually active young people under the age of 25 years are at particular risk of STIs, especially if they have a new sexual partner or have had two or more sexual partners in the last year. Chlamydia is largely asymptomatic in around 70% of women and 50% of men; therefore, referral for appropriate testing is advised if unprotected sex has occurred.

A pharmacy service has the advantage that no appointments are necessary, and in many circumstances pharmacists are available on Sundays and in the evenings (extended hours) when GPs are not normally available. Not all out-of-hours services carry supplies of EHC. In addition, Monday mornings appear to be the time when women will frequently require advice and/or EHC, and this may be easier to obtain in a community pharmacy, without appointment and without taking time off work, than obtaining an appointment with the general practitioner.

Advance provision of EHC, prior to unprotected sexual intercourse occurring, is an area that has been heavily debated. Concerns have been expressed that it may negatively impact on sexual and reproductive health behaviours, undermining the use of more reliable contraceptive methods and leading to increased promiscuity and pregnancy rates. A Cochrane systematic review examined whether advance provision of EHC reduces conception rates and concluded that it does not reduce pregnancy rates when compared with conventional provision, but neither does it impact negatively on sexual and reproductive health behaviours and outcomes. A number of organisations (the Faculty of Family Planning and Reproductive Health Care, the Family Planning Association (FPA) and the World Health Organization) support the advance provision of levonorgestrel to women to increase early use when required. The Royal Pharmaceutical Society has advised that pharmacists may provide an advance supply of levonorgestrel EHC to an individual after assessing whether the EHC is clinically appropriate for that individual and that they are competent and intend to use it appropriately.

### Levonorgestrel (BNF section 7.3.5)

Levonorgestrel, when taken in a large dose in EHC, is believed to act by preventing ovulation or fertilisation in the follicular stage and preventing implantation in the luteal phase of the menstrual cycle. In the normal menstrual cycle the follicular phase is variable in length but usually lasts for the first 14–15 days. If the cycle is longer or shorter than the average 28 days then it is usually the follicular phase that changes. During this phase a number of follicles grow in the ovary and the most mature will produce an ovum capable of being fertilised. The luteal phase has a fairly constant length of 12–16 days and is the second phase of the cycle, beginning after ovulation has taken place. The follicle that releases the ovum is transformed into the corpus luteum and produces progesterone. There is no effect on established pregnancy or on a fetus.

Approximately 85–95% of expected pregnancies can be prevented by a morning-after pill containing a single dose of levonorgestrel 1500 mg when taken within 24 hours of unprotected sex. Between 24 and 48 hours it is expected to be 85% effective, and between 48 and 72 hours the efficacy is about 58%.

The woman should be advised to take the tablet as soon as possible and counselled on adverse effects that she may experience. The adverse effects of levonorgestrel are listed in Box 6.4. The most common adverse effect is nausea and if the woman should vomit within 2 hours of taking the table she should be advised to return to the pharmacy, as she may need to repeat the dose.

### Box 6.4 Adverse drug reactions to EHC

- Nausea
- Vomiting
- Abdominal pain
- Headache
- Breast tenderness
- Irregular menstrual bleeding (bleeding may be earlier or later than usual, and lighter or heavier)
- Spotting (mild, intermittent bleeding during cycle)

## *Advice for missed oral contraceptive pills*

Emergency hormonal contraception can be used in some circumstances when a woman has missed a contraceptive pill. The following guide can be used to determine whether EHC will be necessary or effective.

**Combined oral contraceptives**

EHC is recommended if two or more combined oral contraceptive tablets are missed from the first seven tablets in a packet and unprotected intercourse has occurred since finishing the last packet.

**Progesterone-only contraceptives**

EHC is recommended if one or more progestogen-only contraceptive tablets are missed or taken more than 3 hours late (12 hours if desogestrel) and unprotected intercourse has occurred before two further tablets have been correctly taken. For further guidance on missed pills, including forgotten contraceptive patch, see *British National Formulary* section 7.3.

### Re-consider the case

Before reading further, re-consider the following questions and your initial thoughts on this case.

**Trigger questions**

- What additional information would you need before considering the appropriate management options in this case?
- What issues concern you about this case?
- What health promotion issues affect this case?

**Case study**

A 26-year-old woman asks for a private consultation with the pharmacist and, when comfortably seated in the consultation room, asks for the 'morning-after pill'. She and her partner had an 'incident' with a burst condom last night and she explains that it is really important for her not to get pregnant at the moment as she will be sitting her professional accountancy examinations in the next 12 months.

### Pharmacist opinion

It is appropriate to consider EHC in this situation as the woman is presenting within 72 hours of unprotected sex. It is important to determine whether EHC is appropriate and necessary in this case. Depending where she is in her menstrual cycle, the risk of pregnancy may be low. This needs to be discussed with her but it sounds like she would still want to take EHC 'just to be sure'. The standard questions would be used to check whether she has any contraindications to taking EHC or any conditions that would affect absorption. It is often worth explaining why these questions are being asked and trying to ask them in an interactive way to make the woman more at ease in what may be an already uncomfortable situation. Once the decision has been made to supply EHC, there may be the option of

**Pharmacist opinion** (*continued*)

different routes of supply. If a PGD exists in the area and she meets the inclusion criteria, she may wish to obtain EHC on the NHS, otherwise sale as a P medicine can be made. Before completing the supply, it would be important to sensitively ascertain whether there is any risk of STIs (e.g. does she have a new partner?) and also to advise on where to obtain advice on more reliable methods of contraception than condoms since she is so concerned that she does not conceive at present.

**General practitioner opinion**

There should be two agendas in this situation. The first is to confirm or otherwise that the 'morning-after pill' is appropriate and the second is to discuss options for more reliable forms of contraception. Screening for STIs may also be appropriate.

It is crucial to identify the timing of this 'incident' in relation to her menstrual cycle and whether there have been any other episodes of burst condoms or unprotected sex since her last period. The answers to these questions will have a bearing on whether postcoital contraception is appropriate. She must also be made aware that a postcoital IUD is also an option and can be fitted up to 5 days after the incident.

Hormonal postcoital contraception is more effective when taken soon after the episode of unprotected sex. It can be taken up to 72 hours later but will have a lower efficacy the later it is taken. The woman's period may be earlier or later than expected, but if it has not occurred within 2 weeks, she should take a pregnancy test.

Although the use of condoms is the best way of protecting against STIs, it is variable in its effectiveness as an option for contraception. It would be appropriate then to discuss other options for contraception to be used alongside.

Are there reasons why she is not using any other form of contraception? Are there other health issues? This may be a good opportunity to educate.

**Summary of key points**

| Condition | Management |
|---|---|
| Request for emergency hormonal contraception. | Supply EHC if appropriate, i.e. less than 72 hours since unprotected sex and no contraindications for supply. Advice on ongoing contraception. Assessment for risk of STIs and appropriate referral if necessary. |

**When to refer**

- Unprotected sex more than 72 hours ago
- Under the age of 16 (unless there is a PGD in place that covers it)
- Taking drugs that interact with levonorgestrel
- Absorption difficulties
- Allergy to levonorgestrel

# Pregnancy testing and preconception care

Before reading further, consider the following case and note your initial thoughts.

 **Case study**

A young woman asks for advice on ovulation testing and also the best and most accurate home pregnancy test to use.

**Trigger questions**

- What additional information would you need before considering the appropriate management options in this case?
- What issues concern you about this case?
- What health promotion issues affect this case?

## Management options

The length of time that it takes to conceive is different for everyone and if a couple are having difficulty in getting pregnant then they should be referred to their GP for support. For couples planning a pregnancy there is an opportunity to offer advice on preconception care.

### Ovulation tests

Ovulation and pregnancy tests work on similar principles by detecting hormone levels in the woman's urine. In the case of ovulation tests, the luteinising hormone (LH) surge that occurs 24–36 hours prior to ovulation (see Figure 6.1) is detected. The LH surge triggers ovulation and the women is most fertile for 24–36 hours following the surge. Since ovulation occurs around half way through the menstrual cycle, manufacturers of ovulation tests provide tables of when women should start conducting daily urine tests based on the length of their normal cycle. Manufacturers claim 99% accuracy in detecting the LH surge and predicting ovulation.

It is often suggested that the test be carried out first thing in the morning because urine levels of hormone are highest when urine has been in the bladder for more than 4 hours. Most tests can now be conducted at any time of day, although their sensitivity may be reduced if the woman has emptied her bladder recently.

### Pregnancy tests

Pregnancy tests detect levels of human chorionic gonadotrophin (hCG), which is produced by the developing placenta following implantation of a fertilised egg. hCG is initially produced by the embryo, which becomes implanted around 6 days after conception and then by the placenta once it starts to develop. It reaches detectable levels in a woman's urine around 10–14 days after conception, which is when the woman would normally start her period.

Modern home pregnancy tests are highly sensitive and manufacturers claim over 99% accuracy from the date the period is due. False positive results are very rare but if a test is used before a period is due and a negative result is obtained, there is still a chance that a woman may be pregnant but that the level of hCG is still not high enough for the test to detect, and the woman should be advised to repeat the test on the date she expects her period.

One manufacturer produces a test that indicates an estimate of the number of weeks since conception occurred. This will differ from the number of weeks 'pregnant' that a healthcare professional will use as a pregnancy is formally dated from the first day of the last period, which occurs around 2 weeks before conception.

### Folic acid

Women should be advised to take folic acid supplements before and during pregnancy to reduce the risk of neural tube defects such as spina bifida. They should take 400 micrograms of folic acid daily while trying to conceive, and should continue to take it until the 12th week of pregnancy, while the baby's nervous system develops. Women who are at a high risk of conceiving a child with neural tube defect require a higher daily dose of folic acid, which must be prescribed by a doctor.

As well as taking folic acid supplements, women can be advised to consume foods that are high in folate, such as green leafy vegetables and breads and fortified cereals. Chapter 8 also contains information on folic acid.

### Lifestyle and health advice

A balanced, healthy diet is important when trying to conceive and while pregnant. Pregnant women should avoid foods such as soft cheeses, paté, raw and partially cooked eggs or meat because of the risk of *Listeria* and *Salmonella* infection. Vitamin A supplements and liver, which is high in vitamin A, should also be avoided as vitamin A is associated with an increased incidence of birth defects.

Smoking while pregnant can cause an increased risk of miscarriage, early birth, and reduced birth weight. Women who smoke who are planning a pregnancy should be encouraged to stop before they try to conceive. For further information on smoking cessation see Chapter 4.

When trying to conceive it is best to avoid drinking any alcohol. Current advice is that a woman should also avoid drinking alcohol while pregnant or, if choosing to drink, should consume less than one or two units of alcohol once or twice a week to avoid risk to the baby.

Too much caffeine during pregnancy can cause lower than normal birth weight and may also increase the chances of miscarriage. The Food Standards Agency (FSA) recommends a maximum daily intake of 200 mg of caffeine (equivalent to two mugs of coffee) during pregnancy. Care should be taken to avoid medicines containing caffeine.

The woman should be advised to make sure that she is up to date with vaccinations, such as rubella and varicella.

Preconception care focuses mainly on the woman's health, but men also are advised to cut down on the amount of alcohol that they drink and to avoid smoking as both have been shown to decrease the quality of a man's sperm and to reduce the chances of their partner conceiving.

 **Re-consider the case**

Before reading further, re-consider the following questions and your initial thoughts on this case.

**Trigger questions**

- What additional information would you need before considering the appropriate management options in this case?
- What issues concern you about this case?
- What health promotion issues affect this case?

**Case study**

A young woman asks for advice on ovulation testing and also the best and most accurate home pregnancy test to use.

 Pharmacist opinion

This case presents an opportunity not only for answering the woman's specific questions but also for proactively offering health promotion advice on preconception care and a healthy pregnancy. The

Pharmacist opinion (*continued*)

way that ovulation and pregnancy tests work and how to use them can be explained and she can be reassured of the high levels of accuracy and sensitivity of modern home tests. Price may be an important factor when choosing a test. She can be asked whether she wants advice on preconception care and it would be important to check that she is taking folic acid if she is planning a pregnancy. If she or her partner smokes, there is an opportunity to offer smoking cessation support (see Chapter 4). She can be given literature or leaflets to take away if she prefers but it is obviously important not to force information on people if they do not want it. It may also be worth sensitively inquiring whether she and her partner are have difficulty conceiving and referring her to her GP for support if this is the case.

General practitioner opinion

Further information is needed in this case. Has this lady been trying to conceive? Is she concerned about infertility and if so why? Is she aware of the physiological process of the menstrual cycle and when the optimal time for fertilisation would be?

Trying to conceive a child has the potential to carry an enormous amount of emotion and anxiety. The use of ovulation tests, although it can be helpful, can also cause more confusion and worry.

A woman who has a regular cycle would be able to use an ovulation test to confirm that ovulation has taken place. A negative result, however, would only confirm that ovulation has not occurred at that point in time. It may be useful in identifying a time in which to try to conceive, but by the time the ovulation test picks up a surge in luteinising hormone, there will have been at least a couple of days of missed opportunity.

The presumption here is that this woman is planning a pregnancy. In that case, this would be an ideal time to address preconceptual issues. Important issues to cover would be any history of medical problems that may affect ability to conceive or health during pregnancy, e.g. diabetes mellitus, inflammatory bowel disease, asthma, epilepsy, hypertension. Some of these conditions would require specialist input, ideally before conception. Is she on any medication that would be dangerous to an unborn child? Again, specialist input may be needed here. Other less complicated issues would be to advise about preconception use of folic acid, smoking, alcohol intake and dietary advice. Printed information in this situation would be advisable as there is so much to take in because guidelines change so frequently.

Summary of key points

| Condition | Management |
| --- | --- |
| Health promotion advice on health pregnancy | Folic acid.<br>Lifestyle and health advice – smoking, alcohol, diet, vaccinations. |

**When to refer**

- Difficulty in conceiving
- Coexisting medical conditions requiring close monitoring before conception and during pregnancy

## Bibliography

Canning S *et al.* (2006). Dietary supplements and herbal remedies for premenstrual syndrome (PMS): a systematic research review of the evidence for their efficacy. *J Reprod Infant Psychol* 24: (4) 363–378.

Jepson RG, Craig JC (2008). Cranberries for preventing urinary tract infections. *Cochrane Database Syst Rev* Jan 23; (1): CD001321. doi: 10.1002/14651858. CD001321. pub4. Available at http://mrw.interscience. wiley.com/cochrane/clsysrev/articles/CD001321/frame. html (accessed 30 March 2011).

Jepson RG *et al.* (1998). Cranberries for treating urinary tract infections. *Cochrane Database Syst Rev.* (4): CD001322. doi: 10.1002/14651858.CD001322. Available at http:// mrw.interscience.wiley.com/cochrane/clsysrev/articles/ CD001322/frame.html (accessed 30 March 2011).

Killick SR, Irving G (2004). A national study examining the effect of making emergency hormonal contraception available without prescription. *Hum Reprod* 19: 553–557.

Lewington G, Marshall K (2006). Access to emergency hormonal contraception from community pharmacies and family planning clinics. *Br J Clin Pharmacol* 61: 605–608.

Marston C *et al.* (2005). Impact on contraceptive practice of making emergency hormonal contraception available over the counter in Great Britain: repeated cross sectional surveys. *Br Med J* 331(7511): 271–276.

O'Brien S *et al.* (2011). Diagnosis and management of premenstrual disorders. *Br Med J* 342: d2994. 342: d2994. doi: 10.1136/bmj.d2994.

Peacock A *et al.* (2010). Period problems: disorders of menstruation in adolescents. *Arch Dis Child.* doi: 10.1136/ adc.2009.160853. Available at http://adc.bmj.com/ content/early/2010/06/24/adc.2009.160853.short?rss=1 (accessed 30 March 2011).

Polis CB *et al.* (2007). Advance provision of emergency contraception for pregnancy prevention. *Cochrane Database Syst Rev* Apr 18; (2): CD005497. doi: 10.1002/14651858. CD005497. pub2. Available at www.mrw.interscience. wiley.com/cochrane/clsysrev/articles/CD005497/pdf_ abstract_fs.html (accessed 30 March 2011).

Proctor M, Murphy PA (2001). Herbal and dietary therapies for primary and secondary dysmenorrhoea. *Cochrane Database Syst Rev* (3): CD002124. doi: 10.1002/14651858.CD002124. Available at http://www. cochrane.org/reviews/en/ab002124.html (accessed 30 March 2011).

Royal Pharmaceutical Society of Great Britain (2008). *Practice Guidance: Azithromycin.* London: RPSGB. Available at http://www.rpharms.com/support-pdfs/ azithromycinguid.pdf (accessed 30 March 2011).

Royal Pharmaceutical Society of Great Britain (2010). Practice Guidance: Tamsulosin. London: RPSGB. Available at http://www.rpharms.com/reclassifications/otc-tamsulosin-reference-guide.asp (Member-only content) (accessed 30 March 2011).

Royal Pharmaceutical Society of Great Britain (2010). Supply of Levonorgestrel Oral Emergency Contraception as a Pharmacy (P) Medicine. A Guidance on Professional Practice. London: RPSGB. Available at http://www.rpharms. com/best-practice/oral-emergency-contraception.asp (Member-only content) (accessed 30 March 2011).

Royal Pharmaceutical Society of Great Britain (2011). Practice Guidance: Tranexamic Acid P Medicine. London: RPSGB. Available at http://www.rpharms. com/reclassifications/tranexamic-acid-p-medicine.asp (Member-only content) (accessed 30 March 2011).

Wyatt KM *et al.* (1999). Efficacy of vitamin B-6 in the treatment of premenstrual syndrome: systematic review. *Br Med J* 318: 1375–1381.

## Self-assessment questions

The following questions are provided to test the information presented in this chapter.

*For questions 1–7 select the best answer in each case.*

1. Select which of the following is the most common causative organism of urinary tract infections:
   a. *Mycoplasma pneumoniae*
   b. *Pseudomonas aeruginosa*
   c. *Escherichia coli*
   d. *Neisseria gonorrhoeae*
   e. *Klebsiella pneumonia*

2. Select which of the following is not normally considered a symptom of a lower urinary tract infection (cystitis):
   a. Stinging, burning pain on urination
   b. Urinary urgency
   c. Urinary frequency
   d. Loin pain and tenderness
   e. Strong-smelling urine

3. Select which of the following people are suitable for treatment with potassium citrate:
   a. A 42-year-old woman with symptoms of cystitis who takes lisinopril 10 mg daily
   b. A 40-year-old man with symptoms of cystitis who takes bendroflumethiazide 2.5 mg daily
   c. A 33-year-old woman with symptoms of cystitis who takes gliclazide 50 mg daily and metformin 500 mg three times daily
   d. A 32-year-old woman with symptoms of cystitis who takes ethinylestradiol 30 micrograms/levonorgestrel 150 micrograms daily as a contraceptive
   e. A 67-year-old woman with symptoms of cystitis who takes alendronic acid 10 mg daily

4. Select which of the following organisms is not a sexually transmitted infection:
   a. *Gardnerella vaginalis*
   b. *Chlamydia trachomatis*
   c. *Neisseria gonorrhoeae*
   d. *Treponema pallidum*
   e. *Trichomonas vaginalis*

5. Select which of the following is not a feature of primary dysmenorrhoea:
   a. Starts at or shortly after (6–12 months) the menarche.
   b. Pain typically begins within 24 hours of the onset of menstruation and persists for 8–72 hours.
   c. Periods are usually normal or light.
   d. Other gynaecological symptoms are not usually present.
   e. There may be little response to NSAIDs or COCs.

6. Select which of the following drugs interacts with EHC:
   a. Amoxicillin
   b. Griseofulvin
   c. Fluconazole
   d. Ciprofloxacin
   e. Terbinafine

7. Select which of the following is the hormone which can be detected in the urine of pregnant women and forms the basis for urine testing for pregnancy:
   a. Progesterone
   b. Luteinising hormone
   c. Follicle-stimulating hormone
   d. Human chorionic gonadotrophin
   e. Oestrogen

*For questions 8–10 select from the list below one lettered option that is most closely related to it. Each lettered option may be used once, more than once, or not at all.*
   a. bacterial vaginosis
   b. vaginal candidiasis
   c. trichomoniasis
   d. atrophic vaginitis
   e. vulvovaginitis

8. Usually presents as a red, swollen and irritated vulval area with vaginal discharge which is white and odourless.

9. Is associated with a number of causes of vaginal discharge.

10. May increase the likelihood of infection in some women.

*For questions 11 and 12 select from the list below one lettered option that is most closely related to it. Each lettered option may be used once, more than once, or not at all.*
   a. calcium
   b. magnesium
   c. vitamin $B_6$
   d. vitamin E
   e. Evening primrose oil

11. Has strong evidence supporting its effectiveness in the management of premenstrual syndrome (PMS).

12. Can cause peripheral neuropathy in high doses.

*Questions 13–16: Each of the questions or incomplete statements in this section is followed by three responses. For each question one or more of the responses is/are correct. Decide which of the responses is/are correct and then choose a–e as indicated in the table below.*

| Directions summarised | | | | |
| --- | --- | --- | --- | --- |
| **a** | **b** | **c** | **d** | **e** |
| If 1, 2 and 3 are correct | If 1 and 2 only are correct | If 2 and 3 only are correct | If 1 only is correct | If 3 only is correct |

13. The following medicines can be supplied from a pharmacy without a prescription to treat vaginal candidiasis:
    1 – econazole cream
    2 – miconazole intravaginal cream
    3 – fluconazole capsules

14. The following medicines can be supplied from a pharmacy without a prescription to treat primary dysmenorrhoea in a 14 year old female:
    1 – naproxen tablets
    2 – ibuprofen tablets
    3 – paracetamol and codeine tablets

15. Azithromycin can be supplied from a pharmacy without a prescription to treat:
    1 – laboratory-confirmed infection with *Chlamydia* with symptoms of dysuria, vaginal discharge and dyspareunia
    2 – laboratory-confirmed infection with *Chlamydia* with no symptoms
    3 – a sexual partner of an individual with laboratory-confirmed infection with *Chlamydia*

16. Premenstrual syndrome (PMS):
    1 – is a group of symptoms that is normal in most women who are menstruating
    2 – does not need treatment
    3 – is severely debilitating in around 20% of women who experience it.

*Questions 17–20 consist of two statements linked by the word* because; *decide whether each statement is true or false. If both statements are true then decide whether the second statement is a correct explanation of the first statement. Choose a–e as your answer as indicated in the table below.*

| Directions summarised | | | |
|---|---|---|---|
| | **First statement** | **Second statement** | |
| a | True | True | Second statement is a correct explanation of the first statement |
| b | True | True | Second statement is not a correct explanation of the first statement |
| c | True | False | |
| d | False | True | |
| e | False | False | |

17.

| Cranberry juice is effective in treating urinary tract infections | BECAUSE | Cranberry juice contains substances which prevent the bacteria from adhering to the urethral epithelium |
|---|---|---|

18.

| A woman with symptoms of vaginal thrush who is taking folic acid 400 micrograms daily should not be supplied intravaginal clotrimazole as a P medicine | BECAUSE | Folic acid 400 micrograms prevents neural tube defects in unborn babies |
|---|---|---|

19.

| Tranexamic acid should not be supplied as a P medicine to a woman taking an oral contraceptive | BECAUSE | Tranexamic acid increases the metabolism of oral contraceptives and reduces effectiveness |
|---|---|---|

20.

| EHC can be used within 72 hours of unprotected sexual intercourse | BECAUSE | EHC is between 85% and 95% effective in preventing pregnancy within 24 hours of unprotected sexual intercourse |
|---|---|---|

## Answers

1-c; 2-d; 3-d; 4-a; 5-e; 6-b; 7-d; 8-b; 9-e; 10-d; 11-a; 12-c; 13-e; 14-c; 15-c; 16-d; 17-d; 18-b; 19-c; 20-b

# 7

# Eyes, Ears and Oral Health

*Alyson Brown and Brian Addison*

| This chapter will cover the following conditions: | This chapter will cover the following groups of medicines |
|---|---|
| • Eye Infections<br>• Disorders of the inner, middle and outer ear<br>• Oral candidiasis<br>• Gingivitis<br>• Mouth ulcers<br>• Xerostomia<br>• Halitosis | • Ocular lubricants<br>• Chloramphenicol<br>• Cerumenolytics<br>• Local analgesics<br>• Drugs for oral ulceration<br>  Mouthwashes |

In this chapter we will consider the different minor illnesses that affect the eyes, the ears and the buccal cavity. This chapter will also consider general approaches to dealing with these conditions and the specific groups of drugs that can be used to manage these conditions.

# Eye disorders

Before reading further, consider the following case and note your initial thoughts.

**Case study**

A young man complains of a gritty, red right eye, which he has had 'on and off' for a number of weeks. He explains that the eye is not painful and that he has tried using some eye drops belonging to a friend, but these have not been effective.

**Trigger questions**

- What additional information would you need before considering the appropriate management options in this case?
- What issues concern you about this case?
- Are any alarm symptoms being exhibited that require more urgent treatment or referral?

## Assessing symptoms

There are a limited number of mechanisms which can cause a diseased state in the eye and they can be categorised as disorders of the eyeball or of the eyelids. However, some common symptoms to look for are alteration in visual acuity, redness, pain, discharge and photophobia.

Figures 7.1 and 7.2 show diagrammatic representations of the eye.

Three situations that are relatively easy to recognise and usually present no immediate danger and in most cases can be treated symptomatically in the first instance are:

- Painless red eye
- Disorder of tear formation
- Inflammation of the eyelids.

### Painless red eye

Conjunctivitis is the most common cause of red eye and is an inflammation of the conjunctiva of the

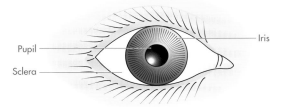

**Figure 7.1**  Anterior view of the eye.

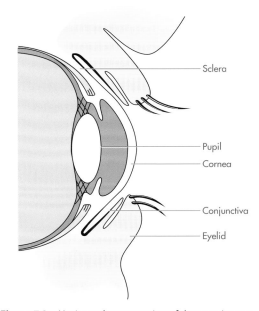

**Figure 7.2**  Horizontal cross-section of the anterior eye.

anterior eye. The conjunctiva is a thin vascular membrane that covers the anterior surface of the eyeball and folds back on itself to form the lining of the eyelid. In wearers of contact lenses, conjunctivitis can be caused by a scratched cornea, a reaction to a lens solution, a poorly fitting lens or corneal drying.

Conjunctivitis commonly affects both eyes, although one may be affected more than the other. If both eyes are affected, and in the absence of any warning signs or symptoms, the conjunctivitis will probably have either an allergic or an infective cause.

In both allergic and infective conjunctivitis the white (sclera) of the eye is red, and this redness extends to the inner surface of the eyelids (Figure 7.3). Pulling

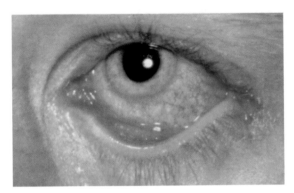

**Figure 7.3** Conjunctivitis.

(Reproduced with permission from St Bartholomew's Hospital/Science Photo Library, SPL M155/117.)

down the lower lid will reveal a red and oedematous conjunctiva covering its inner surface, compared with the pale pink seen in a normal eye. The sufferer will usually complain of an itchiness or grittiness on the surface of the eye.

The commonest cause of allergic conjunctivitis is hay fever and is often seen in young people, in whom any allergic predispositions are more evident. This is more commonly seen in females than males, the cause often being eye cosmetics, although soaps, cleansers and powders applied to the face can also provoke a reaction. In allergic conjunctivitis there is usually a clear watery discharge in addition to an itchy or gritty sensation on the surface of the eye.

In infective conjunctivitis there is usually a discharge that may be purulent in bacterial conjunctivitis but clear and watery in viral conjunctivitis. The exact percentage of infections that are bacterial or viral is not clear and it has been estimated that somewhere between 33% and 78% of infective conjunctivitis cases are bacterial in origin. The most common bacterial cause is *Staphylococcus aureus*. A discharge of pus that collects in the inner corner of the eye or that prevents easy opening of the eyelids on awakening is a sign of bacterial conjunctivitis. This may be unilateral but usually affects both eyes. It can be clinically difficult to distinguish between bacterial and viral conjunctivitis, for although the symptoms and signs are described differently in textbooks there is often confusion clinically.

A unilateral red eye is more likely to be related to a condition within the eye, such as iritis or glaucoma. Iritis is an inflammation of the iris. Associated structures, such as the ciliary body, are often involved (iridocyclitis). The condition may be caused by infection or allergy, or may be the result of systemic disease. Symptoms include pain within the eye, photophobia, visual impairment, and hazy, small, irregularly shaped and unreactive pupils. Iritis may progress to cause cataracts (if the lens is involved) or glaucoma (if the angle at the edge of the ciliary body is eliminated). There is a danger of permanent visual loss unless diagnosis and treatment take place at an early stage.

In such cases the redness typically occurs more around the centre of the eye, close to the iris, and is largely absent from inside the lids, compared with the more peripheral redness of an allergy or infection. However, it is often difficult to distinguish the conditions on this basis.

A subconjunctival haemorrhage (caused by a burst blood vessel) appears as a red spot or may cover the white of the eye (Figure 7.4). Although it can provoke much anxiety in the sufferer, it is harmless and will heal spontaneously without treatment within a few weeks, provided that no accompanying symptoms are present.

### Disorders of tear formation

People who complain of dry eyes may require artificial tears (as eye drops). This condition is seen as a

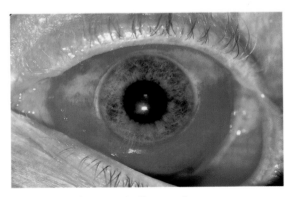

**Figure 7.4** Subconjunctival haemorrhage.

(Reproduced with permission from Science Photo Library, SPL M155/186.)

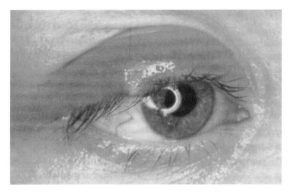

**Figure 7.5** Stye on the upper eyelid.

(Reproduced with permission from Western Ophthalmic Hospital/Science Photo Library, SPL M130/093.)

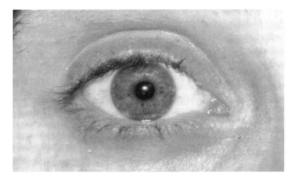

**Figure 7.6** Blepharitis, inflammation of the eyelid.

(Reproduced with permission of Cosine Graphics/Science Photo Library, SPL M155/083.)

complication of certain disorders, such as rheumatoid arthritis (Sjögren syndrome), and in oestrogen deficiency, as occurs in menopausal women. It is wise to refer people with dry eyes to eliminate corneal ulceration or any other pathology.

### Inflammation of eyelids

Inflammation of the margin of one eyelid is likely to be caused by a small abscess or stye, which is an infection of a hair follicle gland at the base of an eyelash (Figure 7.5). The infection can cause redness and irritation around the affected area with possible progression to pain and swelling of the eyelid. Styes are common and often recurrent, the inflammation will be localised at first but may spread to involve the rest of the eyelid, which will become tender and painful. After 1 or 2 days the stye will usually come to a head and may burst, or may simply shrink and resolve. Those that do not resolve may require surgical excision.

Redness and irritation of the eyelid margins (affecting one or both eyes), often with scales adhering to the base of eyelashes, occurs in blepharitis (Figure 7.6). Blepharitis is caused by inflammation of the glands of the margin of the eyelid, most noticeably the eyelash roots. This is commonly associated with seborrhoeic dermatitis or dandruff, or it may be allergic, in which case concurrent conjunctivitis may also be noticed. More rarely, it may be caused by infection. Some eyelashes may be either absent or distorted, sometimes pointing inwards and irritating the surface of the eye. If the cause is infective, pus may be seen discharging from the base of the lashes.

Displacement of the eyelids may be seen, particularly in the elderly. In such cases, the margins of the eyelids do not come together when the eyes are closed. Spasm or atony of the orbital muscles causes the lids either to invert, which is called entropion (Figure 7.7), or to evert, which is called ectropion (Figure 7.8). In the former the lid margins and lashes point inwards and irritate the eye, whereas in the latter the lower lid falls away from the eye, offering it insufficient protection and lubrication.

In both conditions there is an overflow of tears. In ectropion the lower lid may become chronically infected and scarred. In entropion the lashes may fall out and infection may follow. As with ectropion, if it is seen relatively early on, a minor surgical procedure can correct the displacement. If left untreated it may lead to corneal ulceration because of trauma from the inverted lashes and poor lubrication of the tissues. Entropion and ectropion will usually

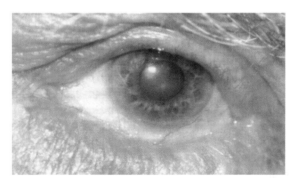

**Figure 7.7** Entropion: the lower eyelid is inverted.

(Reproduced with permission from the Science Photo Library, SPL M155/112.)

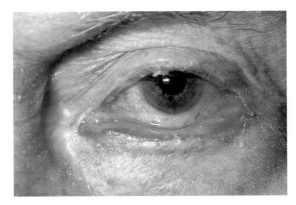

**Figure 7.8** Ectropion of the lower eyelid, where the eyelid falls away from the eye.

(Reproduced with permission from Dr P. Marazzi/Science Photo Library, SPL M155/337.)

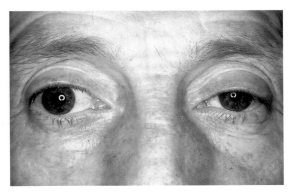

**Figure 7.10** Ptosis.

(Reproduced with permission from the Wellcome Trust Medical Photographic Library.)

have been present for a long time before someone seeks advice for these conditions and they require no urgent treatment, although referral for a medical opinion may be appropriate if the patient is at all anxious or worried.

A hard pea-like lump appearing under the skin of the lid, most commonly the upper lid, away from the margin, will probably be a meibomian cyst (chalazion). These may also be found in the lower lid, and can be visualised by pulling down the lower lid to reveal a small lump resembling an internal stye under the conjunctiva (Figure 7.9). This is an infection of one of the meibomian glands, which are located deep in the cartilaginous tissue on the underside of the lids and secrete fluid on to the conjunctiva.

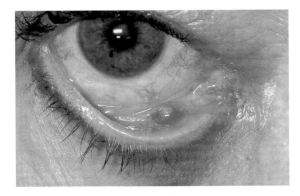

**Figure 7.9** Meibomian cyst (chalazion).

(Reproduced with permission from Dr P. Marazzi/Science Photo Library, SPL M155/258.)

Infection of the outlet of a gland results in blockage and inflammation in the same way that a stye forms. The cyst will normally resolve spontaneously without incident and is generally painless, but may recur from time to time in some people. A persistent cyst may require surgery.

Ptosis, which is a drooping upper eyelid (Figure 7.10), is often a sign of systemic disease, such as myasthenia gravis, and referral is essential. In babies, special measures are needed to rectify the droop to avoid reduced visual input to the brain and blindness. Ptosis is also a sign of Horner syndrome, which is caused by a lesion in the cervical sympathetic nerve, often due to trauma, tumours or bleeds.

## Accompanying symptoms

### Pain

Itchiness, grittiness and soreness on the surface of the eye are common symptoms of minor superficial conditions, such as conjunctivitis. These symptoms should be distinguished from a deep-seated pain arising from within the eye, which indicates possible serious pathology, such as a raised intraocular pressure (glaucoma) or iritis, and requires urgent referral for medical investigation. Similarly, trauma such as flash burns (in welders working with oxyacetylene burners) and corneal injury will cause severe pain. A feeling of grittiness on the surface of one eye only will frequently be caused by a foreign body. It should be relatively easy to distinguish a superficial itching or irritation of the conjunctiva on the eye surface from a more intense pain caused by pathology within the eye itself. Any such pain, which may be accompanied by other symptoms or signs, requires referral for a medical opinion. If severe, referral should be made urgently.

### Nasal symptoms

Conjunctivitis accompanied by nasal symptoms, such as congestion, sneezing and rhinorrhoea, suggests an allergic component to the condition. A sore throat, symptoms of a cold or general malaise may be associated with a viral conjunctivitis, which is usually caused by an adenovirus.

### Visual disturbance

Loss of vision is a medical emergency. Disturbance of vision may be due to the visual component of migraine, in which case it is likely to be recurrent and recognised by the sufferer. The visual disturbances that accompany classic migraine are easily distinguishable from those described here (see Chapter 4).

In conjunctivitis, vision is not significantly affected because the conjunctiva does not cover the cornea and the underlying pupil, and thus light enters and penetrates the eye in the normal manner. Vision may temporarily be affected if the cornea is obscured by fluid or pus. Loss of visual acuity is often accompanied by pain within the eye, but there are exceptions, such as vascular blockage or haemorrhages in the eye, optic nerve damage, temporal arteritis or retinal detachment, which will not be painful.

Double vision accompanied by ptosis and a headache of sudden onset suggests the possibility of an intracranial bleed and requires urgent medical attention.

Bizarre patterns in the field of vision, with haloes seen around bright lights (particularly noticed when coming out of a dark into a lit area, e.g. when leaving a cinema, or driving at night), requires referral, as this is seen in glaucoma and multiple sclerosis (known as optic neuritis in the latter case). In such cases individuals should be advised to seek medical opinion with the suspicion of multiple sclerosis left unstated as the diagnosis may prove to be different and will require careful handling by a clinician.

### Tired eyes

Complaints of tired and sore eyes may be associated with conjunctivitis; in the absence of this condition, a referral to the optometrist may be in order to check for eye strain and any defects in visual acuity.

### Lacrimation

Lacrimation is associated with interrupted drainage of the tear film and in babies requires referral so that the condition can be rectified. In older people it will be seen in ectropion.

### Pupils

It is wise to carry out a simple physical examination of the eyes, especially if a serious condition is suspected. The pupils should be round and equal in size and they should react equally and oppositely to light, such that each will constrict when a light is directed at it. The pupil should remain circular as it constricts; irregularity suggests adhesions due to iritis. This may be a previously diagnosed condition, and therefore it should not automatically be assumed that this is a recent finding. Any inequality or abnormality of size, shape or reaction will suggest serious pathology within the eye and the need for immediate referral. A hazy or cloudy appearance to the iris or pupil may be caused by inflammatory exudate in the anterior chamber (as in iritis) or corneal oedema (as in glaucoma), and therefore requires medical referral.

### Bulging eye

A rare presentation of a bulging eye (proptosis) or of retracted eyelids (upper, lower or both) may be accompanied by symptoms of an overactive thyroid, such as sweating, hot skin, flushing, tremor of the hands or fingers, weight loss despite an increasing appetite, a fast heart rate and a state of physical overactivity. In a mild form it is difficult for the untrained observer to detect, but a gap of white sclera between the iris and the affected lid will be seen if the affected eye is compared with a normal eye. Bulging of one eye, however, raises the possibility of some local pathology behind the eye and both situations require medical appraisal and investigation.

### Headache

Headaches accompanying eye symptoms can occur in glaucoma, migraine and temporal arteritis. The nature of the headache will assist in differentiating these conditions.

## Management options

If an eye condition does not respond to appropriate simple self-medication within 7 days, then medical advice should be sought. This is because some conditions may become chronic, for example blepharitis, and some may require treatment with antibiotics, for example severe infective conjunctivitis.

### Antibacterial eye drops and ointments (BNF section 11.3.1)

The agent of choice for infective conjunctivitis is chloramphenicol, although in most cases simple self-care advice is the preferred option as opposed to antibacterial therapy. Chloramphenicol is active against the bacteria commonly implicated in eye infections, such as staphylococci, streptococci and *Haemophilus influenzae*, and should improve symptoms within 48 hours and completely resolve simple infections within 5 days. Chloramphenicol can be sold to members of the public from pharmacies as eye drops or ointment for the treatment of acute bacterial conjunctivitis in adults and children over 2 years old. The efficacy of eye drops can probably be maximised in the treatment of conjunctivitis by 2-hourly instillation, at least for the first 2 days of treatment. However, most cases of infective conjunctivitis will get better within 1–2 weeks without the use of antibacterial eye drops.

Although the ability to distinguish between viral and bacterial conjunctivitis is recognised as being problematic, the use of antibacterial eye drops in a viral infection is still beneficial. Viral infections will still cause the eye to feel very uncomfortable and therefore the application of an eye drop or ointment will provide some degree of symptomatic relief from this discomfort as well as preventing secondary bacterial infection. It must be noted that chloramphenicol is only licensed for supply to the public from pharmacies for acute bacterial conjunctivitis.

Propamidine is also available in various products that can be sold to members of the public from pharmacies for the treatment of minor eye infections such as conjunctivitis and blepharitis. It has little value in bacterial infections but it has a specific role in the management of the rare, sight-threatening condition *Acanthamoeba keratitis*. This condition is associated with poor lens cleaning and disinfection, especially with soft lenses even if they are replaced frequently.

Care should be taken in contact lens wearers that infection has not been caused by the lens itself, as in the case of corneal abrasion or dendritic ulcer, and some may consider it wise to refer such people to their doctor or optometrist before attempting to treat such cases.

In any case, lenses must be removed for the whole treatment period with antibacterial drops, because they can cause keratitis (infection of the cornea) to develop as a serious complication. Soft lenses also cause accumulation of preservatives, with resulting irritation, and should not be worn until 24 hours after treatment has finished.

Eye ointment containing dibromopropamidine can be used overnight to treat conjunctivitis. It is also suitable as a once- or twice-daily application to the eyelid margins in infective blepharitis and styes, though styes usually resolve spontaneously without the application of antibacterial preparations. However, if there has been a failure to reduce the symptoms of a stye within 7 days or when blepharitis has not responded to appropriate over-the-counter remedies within 7 days, referral for medical opinion would be appropriate as delays may result in the conditions becoming chronic.

Scales or pus adhering to the lid margins can be loosened and lifted by the use of antibacterial eye ointment and by wiping the lid margins with diluted baby shampoo, which is unperfumed and non-irritant.

Simple hygiene measures, such as the use of separate face flannels and towels, may be helpful in preventing the spread of infection to other family members.

### Other anti-inflammatory preparations (BNF section 11.4.2)

The cause of allergic conjunctivitis, such as pollen or cosmetics, should be identified and, where possible, removed. Hypoallergenic preparations will still affect some people and the condition will only clear after total avoidance of cosmetics around the eyes. The symptoms are mediated by histamine receptors in the mucosa of the eye. The use of eye drops containing either an antihistamine alone, such as levocabastine, or a combination product such as antazoline together with a vasoconstrictor such as xylometazoline, is effective in providing fast, symptomatic relief in this condition. The vasoconstrictor will address the engorged lymphatic and fine blood vessels in the conjunctiva, which cause the red, swollen appearance of the eyes. If nasal symptoms are also present, as in allergic rhinitis, oral antihistamines should be recommended in addition to eye drops. Further information on the presentation and management of allergic rhinitis and the use of antihistamines to manage this condition is provided in Chapter 3.

Sodium cromoglicate eye drops, a mast cell stabiliser, give symptomatic relief of allergic conjunctivitis caused by seasonal allergies. While sodium cromoglicate eye drops will give symptomatic relief, they do require to be administered four times a day to maintain their effectiveness and failure to follow this regimen will result in limited efficacy of this product.

### Astringent eye lotions

Eye lotions that contain astringents such as witch hazel are promoted for the treatment of irritation and red eyes. They are best recommended where no specific syndrome exists, for example in cases where someone complains of 'tired eyes' but has no significant conjunctivitis.

### Vasoconstrictor substances

Naphazoline is the principal vasoconstrictor drug in over-the-counter eye drops. In conjunctivitis, a sympathomimetic agent such as this will reduce the injection of the conjunctiva with blood by its vasoconstrictive action. This not only serves a cosmetic function but also reduces the irritation caused by the conjunctival hyperaemia and inflammation. It should not be used if other eye disease is present, such as glaucoma.

### Other measures

A stye may be drawn to a point to facilitate the exudation of pus by applying a hot compress to the lid. This can be done by soaking a clean towel or flannel in hot water and placing it on the closed lid for several minutes each day.

Where blepharitis is associated with seborrhoeic dermatitis or dandruff, treatment of the skin condition may be undertaken at the same time as local treatment of the eyelids.

Where a blockage of the nasolacrimal duct is suspected (as with excessive lacrimation), an attempt can be made to resolve the problem by applying pressure with one finger to the lacrimal sac at the internal corner of the eye and lightly massaging the duct beneath. Failure to release fluid should not be followed by increasing the pressure. If the condition is troublesome, especially in children, an appointment should be made to see their GP.

Generally people should be reminded to take commonsense measures to reduce the irritant effects of environmental substances, such as dust, cosmetics, smoke and chlorine in swimming pools, where this is appropriate.

Preservatives such as benzalkonium chloride used in eye drops can damage contact lenses, and therefore wearers are best advised to refrain from wearing lenses during treatment and for 24 hours afterwards, if possible.

 **Re-consider the case**

Before reading further, re-consider the following questions and your initial thoughts on this case.

**Trigger questions**

- What additional information would you need before considering the appropriate management options in this case?
- What issues concern you about this case?
- Are any alarm symptoms being exhibited that require more urgent treatment or referral?

**Case study**

A young man complains of a gritty, red right eye which he has had 'on and off' for a number of weeks. He explains that the eye is not painful and that he has tried using some eye drops belonging to a friend, but these have not been effective.

### Pharmacist opinion

It would be important to establish initially that this man is not experiencing any other symptoms such as alteration in visual acuity, photophobia or pain. By simply looking at the affected eye it will be obvious if there is redness, inflammation and possible discharge. If no discharge is present, then it would be prudent to inquire about this point to ensure that the absence of any discharge is not because it has been cleaned up. In examining the right eye it should be compared to the man's left eye to establish whether this is a condition affecting just one eye (unilateral) or both eyes (bilateral).

In examining the eye it is important to establish which part of the eye is red. By pulling down the lower eye lid it will be possible to establish whether both the sclera and conjunctiva are red. If this is the case then the likely explanation, assuming the absence of any warning signs, is that he is suffering from conjunctivitis. The description of a gritty feeling in the eye would also support this explanation, assuming that it is not being caused by a foreign body.

It is difficult based on the case described to establish whether this is an allergic or infective conjunctivitis, as typically these present in a similar fashion. The one feature that can help indicate whether there is an allergic or infective cause would be the nature of any discharge. A clear, watery discharge would be associated more with an allergic cause, although this can also be the case in viral conjunctivitis, whereas a purulent discharge is more commonly seen in bacterial conjunctivitis.

The description in this case of the symptoms being experienced as 'on and off' for a few weeks is also worthy of consideration. This may suggest that an allergic cause is more likely as the condition has not resolved and is persisting. It would not be uncommon if there was an allergic cause to the conjunctivitis for other signs and symptoms of allergy to be present, e.g. sneezing and/or rhinorrhoea. Equally, these symptoms could also be present if the man was suffering from a cold, considering the ability of infections of the nasal mucosa to extend through the nasolacrimal duct.

It would also be important to establish what eye drops he has been using that belong to his friend and importantly how long these have been opened. The potential that this man may be re-infecting his eye with these eyedrops needs to be borne in mind and investigated thoroughly.

An important consideration in anyone complaining of an eye disorder is whether they are contact lens wearers. The use of contact lenses can cause a number of eye conditions but also some products can have a detrimental effect on the contact lenses themselves. For further information regarding drug treatment and contact lenses see *BNF* section 11.9.

In this case it would be important to establish whether this man does wear contact lenses as given the duration of his symptoms he would be best advised to seek the advice of an optician or optometrist. *Acanthamoeba keratitis* is a sight-threatening eye condition that is associated with ineffective contact lens cleaning and disinfection and requires specialist medical treatment.

Assuming that there are no alarm symptoms that require investigation in this man, it would be appropriate to advise the use of chloramphenicol if bacterial conjunctivitis is suspected, or if an allergic cause is suspected then a product containing an antihistamine or mast cell stabiliser.

### General practitioner opinion

These symptoms might suggest a viral conjunctivitis. Supportive features would include other viral symptoms, e.g. sore throat, coryza. The intermittent nature of these symptoms would point to a possible allergic element. Further questioning may reveal a specific allergen, usually pollen, but the condition may

General practitioner opinion (*continued*)

be work related. A history of hay fever or atopy would further support a diagnosis of an allergic conjunctivitis. Identifying the drops that were ineffective would be helpful in coming to a diagnosis. Any visual disturbance, more significant pain, or photophobia might suggest other causes and would need referral.

Viral conjunctivitis is self-limiting and does not require treatment. Allergic conjunctivitis can be successfully treated with antihistamines, although local topical treatment is also available and may be more acceptable.

 Summary of key points

| Condition | Management |
| --- | --- |
| Bacterial conjunctivitis is characterised by a redness of the sclera and conjunctiva of the eye along with a gritty sensation and purulent discharge. | Chloramphenicol eye drops or ointment for 5 days. |
| Allergic conjunctivitis is characterised by a redness of the sclera and conjunctiva of the eye along with a gritty sensation. | Sodium cromoglicate gives symptomatic relief from seasonal allergies. Eyedrops that contain naphazoline or levocabastine (either alone or in combination): • Naphazoline can be used to reduce the irritation of an inflamed conjunctiva • Levocabastine is an antihistamine that will provide fast, symptomatic relief |
| Subconjunctival haemorrhage is caused by a burst blood vessel. | Heals spontaneously within a few weeks and requires no treatment unless there are accompanying symptoms. |
| Blepharitis is characterised by a redness and inflammation of the margins of the eyelids. | Dibromopropamidine eye ointment applied to the eyelid margins. |
| Styes are characterised by a localised inflammation of the eyelid. | Dibromopropamidine eye ointment can be used in the treatment of styes, but they usually resolve spontaneously. |

 When to refer

- Pain within the eye (in contrast to superficial itchiness, grittiness or soreness)
- Disturbance in vision
- Pupils appear abnormal or uneven
- Pupils have abnormal or uneven reaction to light
- Upper eyelid drooping (ptosis)
- Recurrent lump under upper eyelid
- Recurrent subconjunctival haemorrhage
- Babies under 3 months old or babies with a squint
- Existing eye disease
- Bulging of eyes (proptosis)
- Dry eyes (unless previously seen by a doctor)
- Any associated headache
- Systemically unwell
- Specific genitourinary symptoms suggesting the possibility of chlamydial infection
- Recent long-haul travel in someone whose symptoms are not resolving

# Ear disorders

Before reading further, consider the following case and note your initial thoughts.

**Case study**

A woman asks your advice regarding her 8-year-old daughter who has had earache for two nights that has caused some sleep disturbance. Her child has described a sensation of something in the ear, but the mother also suspects that she has developed some hearing loss as she has noticed recently that she often has to repeat herself when speaking to her daughter.

**Trigger questions**

- What additional information would you need before considering the appropriate management options in this case?
- What issues concern you about this case?
- Are any alarm symptoms being exhibited that require more urgent treatment or referral?

## Assessing symptoms

Symptoms in the ear can be classified as disorders of the outer, middle or inner ear. The inner ear is continuous with the upper respiratory tract, being connected by the Eustachian tube, which functions to equalise pressure in the ear; thus symptoms in the ear are often associated with upper respiratory tract disorders and are common in children. A diagram of the ear is shown in Figure 7.11.

### Deafness

Deafness can be caused by obstruction in the external ear canal, inflammation in the middle or inner ear, or a disturbance of the auditory nerve. Deafness can be tested with a tuning fork to determine whether it is conductive or perceptive. Conductive deafness is caused by failure of conduction of sound waves. Normally, sound waves enter the ear canal and cause the eardrum to vibrate, which then moves

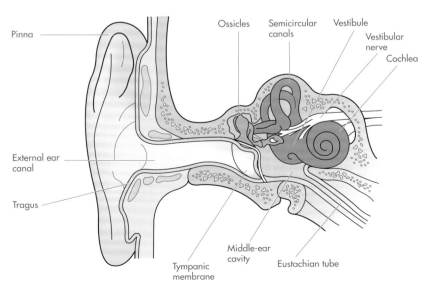

**Figure 7.11** Diagram of the ear.

the chain of ossicles to transmit the vibrations to the cochlea in the inner ear. Perceptive deafness is failure of the system beyond this point, such as the cochlea failing to transmit the vibrations and stimulate the auditory nerve or the nerve itself failing to transmit impulses so that the sound can be appreciated in the brain. Deafness is therefore to be expected when the ear canal is blocked by wax, debris, a furuncle (boil) or a discharge (as from an infection), and in otitis media (chronic and acute), Eustachian catarrh and barotrauma.

Wax is produced in every ear in varying amounts. If it accumulates in the ear canal it may dry and harden to form a solid plug, which can obstruct the canal. This prevents the transmission of sound waves to the eardrum and results in hearing impairment.

Secretory otitis media, also known as glue ear or chronic or serous catarrhal otitis media, is a condition mainly of children. The middle-ear space becomes full of a sticky effusion (hence the term 'glue ear'), the escape of which is impeded by some obstruction or defect in the Eustachian tube. It is symptomless, apart from impairment of hearing that is insidious in onset and is often undiagnosed for some time (it may persist for several weeks or months) and may only be recognised when a child is observed to be failing at school because he or she cannot hear properly. Secretory otitis media may be suspected following frequent and recurrent middle-ear infections.

Otitis externa is inflammation of the skin of the pinna or external ear canal and may be infective or reactive. The infective type is caused by bacteria, viruses or fungi. An exudate is discharged, which may block the external ear canal. In the reactive type the condition is seen as a form of dermatitis, which may be atopic or contact, most commonly related to wearing of earrings. Often dermatitis will become infected, and the two types of otitis externa will coexist. The ear canal will be sore and itching in either type, but in the purely reactive type the skin will usually be dry, red, and sometimes scaly. Otitis externa can also develop into a chronic condition that is symptomatic from time to time.

Acute otitis media is a bacterial (the main pathogen is streptococcal) or viral infection of the middle ear that generally lasts for less than one week, causing pain, discharge and often fever. It often follows an upper respiratory infection such as the common cold and children are most commonly affected. Frequent upper respiratory infections and attacks of otitis media in children may be associated with the development of a persistent catarrhal problem. Perforation of the eardrum may occur, in which case the release of pressure relieves the pain, but the discharge will persist. Chronic suppurative otitis media is more common in adults than in children and usually follows perforation of the eardrum in acute otitis media, resulting in superinfection with other bacteria. Recurrent episodes of otitis media may be associated with swimming and water sports.

As might be expected, infections of the middle ear (otitis media) are more common in winter because of the association with upper respiratory infections. In the summer, such infections may result from swimming, diving and air travel. Symptoms may not become significant until several days after acquiring the infection, and sufferers should be questioned about their activities, especially after a holiday.

Blockage of the Eustachian tube causes air to be absorbed from the middle ear, resulting in the eardrum being drawn in. The main symptom is transient pain and deafness, which usually resolves within a few days. It may follow a respiratory infection such as the common cold (usually in children – Eustachian catarrh) or mechanical pressure factors such as diving and rapid descent in an aircraft (often in adults – barotrauma). In such circumstances the air pressure outside the middle ear is greater than that inside and the air is sucked up the Eustachian tube, which then occludes. Eustachian catarrh usually lasts less than one week, but occasionally it may continue and develop into a chronic catarrhal state; repeated barotrauma in frequent air travellers can have the same effect.

Otitis media and Eustachian catarrh can also be caused by swimming, diving and air travel, when pressure differentials between the middle-ear cavity and the outside can suck fluid and microorganisms from the nasopharynx through the Eustachian tube.

Deafness with no apparent cause in young adults may be due to otosclerosis or may be industrial deafness, a permanent result of long-term unprotected exposure to high levels of noise, mostly from machinery. Otosclerosis is a cause of deafness in which there is deposition of new bone around one of the ossicles (the stapes) in the middle ear, preventing conduction of the vibrations of the eardrum to the cochlea. It usually begins unilaterally, mainly in young adults, and it may be some years from its onset before deafness is noted. Tinnitus is sometimes present and there is often a family history.

### Pain

Pain may be associated with a furuncle (boil) in the external ear canal and sufferers will complain that it is painful when the pinna is pulled upwards and back (as when an observer attempts to examine the ear) or when the tragus is pressed. However, when the boil bursts the pain will subside, and otherwise it is not a major feature of otitis externa. Problems caused by ear wax do not generally produce pain, and it is rarely a major feature of glue ear. Earache is complained of by the majority of people with otitis media – this is the commonest cause of earache in children. Earache may or may not be a feature of Eustachian catarrh and occurs in chronic suppurative otitis media only if the drum perforates. Pain may be experienced during descent in an aircraft (barotrauma), particularly if the sufferer has catarrh. Earache should generally be regarded as a referable symptom.

## Accompanying symptoms

### Cold, sore throat

Infection easily passes from the mouth and nasopharynx to the ear via the Eustachian tube, and ear infections may therefore be the result of bacterial or viral infection.

### Redness, swelling and discharge

Redness, swelling and a discharge are common features of a furuncle in the ear canal, but may also reflect an infective dermatitis in the canal. A discharge may be seen in both acute and chronic types of otitis media.

### Bleeding and bruising

Bleeding in the pinna is often copious and may not respond to the application of pressure, therefore referral for medical treatment would be required in this situation. In addition, any trauma to the pinna, with or without external bleeding, may result in large haematomas between the skin and the cartilage. These should be assessed by a doctor to determine whether they require surgical drainage to prevent fibrous scarring, which can result in the familiar 'cauliflower ear'. Any blood discharged into the ear canal requires a medical opinion to exclude perforation of the eardrum if the bleeding does not appear to arise from the canal itself.

### Itching

Itching or irritation of the ear canal or pinna usually represents a form of dermatitis, which can be treated with non-prescription topical preparations. It may sometimes be caused by the presence of a discharge in the canal.

### Red eardrum

Using an auriscope to examine the ear (a relatively simple skill to learn) allows the differentiation of many ear conditions by the assessment of the state of the tympanic membrane (eardrum). It appears normal in otitis externa, is often normal in glue ear, but is red in otitis media or following trauma. This is important, because the instillation of ear drops is contraindicated when the drum is perforated. Often the drum cannot be seen during examination with an auriscope because of occlusion by a discharge or wax.

### Fever and malaise

Otitis externa does not usually produce any signs of systemic disturbance, even in the case of a furuncle in the ear canal, unless the infection is severe. Fever is generally a sign of infection and is common in children with otitis media; it is often accompanied by vomiting. It is also a common sign of teething in babies with earache.

### 'Something in the ear'

Although someone may describe occlusion of the ear canal and the associated deafness as a feeling of 'something in the ear', it should be remembered that foreign bodies can also be real rather than imaginary. They can cause anxiety and, in the case of live insects, acute pain and appalling irritation as they struggle and flap their wings.

### Neck stiffness

Neck stiffness associated with symptoms in the ear requires referral for medical investigation to exclude the rare cases of an abscess in the mastoid air cells, or thrombosis of the adjacent cavernous venous sinus, the associated inflammation spreading to involve the meninges or even the brain.

### Tinnitus

Tinnitus is the complaint of an extraneous noise arising in the ear or anywhere in the head. It is usually described as ringing, buzzing, hissing or even pulsating. It may be a symptom of any disorder of the ear. It can be an accompaniment of senile deafness, otosclerosis, industrial deafness, Ménière's disease or drug toxicity (e.g. high-dose aspirin, furosemide, and gentamicin).

### Vertigo

Vertigo is best described as a sensation of the room spinning around the sufferer. It should be distinguished from unsteadiness on the feet (as occurs, for example, in muscle weakness or Parkinson disease) or light-headedness (a feeling of dizziness, as in postural hypotension, which may be associated with some drugs, particularly antihypertensive drugs in older people).

Vertigo may occur briefly during an ear infection associated with an upper respiratory tract infection, and in such cases the symptom will resolve in a few days. Disturbances of the inner ear can cause vertigo, the most important causes being Ménière's disease, vestibular neuronitis and positional (postural) vertigo. The symptoms of Ménière's disease are caused by increased pressure of the fluid in the labyrinth (the organ of balance). The cause of the condition is not understood and sufferers experience attacks of vertigo that either persist or recur and become more severe. This can also be accompanied by tinnitus and a perceptive deafness. Vertigo is a referable symptom if it occurs at some time of the day for more than a few days. People with positional vertigo will often have momentary vertigo when getting out of bed.

Vestibular neuronitis is also known as epidemic vertigo; this condition presents as an attack of vertigo associated with a febrile upper respiratory infection. It is probably a viral invasion of the ear and usually resolves within a few days with bed rest. Hearing is not affected, unlike with Ménière disease.

## Management options

The severity of symptoms will determine the need for and the urgency of referral. Any severe pain in the middle ear is distressing and requires referral for medical appraisal and an examination with an auriscope. If a lesion causing discomfort in the external ear is visible, then a judgement based on the severity of the symptoms and the possible diagnoses must be made. Thus, dermatitis on the pinna may be itching and uncomfortable, but may be treated with non-prescription creams in the first instance without the need for referral. On the other hand, an isolated blister, ulcer or unusual lesion on the pinna, which is growing in size but causing only minimal itch, should be tactfully but firmly referred for medical appraisal so that malignancy can be excluded.

The pinna has an abundant blood supply therefore trauma to the pinna can result in profuse bleeding. The ear should be compressed with a clean pad and the individual sent to a hospital Accident and Emergency department

### Problems of the external ear

Dry skin on the pinna can be treated with an emollient such as aqueous cream, emulsifying ointment or a similar proprietary preparation. If the skin of the external ear canal is affected, olive oil may be more convenient to use. If there is a contact dermatitis caused by sensitivity to earrings, individuals should be encouraged to wear nickel-free earrings or to use a proprietary clear lacquer to coat the earrings, so that the nickel is not in contact with the skin. Topical hydrocortisone should also be used in such a case of contact dermatitis, provided there is no infection present. If an infection is suspected or the lesion is not showing signs of improvement after 7 days, referral for medical appraisal should be advised so that an evaluation for the need for antibiotics can be undertaken.

Many cases of otitis externa affecting the external ear canal are aggravated by water and by scratching. These factors, and poor cleaning of the ear, will predispose to infection. The sufferer should be advised either to avoid swimming or at least to use earplugs when doing so, to dry the ears gently but thoroughly, and to perform an aural toilet before instilling drops into the ear canal. The removal of debris from the ear canal and the maintenance of a clean, dry environment will deter invasion by pathogenic organisms. Cleaning should be done with cotton-wool buds, which should be used once and then disposed of. The cotton wool should be gently rotated along the entire length of the canal.

Although it is necessary to keep the ear canal dry, it should not be occluded with a plug (except when swimming) if there is any exudate, as this will only serve to keep the exudate inside and provoke further irritation. The use of an appropriate proprietary preparation or aluminium acetate solution should assist in drying up excess moisture when there is a wet dermatitis either on the pinna or in the ear canal and such a preparation can be used prophylactically. Aluminium acetate solution may also be a useful astringent for itching otitis externa.

Adults should be told not to poke hard objects, such as hairgrips or matchsticks, down the ear canal as they may scratch the canal and promote infection, and there is also a small risk that the eardrum may become perforated. Fretful children who writhe are at risk of damage to the ear during cleaning. They are best dealt with by sitting the child sideways on the parent's lap while another person performs the cleaning procedure. One parental arm can be placed around the child's shoulders and the other around its head, holding it against the parent's chest.

Furuncles in the ear canal are difficult to treat, but some relief can be obtained by the application of a hot flannel and oral analgesics.

### Middle-ear conditions

For most people with acute otitis media a no-antibiotic or delayed antibiotic regimen should be advised, which can also be supported with oral analgesics and nasal vasoconstrictor drops. The pharmacist can advise on their choice and usage, although ear drops containing analgesics are unlikely to have any advantage over oral analgesics.

Episodes of acute otitis media accompanying chronic glue ear will be similarly treated with antibiotics and decongestants. In children, radical treatment of glue ear takes the form of myringotomy (incision of the eardrum) and drainage of the effusion. The cavity is then kept dry by inserting a grommet in the hole in the drum, and this remains in place for several months.

### Cerumenolytics (BNF section 12.1.3)

Water- or oil-based ear drops can be used to dissolve excess wax; the key active ingredients found in such ear drops are choline salicylate, urea hydrogen peroxide, almond oil, arachis oil and sodium bicarbonate. They are not always successful and take several days to produce their effect. However, they do facilitate ear irrigation, which may have to be resorted to by the doctor or practice nurse if the drops alone are not effective within one week. Problems may arise if drops are instilled into an ear with a perforated drum, as this may cause irritation or pain and perhaps infection of the middle ear.

It is often impossible to visualise the eardrum using an auriscope when there is a large amount of wax in the canal, and the doctor then has to rely on taking a brief history to assess the likelihood of a perforated eardrum. This can be achieved by establishing whether there has been a recent ear infection, history of perforation or a chronically discharging ear.

Perforation may have occurred recently without being diagnosed by a doctor, and therefore the presence of any discomfort or pain should be excluded, especially after diving or any other water sports or air travel. If any discomfort or pain has been experienced recently, especially if this has been when instilling ear drops, then a medical opinion should be sought.

Some cerumenolytics will sometimes cause ear wax to swell at first, and people using these products should be warned that deafness may worsen initially.

Several proprietary drops contain wetting agents, such as docusate, which may be helpful. On the other hand, some contain potential irritants such as chlorobutanol and paradichlorobenzene.

Their use is contraindicated in the presence of otitis externa and their use should be discontinued if any discomfort is felt.

It is difficult to assess the comparative efficacy of cerumenolytics from the literature, and many doctors hold the view that simple generic preparations, such as olive or almond oil, are satisfactory, although care must be taken specifically with the use of almond oil in someone who has or suspects they have an allergy to nuts. Sodium bicarbonate ear drops may also be effective in facilitating the removal of wax from the ear canal, but do have the potential to cause dryness of the ear canal.

To aid irrigation, the ear wax can be softened on the day of irrigation using a softening remedy, although for wax that is hard and impacted the remedy can be instilled into the affected ear twice a day for a few days prior to irrigation. It is important when using oil remedies such as olive oil and almond oil to allow them to warm to room temperature before use.

### Removal of foreign bodies

Removal of foreign bodies from the ear (usually of a child) is best left to an expert unless the object is easy to grip with either fingernails or forceps and the pharmacist is particularly dextrous. This is because the eardrum is easily damaged and the object can be inadvertently pushed further into the canal. If there is a live insect in the canal, a few drops of olive oil should cause the speedy demise of the intruder, whose remains can be removed by syringing. If the insect has stung the person, producing oedema and occlusion of the ear canal, referral to an Accident and Emergency department is necessary.

### Eustachian catarrh

Measures can be taken to prevent and treat Eustachian catarrh or barotrauma. The aim is to force air up the Eustachian tube to allow ventilation of the middle ear. Sucking sweets, swallowing, using earplugs or the Valsalva manoeuvre are all useful tactics to promote the ventilation of the middle ear. The Valsalva manoeuvre involves pinching the nose, closing the mouth and then trying to breathe out.

Both Eustachian catarrh and barotrauma can be treated with oral or topical nasal decongestants such as pseudoephedrine tablets or ephedrine nasal drops. If drops are used, the sufferer should be told to lie down with the head extended and to remain in that position for 5 minutes after instillation so that the drops will travel down and backwards to the postnasal space and the oropharynx, where the entrance to the Eustachian tube lies. Oral analgesics and local warming may also give symptomatic relief.

**? Re-consider the case**

Before reading further, re-consider the following questions and your initial thoughts on this case.

**Trigger questions**

- What additional information would you need before considering the appropriate management options in this case?
- What issues concern you about this case?
- Are any alarm symptoms being exhibited that require more urgent treatment or referral?

**Case study**

A woman asks your advice regarding her 8-year-old daughter who has had earache for two nights that has caused some sleep disturbance. Her child has described a sensation of something in the ear, but the mother also suspects that she has developed some hearing loss as she has noticed recently that she often has to repeat herself when speaking to her daughter.

### Pharmacist opinion

The first observation to make in this case is that it is a presentation of earache in a child and therefore the more common ear conditions that occur in children need to be considered, e.g. acute otitis media.

A simple examination of the outer ear can yield some clues that may add to the history being presented. Sufferers of earache may complain that the pinna and tragus are painful when touched and this can impede auriscopic examination of the ear canal. In examining the ear, any discharge should be noted and if not seen it should be inquired after to confirm its absence. Chronic suppurative otitis media is more likely to be seen in adults than in children and usually following perforation of the eardrum.

It would be important to establish whether the earache was in both ears or just one ear and whether they suspected deafness was real. If the child permits it, careful examination of the ear canal would be appropriate to confirm whether or not the ear canal was occluded by wax or a foreign object. Extreme care is needed when examining the ear canal to ensure that any object within the ear canal is not pushed deeper into the ear, risking perforation of the eardrum.

Treatment with oral analgesia, e.g. paracetamol or ibuprofen, appropriate for an 8-year-old child would be the main course of action that could be taken in this case until a definitive diagnosis was made. While products to soften and facilitate the removal of ear wax are relatively safe to use, their use would not be recommended until impacted wax was identified as being the cause of the earache and deafness.

### General practitioner opinion

There are several differential diagnoses here, which require more information to distinguish between them. Firstly, is this unilateral or bilateral pain? If there is a history of high temperatures and feeling generally unwell, this would support a diagnosis of otitis media. These symptoms with no systemic features may be caused by impacted ear wax, otitis externa or foreign body. Examination of the ear canal using an auriscope would pick up the presence of impacted wax instantly. Examination may also identify the presence of a foreign body, although this may be less obvious.

Otitis externa is an infection of the skin of the ear canal, which may extend to the pinna itself. Risk factors include pre-existing skin conditions, e.g. eczema, regular swimming, and regular use of hairspray. Treatment is topical with antibiotic combined with steroid.

### Summary of key points

| Condition | Management |
|---|---|
| Secretory otitis media is characterised by insidious deafness. | May require treatment with antibiotics or surgery. |
| Acute otitis media is characterised by pain, discharge from the ear and fever. | May require treatment with antibiotics. |
| Eustachian catarrh is characterised by transient pain and deafness. | Sucking sweets, swallowing, using earplugs or the Valsalva manoeuvre. Oral or nasal decongestants such as pseudoephedrine or ephedrine. |
| Impacted wax is characterised by the feeling of something in the ear and possibly a degree of deafness. | Water- or oil-based cerumenolytics can be used to soften and loosen accumulations of wax in the ear canal. Their use on their own may be sufficient or the ear may also require syringing. |

**When to refer**

- History or suspicion of a perforated eardrum
- Abnormal lesion/blister/ulcers
- Persistent vertigo
- Tinnitus
- Eustachian catarrh before air travel
- Foreign body in ear canal (even if only a suspicion)
- Discharge from the ear canal
- Contraindication to use of ear drops such as dermatitis, erythema or irritation in the ear canal
- Persistent wax
- Pain within the ear
- Profuse bleeding from or bruising of the pinna (refer to Accident and Emergency department)
- Any trauma or swelling of the pinna
- Redness of the pinna, unless due to allergic eczema
- Reported ear problems that are accompanied by nausea and vomiting or nick stiffness

## Oral health

Before reading further, consider the following case and note your initial thoughts.

**Case study**

A 20-year-old man asks for advice because he has had a painful mouth for the last 3 days.

**Trigger questions**

- What additional information would you need before considering the appropriate management options in this case?
- What issues concern you about this case?
- Are any alarm symptoms being exhibited that require more urgent treatment or referral?

### Assessing symptoms

In the case of someone presenting with oral pain, it is always useful to ask to examine the area that is painful. This will allow you to use what you see to aid in making a diagnosis and deciding whether to treat or refer.

It is important to assess the location of the pain as different conditions will present with pain in different areas. Pain is common with mouth ulcers and they can occur anywhere within the oral cavity. Sufferers will often comment that certain foods can aggravate the pain and the uncomfortable feeling they experience. The most common type of ulcer is the minor aphthous ulcer, which usually appears as small yellow areas that are often surrounded by an inflamed area that may be red and sometimes swollen. Ulcers can occur on their own but commonly up to five can occur at any one time. Minor aphthous ulcers are usually self-limiting and resolve within 10 days. Major aphthous ulcers and herpetiform ulcers are less common and both can take several months to heal. Major aphthous ulcers are usually larger and can be 10 mm or more in diameter. Usually only one or two will appear at a time; however, these can be particularly painful and may be very troublesome. Herpetiform ulcers tend to be very small in size; however, many tend to appear at the same time, and they can often join together to form irregular shapes. Ulcers are usually easy to identify on investigation and often sufferers will have had similar symptoms before. Ulcers are more common in women than in men and although the cause is not known, ulcers can present in relation to other factors, such as changes in hormones, injury, ex-smokers, a lack of iron and anxiety or stress. Some medicines are also known to cause mouth ulcers, such as anti-inflammatory drugs and nicotine replacement therapy, and this should always be investigated during the course of a consultation.

Oral thrush can also present with a painful mouth that can affect eating and drinking if particularly painful and taste can also be altered in some cases. The classic symptom of oral thrush is the white spots that develop on the inside of the mouth and these can form plaques if they join together. It is usually possible to remove the spot; however, underneath will be red and some bleeding may occur around the area from where the spot has been removed. Oral thrush is caused by a yeast infection called *Candida*, however it is not contagious and cannot be passed to other people. This infection can also be present and affect the vaginal area, the nappy area and occasionally under the nails. Box 7.1 summarises some factors that predispose to oral thrush.

Pain is also a presenting symptom for gingivitis, where there is inflammation of the gums caused by bacteria. Other symptoms such as swelling, redness and bleeding are also usually present and often the breath can become foul-smelling.

---

**Box 7.1  Predisposing factors for oral thrush**

- Age – oral thrush is common in young babies and will often present with nappy rash.
- Having dentures – particularly if the dentures are not fitted correctly or if good hygiene advice is not followed.
- Antibiotics use – antibiotics affect the normal bacteria that live in the mouth and allow the *Candida* to grow much more easily.
- Steroid and inhaler use.
- Diabetes.
- Anaemia.
- Individuals who are immunocompromised.
- Smoking.

---

Toothache is a common presenting complaint. Sufferers of toothache will typically complain of continuous pain, usually throbbing in nature. The pain may be exacerbated by hot, cold or sweet foods or drinks and some sufferers may have difficulty discerning which tooth is causing the pain. In many instances there may be an obviously carious or broken tooth. Toothache may also arise as a result of a lost restoration (filling), or from a heavily or recently restored tooth. Sufferers may also comment that their outer cheek looks swollen around the painful area, and this may also be visible on investigation. Chapter 4 deals with analgesics in more depth.

## Accompanying symptoms

### Fever

A fever will often be present if an infection is the cause, and also in a child if they are teething. It may be appropriate to refer an adult with a fever for further investigation if an infection is suspected. For children, where teething is suspected, other symptoms such as drooling and red cheeks are also usually present and so symptomatic management would be appropriate.

### Bleeding

Bleeding is one of the symptoms that presents with gingivitis, and this condition needs to be diagnosed by a medical practitioner or a dentist in order to ascertain the cause and an appropriate course of treatment. Any bleeding in the mouth should be referred for investigation, unless it is suspected that a minor injury has caused it, for example if the tongue has been 'bitten'.

### Dry mouth (xerostomia)

Dry mouth can occur as the result of medication use; however, it can also occur due to damage to the salivary glands or due to dehydration or can be anxiety related. Dry mouth causes difficulties in chewing and tasting food, which therefore can impact upon appetite and nutritional intake, so resolution or management of the dry mouth is important to ensure that nutritional intake is not compromised.

Simple advice can be given to minimise the effects of dry mouth, such as sucking sugar-free sweets, or drinking regular sips of water or pineapple juice. However if it is suspected that medication is the cause, then referral to a relevant practitioner is necessary for further investigation. Lip dryness and occasionally cracking are also symptoms associated with xerostomia, which are due to the lack of saliva and general dryness of the area.

### Halitosis (bad breath)

The most common cause of bad breath is bacteria present in the mouth, which can occur due to infection, plaque or, in cases of poor oral hygiene, the build-up of food in the mouth. Sufferers will sometimes present with bad breath that occurs mainly in the morning and this is usually caused by the mouth becoming dry overnight. In this case, after a period of time it will clear owing to normal salivary function being resumed after waking or after eating breakfast. Sometimes medication, including nitrates and chemotherapy, can also cause bad breath and where this is thought to be the cause referral will be necessary.

### Smoking

Smokers are predisposed to a number of oral conditions as smoking affects the normal bacteria within the mouth, leaving smokers particularly susceptible to infections. This is also applicable to smokers who have recently quit smoking as the oral bacteria will have to readjust.

## Management options

For all oral health conditions, good oral hygiene is important in both the prevention and treatment of these conditions. It is also important to appreciate the interaction between diet and oral health, a balanced and varied diet reduces the risk of nutritional deficiencies, which show as symptoms in the mouth – e.g. angular stomatitis with B vitamin deficiencies, and dental caries with vitamin A deficiencies.

It is important that teeth are brushed regularly and it is recommended that teeth should be brushed at least twice a day. A soft brush should be used as well as a fluoride-containing toothpaste, unless fluoride is added to the water in their area. Toothbrushes should be replaced regularly. Flossing is also advised to clean the areas where a toothbrush does not reach.

As well as good oral hygiene measures, mouthwashes can be used on a daily basis with the aim of killing the bacteria that cause halitosis. Tongue cleaning may also be appropriate as the tongue may have a coating on it that contributes to the 'bad breath'. Although a toothbrush can be used to do this, tongue cleaners are also available that are more effective at removing the coating. If drug treatment is suspected to be causing symptoms of halitosis then the individual should be referred to their doctor for discussion about their treatment.

Smokers should be advised to quit smoking as not only does smoking increase the risk of gum disease but other common conditions like mouth ulcers are more common in those who smoke. Nicotine replacement therapy is available to aid smoking cessation, or other products such as bupropion and varenicline are available from the general practitioner (see Chapter 4).

It is important that individuals have regular dental checks, preferably at least once every year, where general oral health can also be observed.

If gingivitis is suspected, then general oral hygiene advice can be given; however, a referral is necessary to a doctor or dentist for an accurate diagnosis and appropriate treatment, as in severe cases antibiotics may be required to treat the bacterial infection.

General dietary advice will also help to alleviate a sore mouth, ensuring that nutritional intake is not compromised. Measures such as keeping the mouth fresh and clean, drinking plenty of fluids, eating soft, moist or liquidised foods that are easier to chew and swallow, or adding moisture to food using sauces and gravies and avoiding foods that hurt or irritate the mouth are all general measures that can be advised.

### Drugs for oral ulceration and inflammation (BNF section 12.3.1)

Symptomatic treatment such as a topical analgesic can be advised if ulcers are painful, for example, benzydamine spray or oral rinse. A barrier paste such as carmellose sodium can also be used to protect the ulcer and promote healing.

Various products containing a corticosteroid such as triamcinolone, betamethasone or hydrocortisone are useful in some forms of oral ulceration. In aphthous ulcers a corticosteroid is more effective in the prodromal phase.

Benzydamine mouthwash can be used to reduce pain in the oropharynx and it is thought it may also promote healing. Although mouthwashes can be used to maintain good oral hygiene, they will not prevent the occurrence of mouth ulcers.

## Oropharyngeal anti-infective drugs (BNF section 12.3.2)

Miconazole oral gel is the first-line treatment for oral thrush and should be used for 7 days. Treatment should be continued for 48 hours after symptoms have resolved. It is important that this product is used after a meal and a small amount should be applied to the affected area using a clean finger four times a day. Individuals should also be advised not to eat or drink for 30 minutes after application.

Other products such as nystatin and fluconazole may be prescribed by a doctor but this requires referral.

Miconazole treatment is also appropriate in babies, but it is only licensed for babies over 4 months of age. Any baby younger than this should be referred for treatment. If the baby is being breast fed, the mother should be advised that thrush can also affect the nipple area and referral would be appropriate if this happens. For bottle-fed babies, ensure that the parent is aware of good practice for cleaning bottles and that bottles are fully sterilised prior to use.

## Mouthwashes, gargles and dentrifices (BNF section 12.3.4)

Chlorhexidine mouthwash is a widely available mouthwash; it can stain the teeth during use, but this is not permanent. It is usually used twice daily and users should be advised to rinse the mouth for around 1 minute at each use. Dentures can be left to soak in the solution for 15 minutes twice daily. It is important to advise anyone using chlorhexidine mouthwash that it may be incompatible with some toothpastes and so at least 30 minutes should be left between using the mouthwash and brushing the teeth with toothpaste.

## Treatment of dry mouth (BNF section 12.3.5)

Artificial saliva treatments are available, although most are no more effective than the above measures and indeed one study has shown that sugar-free chewing gum is as effective as artificial saliva products. Chewing sugar-free chewing gum after meals is also an option for the treatment of halitosis. It is thought that the chewing increases the saliva flow, which in turn helps to break down and remove any remaining food left in the mouth after the meal.

The underlying cause should be identified and treated first. Where this is not possible, symptomatic treatment and general measures can be advised. Box 7.2 lists some measure that can help with dry mouth.

Anyone with persistent dry mouth despite implementing good oral hygiene and using the above general advice should be referred to their GP for further investigation, particularly where drug treatment is thought to be the cause.

---

**Box 7.2   Measures to help with dry mouth**

- Drinking small amounts of cool drinks frequently.
- Chewing sugar free chewing gum or sucking on pastilles or ice cubes.
- Lip moisturisers can be used to prevent drying and cracking of the lips.

---

 **Re-consider the case**

Before reading further, re-consider the following questions and your initial thoughts on this case.

**Trigger questions**

- What additional information would you need before considering the appropriate management options in this case?
- What issues concern you about this case?
- Are any alarm symptoms being exhibited that require more urgent treatment or referral?

**Case study**

A 20-year-old man asks for advice because he has had a painful mouth for the last 3 days.

### Pharmacist opinion

In people of this age, mouth pain is often caused by mouth ulcers. These can often be seen during a simple examination of the mouth and usually appear as yellow spots, often with inflamed areas around them on the inside of the cheek. Individuals may present with only one ulcer or up to five may occur at any one time. Although ulcers are usually self-limiting to around 7–10 days, symptomatic treatment such as products containing a local anaesthetic can be offered to this man. A mouthwash could also be suggested as a suitable option for treatment, which will help ease the pain. If the ulcers are recurring despite treatment and good oral hygiene, then referral may be appropriate to rule out any underlying causes. Pain may also present with gingivitis, but this would usually be limited to the gum area where the infection has caused inflammation and a simple examination of the mouth would allow this to be investigated.

### General practitioner opinion

This is quite an unusual situation in the general practice setting. Questions to ask would be: Is it a generalised pain or local to a specific area of the mouth? Has this pain occurred before? Are there any dental problems? Is the sufferer using regular medications or inhalers?

Differential diagnoses here would include simple mouth ulcers, dental problems, hygiene issues, oral thrush, and ulcers related to chronic disease.

Examination of the mouth and pharynx is simple and may reveal very clearly the cause of pain.

### Summary of key points

| Condition | Management |
| --- | --- |
| Mouth ulcers are common and occur as yellow spots on the inside of the mouth, often accompanied by pain and sensitivity. | Good oral hygiene is recommended in all cases of mouth ulcers and people with mouth ulcers should be advised to avoid aggravating foods. Mouthwashes can be used to reduce pain and symptomatic treatment such as local analgesia is also available. |
| Oral thrush is characterised by 'white spots' seen on the inside of the mouth. | Miconazole gel is available to treat oral thrush and should be used for 7 days. Children under 4 months should be referred for treatment. |
| Gingivitis is caused by bacteria that subsequently cause inflammation of the gums. | Referral is necessary to make a diagnosis. Good oral hygiene should be advised, but in some cases antibiotic therapy is necessary to treat the infection. |

### When to refer

- Unexplained ulceration lasting longer than 3 weeks
- Oral symptoms are lasting longer than 6 weeks and a diagnosis cannot be made
- Suspected underlying pathology
- Suspected gingivitis
- Failure of treatment or no improvement of symptoms
- Children under 4 months of age with oral thrush
- Persistent bleeding of the gums
- Ill-fitting dentures causing oral pain or irritation

# Bibliography

Bandolier (2004). Treating earwax – a systematic review. *Bandolier 130*. Available from: http://www.medicine.ox.ac.uk/bandolier/painres/download/Bando130.pdf (accessed 31 March 2011).

Doughty MJ (2002). Levocabastine, a topical ocular antihistamine available as a pharmacy medicine – a literature review. *Pharm J* 268: 367–370.

Douglas G, Nicol F, Robertson C, eds (2005). *MacLeod's Clinical Examination*. Edinburgh: Churchill Livingstone.

Everitt H, Little P (2002). How do GPs diagnose and manage acute infective conjunctivitis? A GP survey. *Fam Pract* 19: 658–660.

Hand C, Harvey I (2004). The effectiveness of topical preparations for the treatment of earwax: a systematic review. *Br J Gen Pract* 54(508): 862–867.

Kumar P, Clark M, eds (2005). *Clinical Medicine*. London: Elsevier Saunders.

Little P *et al.* (2001). Pragmatic randomised controlled trial of two prescribing strategies for childhood acute otitis media. *Br Med J* 322: 336–341.

National Institute for Health and Clinical Excellence (2011). *Clinical Knowledge Summary: Conjunctivitis – Infective*. London: NICE. Available from: http://www.cks.nhs.uk/conjunctivitis_infective/background_information/prevalence (accessed 31 March 2011).

Owen CG *et al.* (2004). Topical treatment for seasonal allergic conjunctivitis: systematic review and meta-analysis of efficacy and effectiveness. *Br J Gen Pract* 54: 451–456.

Rose P (2007). Management strategies for acute infective conjunctivitis in primary care: a systematic review. *Expert Opin Pharmacother* 8(12): 1903–1921.

Scully C, Shotts R (2000). ABC of oral health: mouth ulcers and other causes of orofacial soreness and pain. *Br Med J* 321: (7254) 162–165.

# Self-assessment questions

The following questions are provided to test the information presented in this chapter.

*For questions 1–7 select the best answer in each case.*

1. Select which is the most common cause of a red eye:
   a. Blepharitis
   b. Conjunctivitis
   c. Stye
   d. Iritis
   e. Glaucoma

2. Select which of the following is the most common causative organism of bacterial conjunctivitis:
   a. *Mycoplasma pneumoniae*
   b. *Escherichia coli*
   c. *Streptococcus pneumoniae*
   d. *Staphylococcus aureus*
   e. *Klebsiella pneumoniae*

3. Select which of the following acts to equalise pressure in the middle ear:
   a. Eustachian tube
   b. Tympanic membrane
   c. Tragus
   d. Pinna
   e. Ossicles

4. Select which of the following would not require referral for medical treatment:
   a. Suspected perforated eardrum
   b. Tinnitus
   c. Eustachian catarrh
   d. Trauma to the pinna
   e. Persistent vertigo

5. Select which of the following is most likely to precede acute otitis media:
   a. Allergic conjunctivitis
   b. Tinnitus
   c. Vertigo
   d. Common cold
   e. Barotrauma

6. Select which of the following does not describe minor aphthous ulcers:
   a. Ulcers usually resolve within 10 days
   b. Ulcers are usually more than 10 mm in diameter
   c. Pain is a common presenting symptom
   d. They occur more commonly in women
   e. Stress and smoking are thought to be contributing factors

7. Select which of the following would not require referral:
   a. A 3-month-old baby presenting with symptoms of oral thrush
   b. A woman who is taking prednisolone tablets and complaining of mouth ulcers occurring regularly
   c. Someone who has dentures presenting with painful gums
   d. A 20-year-old man presenting with four small mouth ulcers
   e. A man who is complaining of sore and bleeding gums

*For questions 8–10 select from the list below one lettered option that is most closely related to it. Each lettered option may be used once, more than once, or not at all.*
   a. deafness
   b. pain
   c. itching
   d. bleeding and bruising
   e. fever

8. Is caused by an obstruction in the external ear canal.

9. Is a common sign of infection in otitis media.

10. Is associated with a furuncle in the external ear canal.

*For questions 11 and 12 select from the list below one lettered option that is most closely related to it. Each lettered option may be used once, more than once, or not at all.*

    a. chlorhexidine
    b. miconazole
    c. artificial saliva
    d. benzydamine
    e. sugar free chewing gum

11. Is first line treatment for oral thrush.

12. Can be advised for individuals who have symptoms of halitosis.

*Questions 13–16: Each of the questions or incomplete statements in this section is followed by three responses. For each question one or more of the responses is/are correct. Decide which of the responses is/are correct and then choose a–e as indicated in the table below.*

| a | b | c | d | e |
|---|---|---|---|---|
| If 1, 2 and 3 are correct | If 1 and 2 only are correct | If 2 and 3 only are correct | If 1 only is correct | If 3 only is correct |

13. The following are appropriate treatments for bacterial conjunctivitis:
    1 – chloramphenicol eye drops
    2 – chloramphenicol eye ointment
    3 – levocabastine eye drops

14. The following are appropriate treatments for the removal of ear wax:
    1 – sodium bicarbonate
    2 – urea hydrogen peroxide
    3 – almond oil

15. The following are measures for ensuring good oral hygiene:
    1 – use a hard toothbrush
    2 – brush the teeth at least twice daily
    3 – use a fluoride toothpaste if fluoride is not added to the water supply

16. The following is appropriate advice for individuals presenting with xerostomia:
    1 – use a moisturiser to prevent cracking of the lips
    2 – drink small amounts of cool drinks frequently
    3 – use sugar-free chewing gum

*Questions 17–20 consist of two statements linked by the word* because; *decide whether each statement is true or false. If both statements are true then decide whether the second statement is a correct explanation of the first statement. Choose a–e as your answer as indicated in the table below.*

## Directions summarised

| | First statement | Second statement | |
|---|---|---|---|
| a | True | True | Second statement is a correct explanation of the first statement |
| b | True | True | Second statement is not a correct explanation of the first statement |
| c | True | False | |
| d | False | True | |
| e | False | False | |

17.

| | | |
|---|---|---|
| Individuals presenting with symptoms of inflammation and bleeding of the gums should be referred | BECAUSE | Individuals who are suspected to have gingivitis need to be referred for an accurate diagnosis |

18.

| | | |
|---|---|---|
| Babies who are under 1 year should be referred to the doctor if they have symptoms of oral thrush | BECAUSE | Products used to treat oral thrush are only licensed for use over 1 year of age |

19.

| | | |
|---|---|---|
| A person complaining of a deep-seated pain in the eye should be referred to their general practitioner | BECAUSE | Deep-seated pain in the eye can be a sign of raised intra-ocular pressure |

20.

| | | |
|---|---|---|
| A person with a perforated eardrum should always be referred to their general practitioner | BECAUSE | Perforated eardrums can lead to chronic infection of the ear |

## Answers

1-b; 2-d; 3-a; 4-c; 5-d; 6-b; 7-d; 8-a; 9-e; 10-b; 11-b; 12-e; 13-b; 14-a; 15-c; 16-a; 17-a; 18-e; 19-a; 20-a

# 8

# Nutrition

*Susan Lennie*

| This chapter will cover the following conditions: | This chapter will cover the following groups of medicines: |
| --- | --- |
| • Malnutrition<br>• Hyperlipidaemias | • Iron products<br>• Folic acid<br>• Minerals, vitamins and multivitamins<br>• Oral rehydration therapy<br>• Statins<br>• Dietary supplements |

In this chapter we will consider nutritional disorders and conditions that may be encountered in community pharmacy, and may merit pharmacological intervention in their management.

## Malnutrition

By definition, malnutrition includes any deviation from what is considered 'normal' nutrition. Con-trary to popular belief, therefore, overweight and obese individuals are also classed as malnourished. This section will explore the assessment of nutritional status, and consider undernutrition and nutritional deficiencies and the pharmaceutical products that can be used in their management. Consideration of overweight and obesity can be found in Chapter 4.

Before reading further, consider the following case and note your initial thoughts.

**Case study**

A 27-year-old woman attends the pharmacy and reports feeling fatigued for the last few weeks; she feels she looks drawn and pale. Her appetite has been a little poor. She asks whether there are any supplements that you could recommend that would help her increase her energy levels. In particular, she is concerned about her iron levels as she has a history of anaemia. You observe that she is slim and has a pale and dull complexion with dark circles under her eyes.

**Trigger questions**

- What additional information would you need before considering the appropriate management options in this case?
- What issues concern you about this case?
- Are any alarm symptoms being exhibited that require more urgent treatment or referral?

## Assessing symptoms

Fatigue is a very non-specific term used to describe either physical or mental weakness or tiredness. Although it may be present in a range of medical conditions or as a side effect of various medications, other factors such as recent exercise, lifestyle, lack of sleep and work pressures render it too vague in itself to be a useful diagnostic criterion.

Pallor describes a paleness of the skin. It can develop suddenly or gradually, depending upon the cause, which may include emotional shock or stress, illness, stimulant use, lack of exposure to sunlight, anaemia, or genetics, but is generally not clinically significant.

Appetite refers to the psychological desire for food. Deterioration in appetite (poor appetite) may present in physical illnesses, during periods of emotional stress, or as a result of drug treatment. A reduced appetite may not necessarily limit food intake to a large extent because hunger – which is the unpleasant physiological drive for food – or habit may ensure that nutritional needs are met.

It is important for the community pharmacist to identify individuals whose food intake is significantly restricted and to explore the possible reasons for the restriction. This will aid in deciding whether a referral to the GP is required.

In some cases, deliberate restriction of food intake, as in the cases of anorexia nervosa and bulimia nervosa, may be suspected. The SCOFF questions (Box 8.1) are a simple screening tool to aid in

> **Box 8.1    The SCOFF questions (Morgan *et al* 2000)**
>
> - Do you make yourself **S**ick because you feel uncomfortably full?
> - Do you worry you have lost **C**ontrol over how much you eat?
> - Have you recently lost more than **O**ne stone in a 3-month period?
> - Do you believe yourself to be **F**at when others say you are too thin?
> - Would you say that **F**ood dominates your life?

the identification of these eating disorders and may be appropriate for use in a one-to-one consultation. One point is scored for every 'yes' answer. A score of ≥2 indicates a likely case of anorexia nervosa or bulimia nervosa.

## Other considerations

It is often useful to obtain a weight history to determine the significance of any weight loss that has been reported. This is usually presented as a percentage of usual body weight and calculated using the formula:

$$\% \text{ weight loss} = \frac{\text{usual weight(kg)} - \text{current weight(kg)}}{\text{usual weight(kg)}} \times 100$$

In 2007 the Parenteral and Enteral Nutrition Group provided guidance on the interpretation of

| Table 8.1 | Weight loss as a percentage of pre-illness weight and interpretation (Todorovic and Micklewright, 2007) |
|---|---|
| <5% | Not significant unless likely to be on-going |
| 5–9% | Not serious (unless rapid/ already malnourished) |
| 10–20% | Clinically significant: nutritional support |
| >20% | Severe: long terms aggressive nutritional support |

The more rapid the decline in weight, the greater the proportion of lean: fat tissue that is lost and the more significant the loss. Very rapid weight loss (within days rather than weeks) is most likely to be fluid.

percentage weight loss to determine action that may need to be taken (see Table 8.1).

Diarrhoea and vomiting are also other symptoms that may present and these are considered in more depth in Chapters 2 and 4.

## Assessing nutritional status

To obtain a full picture of nutritional status, one must consider both adipose tissue stores and nutrient stores within the body. The assessment of each of these can vary in complexity, with simple but often non-specific tests or observations being available to the pharmacist.

The body mass index (discussed in Chapter 4) is a simple tool to assess and classify body fatness. At a BMI of <18.5 kg/m2, an individual is considered to be underweight and is likely to require dietary advice or support to restore body weight to within normal ranges. However, a poor nutritional status involving nutritional deficiencies or protein-energy malnutrition may exist at any level of BMI. Indeed, the 'well-nourished' appearance often causes healthcare professionals to assume good nutritional status when in fact the opposite may be true. Therefore it is essential to consider the wider picture.

'MUST' is a five-step screening tool for use in hospitals, community and other care settings by all care workers, to identify adults who are malnourished, at risk of malnutrition (undernutrition), or obese. Contained within the tool (Figure 8.1) are management guidelines, that can be used to develop a care plan. The community pharmacist may wish to use this tool as a simple screening method to determine suitability for supply of supplements containing protein and energy or the need for referral to the GP.

(The Malnutrition Universal Screening Tool ('MUST') is reproduced here with the kind permission of the British Association of Parenteral and Enteral Nutrition. For further information on 'MUST' see www.bapen.org.uk.)

Through a balanced, varied diet, such as one that follows the principles of the Eat Well Plate (see Chapter 4), an individual is generally likely to meet all of their micronutrient requirements. There are some circumstances, such as during pregnancy and lactation, when micronutrient requirements change, but for the most part the body has adaptive responses that alter absorption to ensure that micronutrient needs are still met. Increasingly, however, the general population are turning to supplementing their diet with vitamins and minerals in the belief that 'more is better', or as an alternative to improving overall diet quality. The former group are generally classified as the 'worried well'; however, care needs to be taken to ensure that supplement use does not lead to toxicity. In the latter group, supplements may be beneficial, but dietary advice should always be provided as the complex matrix of foods provides many health benefits beyond the direct effect of vitamins and minerals.

Nutritional deficiencies may arise as a result of both organic and inorganic causes and determination of precipitating factors is essential to ensure that treatment does not inappropriately mask any underlying major disease. Observation of symptoms is not necessary for a nutritional deficiency to be present, and in many cases symptoms only appear at extreme levels of deficiency. The appearance of clinical symptoms in adults is likely to suggest a chronic state of deficiency. In children clinical symptoms may develop much more quickly because of their lower body stores.

Some dietary choices may increase the risk of nutritional deficiencies arising, particularly when individuals embark on dietary changes without fully exploring the necessary steps required to ensure that a balanced intake is still maintained. For example, in the 2009 UK Food Standards Agency 'Public Attitudes to Food Issues' survey, 3% of respondents stated that they were fully vegetarian, with a further

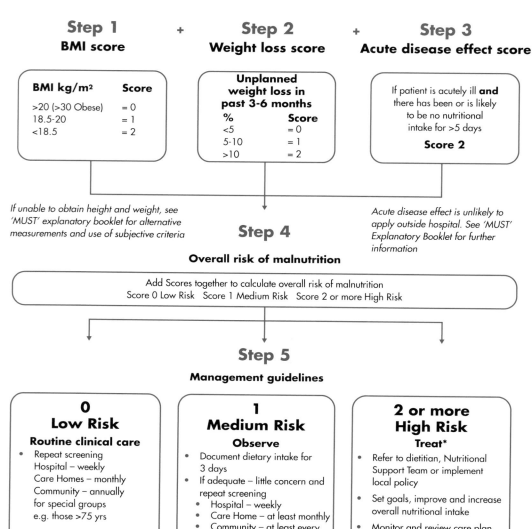

**Step 1**
**BMI score**

| BMI kg/m² | Score |
|---|---|
| >20 (>30 Obese) | = 0 |
| 18.5-20 | = 1 |
| <18.5 | = 2 |

+

**Step 2**
**Weight loss score**

Unplanned weight loss in past 3-6 months

| % | Score |
|---|---|
| <5 | = 0 |
| 5-10 | = 1 |
| >10 | = 2 |

+

**Step 3**
**Acute disease effect score**

If patient is acutely ill **and** there has been or is likely to be no nutritional intake for >5 days

**Score 2**

*If unable to obtain height and weight, see 'MUST' explanatory booklet for alternative measurements and use of subjective criteria*

*Acute disease effect is unlikely to apply outside hospital. See 'MUST' Explanatory Booklet for further information*

**Step 4**

**Overall risk of malnutrition**

Add Scores together to calculate overall risk of malnutrition
Score 0 Low Risk   Score 1 Medium Risk   Score 2 or more High Risk

**Step 5**

**Management guidelines**

**0**
**Low Risk**

**Routine clinical care**
- Repeat screening
  Hospital – weekly
  Care Homes – monthly
  Community – annually
  for special groups
  e.g. those >75 yrs

**1**
**Medium Risk**

**Observe**
- Document dietary intake for 3 days
- If adequate – little concern and repeat screening
  - Hospital – weekly
  - Care Home – at least monthly
  - Community – at least every 2-3 months
- If inadequate – clinical concern – follow local policy, set goals, improve and increase overall nutritional intake, monitor and review care plan regularly

**2 or more**
**High Risk**

**Treat***
- Refer to dietitian, Nutritional Support Team or implement local policy
- Set goals, improve and increase overall nutritional intake
- Monitor and review care plan Hospital – weekly
  Care Home – monthly
  Community – monthly
- Unless detrimental or no benefit is expected from nutritional support e.g. imminent death.

**All risk categories:**
- Treat underlying condition and provide help and advice on food choices, eating and drinking when necessary.
- Record malnutrition risk category.
- Record need for special diets and follow local policy.

**Obesity:**
- Record presence of obesity. For those with underlying conditions, these are generally controlled before the treatment of obesity.

**Re-assess subjects identified at risk as they move through care settings**
See The 'Must' Explanatory Booklet for further details and The 'Must' Report for supporting evidence.

**Figure 8.1**   BAPEN Malnutrition Universal Screening Tool (MUST).

5% stating they were partly vegetarian. Without appropriate planning, vegetarian diets may increase risk of deficiencies in a range of nutrients, including vitamin B$_{12}$, iron and calcium.

## Management options

Various vitamin and mineral preparations are available without prescription; however, caution should be shown when supplying these products. Individuals should always be encouraged to ensure a balanced diet, which should provide all necessary vitamins and minerals. However, there may be some cases where additional supplementation is appropriate, either of single vitamins or minerals or, more likely, multivitamins with or without minerals. Indeed, research continues to identify benefits of specific supplementation.

### Oral iron (BNF section 9.1.1.1)

Iron is an oxygen carrier in haemoglobin in blood and myglobin in muscle. It is required for a number of metabolic processes, including having a central role in cell energy metabolism and an essential component of some enzymes. The human body has no mechanism for iron excretion, so body stores are primarily regulated by absorption. Typical absorption from a balanced diet is approximately 15%, but mechanisms exist to increase this in various situations, such as during pregnancy, and decrease it when there is sufficiency.

Iron deficiency anaemia is very common throughout the world, and is particularly found in women. It is usually slow in producing clinical signs, so haematological tests such as serum ferritin, transferrin or haemoglobin levels are usually used to assess depletion. As haemoglobin levels fall, sufferers may present with pallor, breathlessness and fatigue.

Dietary iron exists in haem and non-haem forms. Haem iron is found in animal foods, for example red meat, offal and, to a lesser extent, poultry and fish. Although it is being consumed in small quantities, haem iron is absorbed well by the body and generally contributes 20–30% of absorbed iron (though not in vegetarians and vegans). Non-haem iron, found in grain products, fortified breakfast cereals, green leafy vegetables, pulses, dried fruits, nuts and seeds, is much less efficiently absorbed and benefits from enhanced absorption in the presence of vitamin C-containing foods such as fruit, fruit juices and potatoes.

Where dietary intake is insufficient or clinical signs of deficiency exist, supplementation may be required in addition to basic dietary advice. Oral iron supplements are classed as P medicines and as such can be supplied from pharmacies without a prescription. Oral iron is available in three different salts; sulphate, fumarate and gluconate. The choice of which salt to use is less important: the effectiveness of oral iron supplementation is related to the dose of elemental iron provided by the product. However, it is also related to the incidence of gastrointestinal side effects; the higher the dose of elemental iron, the higher the risk of experiencing side effects.

Given the slow onset of clinical signs of iron deficiency anaemia, it is important to establish an accurate diagnosis before commencing oral supplementation to ensure that this does not mask the signs of another disease state such as megaloblastic anaemia. Therefore, the supply of oral iron supplements from the pharmacy is best restricted to those with an established diagnosis, e.g. in women who know that they develop iron deficiency anaemia due to heavy bleeding during their periods.

### Calcium supplements (BNF section 9.5.1.1)

Calcium is the most abundant body mineral and is necessary for the maintenance of skeletal structures and for other cellular roles. Calcium requirements are increased during the growth periods of infancy and adolescence. Requirements fall after peak bone mass has been achieved at around 25 years of age, so maximising dietary calcium intake before this time is extremely important in reducing the risk of osteoporosis later in life. Calcium absorption is enhanced by lactose, so milk and dairy products provide the highest bioavailability of calcium. However, calcium is also found in fish containing soft bones (e.g. tinned sardines or pilchards), green leafy vegetables (except spinach, which inhibits calcium absorption owing to a high oxalate content), cereals and cereal products, nuts, pulses and seeds, calcium-enriched soya drinks and tap water in hard-water areas. Vitamin D also enhances the absorption of calcium

Calcium supplements are usually only required when dietary intake is insufficient. This may be seen in those individuals who avoid milk and dairy products and do not adequately increase their calcium intake from non-dairy sources, or in those with higher requirements, such as in coeliac disease.

Oral calcium supplements are also classed as non-prescription medicines and therefore can be supplied from pharmacies without a prescription. They are predominantly available as calcium carbonate, but other salts are also available. The various calcium supplement products vary in the amount of calcium that they provide. Vitamin D is often taken in conjunction to enhance absorption.

### Phosphorus and zinc (BNF sections 9.5.2 and 9.5.4)

Other minerals, such as phosphate and zinc, are also available to supply as non-prescription medicines. Deficiency is unlikely in healthy individuals, and identification of any deficiency would usually involve a medical practitioner who would instigate treatment related to the underlying cause.

### Single vitamins (BNF section 9.6)

Vitamins are used for the prevention and treatment of specific deficiency states, or where the diet is known to be inadequate. In the community pharmacy, it is unlikely that sufficient evidence would exist to supply single vitamins as dietary supplements. Indeed, particular preparations, such as those containing vitamin A, may actually be harmful to individuals if taken at higher than recommended levels.

### Vitamin B group (BNF section 9.6.2)

Vitamin $B_{12}$ (cobalamin) is involved in the recycling of folate coenzymes and valine metabolism. Deficiency of vitamin $B_{12}$ causes pernicious anaemia, presenting with neurological symptoms and damage, and megaloblastic anaemia similar to that seen in folate deficiency.

The main contributors to dietary vitamin $B_{12}$ are milk and dairy products, fortified breakfast cereals, and meat and meat products. Dietary deficiency is rare as vitamin $B_{12}$ can be stored within the liver; therefore, presentation with vitamin $B_{12}$ deficiency usually indicates a problem, most likely linked to intrinsic factor production in the stomach, requiring further investigation.

Cyanocobalamin is the only oral form of vitamin $B_{12}$ but there is little place for its use. The *British National Formulary* advises that this drug is less

suitable for prescribing and where there is a vitamin B deficiency treatment should be with hydroxocobalamin injection, which is only available on prescription.

### Folate (BNF section 9.1.2)

The term 'folate' refers to the compounds derived from folic acid. Folate is part of the vitamin B complex ($B_9$) and has two known important biological roles. It acts as a cofactor for enzymes essential in the synthesis of DNA and RNA, and is required in the transfer of methyl groups in the amino acid methylation cycle, a key step in the recycling of homocysteine back to methionine. Humans are unable to synthesise folate and therefore must rely on exogenous sources to provide it. Rich dietary sources of folate include liver, green leafy vegetables, such as kale and spinach, and also fortified cereal products. Natural sources of folate, from food, require conversion from polyglutamates to monoglutamates in the upper small intestine in order to be absorbed. However, synthetic folic acid supplements contain only monoglutamates and therefore are more stable and provide better bioavailability, although they are metabolised slightly differently from folate.

There are a number of factors that may increase the risk for low folate status. These include: smoking; non-use of vitamin-mineral supplements when dietary intake is low; pregnancy; oral contraceptive use; and high parity. Deficiency can cause megaloblastic anaemia.

Folic acid is available in two different tablet strengths; 400 microgram and 5 milligram tablets. The 5 milligram tablet is only available on prescription, but the 400 microgram strength can be supplied by pharmacies provided the daily dose does not exceed 500 micrograms.

The most common use for the 400 microgram strength tablet is as a supplement taken by women before and up to the twelfth week of pregnancy to reduce the risk of conceiving a child with neural tube defects. The 400 microgram dose is only appropriate for women who are at a low-risk of conceiving a child with neural tube defects. Box 8.2 describes the situations where there is a higher risk of conceiving a child with neural tube defects and women who fall into this group should be advised to take a 5 milligram dose of folic acid, which would require to be prescribed on a prescription.

**Box 8.2** **Higher-risk groups for conceiving a child with neural tube defects**

**Woman**

- Has coeliac disease (or other malabsorption state)
- Has diabetes mellitus
- Has sickle-cell anaemia
- Is taking antiepileptic drugs

**Couple**

- Either partner has a neural tube defect
- Either partner has a family history of neural tube defect
- A previous pregnancy affected by a neural tube defect

### Multivitamins (BNF section 9.6.7)

Multivitamin preparations, with and without minerals, are also available and these products are more likely to be requested by the general public than single vitamins. They may be useful for generalised dietary inadequacies; however, routine supplementation has not been shown to be beneficial.

Particular populations, such as children aged 6 months to 5 years, require extra vitamins A, C and D; however, this may need to commence earlier if the mother's vitamin status during pregnancy was considered to be low. Multivitamin preparations containing vitamins A, B group, C and D are available in a liquid formulation as drops and are suitable for this population. Pregnant and breastfeeding women are also recommended to take additional vitamin D but this usually should be taken as a multivitamin preparation (excluding vitamin A).

### Oral preparations for fluid and electrolyte imbalance (BNF section 9.2.1)

If vomiting or diarrhoea is present, it is important to advise steps to prevent or correct dehydration. In mild cases, for adults, increased fluids, including salty soups and fruit juices, may suffice. However, in children, and in the management of severe vomiting or diarrhoea in adults, oral rehydration solutions are important products. They contain electrolytes and glucose, which are actively absorbed across the intestinal epithelium, taking water and chloride with them. The products are sold as sachets of powders that require mixing with water according to the manufacturer's instructions (to prevent overloading). They are particularly suitable for babies and children. However, for the mild degree of dehydration suffered by babies and children who commonly present to pharmacists, they are not essential and water alone will provide the necessary degree of hydration. A simple rule of thumb is to give one cupful of solution for every loose stool to babies under 1 year and two cupfuls for older children.

### Other dietary supplements

In cases where poor nutritional intake or weight loss is apparent but appears to be short term or have no unexplained underlying factors, it may be appropriate to recommend an energy and protein supplement. Various products exist on prescription, but the pharmacist may wish to supply first-line non-prescription products such as Build Up or Complan. These are available as powdered supplements reconstituted with milk or water, into shakes or soups, and can be consumed between meals as supplements or, on occasion, can replace meals when appetite is poor. They provide a range of vitamins and minerals, as well as energy and protein; however, they are not adequate to meet full macro- and micro-nutrient requirements.

**Re-consider the case**

Before reading further, re-consider the following questions and your initial thoughts on this case.

**Trigger questions**

- What additional information would you need before considering the appropriate management options in this case?

**Re-consider the case** (*continued*)

- What issues concern you about this case?
- Are any alarm symptoms being exhibited that require more urgent treatment or referral?

**Case study**

A 27-year-old woman attends the pharmacy and reports feeling fatigued for the last few weeks; she feels she looks drawn and pale. Her appetite has been a little poor. She asks whether there are any supplements that you could recommend that would help her increase her energy levels. In particular, she is concerned about her iron levels as she has a history of anaemia. You observe that she is slim and has a pale and dull complexion with dark circles under her eyes.

Dietitian opinion

The age of this woman, her clinical symptoms, and the history of anaemia are all suggestive that iron deficiency anaemia is present; however, clarification with a GP is advisable. The underlying reasons for iron deficiency may lie in poor dietary intake or high menstrual blood losses, or may indicate a more sinister pathology. Her poor appetite should be explored to determine whether this has impacted upon her nutritional intake, and whether this is simply a product of her recent fatigue. Any recent weight loss should be quantified, and BMI calculated. If necessary, she may benefit from short-term use of energy and protein supplements such as Build Up or Complan, but any significant unexplained weight loss is likely to indicate a need for referral to the GP.

If iron supplements have previously been used, then a non-prescription supply may be appropriate, and is the most effective treatment for iron deficiency anaemia; however, dietary iron intake should also be explored. Recommendations for increasing consumption of fortified breakfast cereals, red meat (if no dietary restriction) and green leafy vegetables should be made. This woman should also be made aware that iron supplementation can increase constipation symptoms, so adequate fluid and fibre intake should be encouraged. If diet quality appears generally inadequate, she may prefer a multivitamin with iron preparation, but a focus on improving diet quality should again be emphasised.

Pharmacist opinion

In consulting with this woman it would be important to establish what is of most concern to her. Individuals often present in pharmacies with a history that appears vague and unspecific, and quite often looking for a 'tonic' to 'pick them up'.

Anaemias are the most common nutritional deficiencies, but determination of the specific type of anaemia is essential prior to initiating treatment. These may include iron deficiency anaemia, pernicious anaemia or megaloblastic anaemia. Certainly her description of feeling fatigued and her physical appearance of being pale are consistent with the presence of iron deficiency anaemia. However,

Pharmacist opinion (*continued*)

without a confirmed diagnosis and obvious cause she should be referred to her GP for a blood test to confirm whether she has iron deficiency anaemia.

In the absence of any specific reasons explaining these symptoms it would be inappropriate to recommend the use of individual vitamins or minerals. Assuming that the woman has a healthy balanced diet and has no malabsorption state, there is no need for supplementation of specific vitamins or minerals.

General practitioner opinion

Fatigue is probably the most common symptom presented to the general practitioner. It is important to note that this woman has a history of anaemia, but it is also important to understand her day-to-day life. Does she have children? Does she work and if so what type of work does she do? Is she studying for exams? Are any areas in her life causing stress? Why does she think she has lost her appetite? Does she have any sleeping problems? The answers to these questions will build up a broader picture of who this patient is and may reveal some reasons why she may feel fatigued.

A screening blood test is advisable in this case and would include a full blood count and thyroid function tests. If ferritin had been low previously, it would be worth including this in the initial tests. If iron deficiency was revealed in these screening tests, further action would be taken to identify the cause, e.g. coeliac disease, inflammatory bowel disease, poor dietary intake, heavy menstruation.

## Hyperlipidaemias

Cardiovascular disease is the major cause of death in the United Kingdom, being responsible for one-third of deaths. Cardiovascular disease comprises heart disease, stroke and circulatory disease, of which coronary heart disease (CHD) is the main form. The mortality rates for coronary heart disease have been falling in the last 25 years.

There are a number of modifiable and non-modifiable risk factors for cardiovascular disease and the reduction of modifiable risk factors should be undertaken as a holistic approach aimed at promoting healthy living.

Although hyperlipidaemias themselves are not strictly considered a minor illness, the reclassification of simvastatin to permit its supply without a prescription from pharmacies makes it worthy of consideration in this book. Its inclusion in this chapter recognises the importance of dietary modification in modifying the risk factors of those at low or moderate risk.

Before reading further, consider the following case and note your initial thoughts.

Case study

A 47-year-old man comes in to your pharmacy concerned about his cholesterol level. His older brother recently died of a myocardial infarction, at the age of 50, and he is concerned about his own cardiovascular disease risk. He reports that his GP measured his cholesterol about 6 months ago and it was slightly raised. He was advised to stop smoking, cut down his fat intake and lose a little weight, but

**Case study** (*continued*)

unfortunately he has not been very successful with these targets. You measure his weight and height at 102 kg and 1.79 m respectively.

**Trigger questions**

- What additional information would you need before considering the appropriate management options in this case?
- What issues concern you about this case?
- What health promotion issues affect this case?

## Assessing suitability for supply

The risk factors for cardiovascular disease are listed in Table 8.2.

### Non-modifiable risk factors

There are some risk factors that cannot be altered, such as age, male sex, pre-existing cardiovascular disease, family history and ethnicity.

In terms of age, CHD increases as both men and women get older, becoming significant in those over 55 years of age. This coincides with the increase in risk of CHD in women after the menopause, when the protective effect of the female sex hormones declines. The average age of the menopause is 51 years. An earlier menopause is associated with a higher risk of CHD than for other women of the same age. More recent evidence has shown that hormone replacement therapy is not protective against cardiovascular disease as previously thought. How-ever, men at any age are at a higher risk of CHD than women.

Coronary heart disease tends to run in families, and families with a number of members affected by cardiovascular disease at an early age have a higher risk than others. The increased risk of an individual with a close family member who has had CHD is estimated to be 1½ times greater than in an individual who has not.

Ethnicity also increases the risk of CHD, with people from the Indian subcontinent (India, Pakistan and Bangladesh) having an increased risk of CHD, estimated to be about 1½ times that of an individual who is not from that part of the world.

### Modifiable risk factors

As Table 8.2 demonstrates, there are a number of modifiable risk factors for cardiovascular disease.

The incidence of cardiovascular and coronary heart disease is about 50% higher in smokers than in non-smokers. Passive smoking is said to increase the risk by about 25%. Five years after cessation of smoking, the risks of CHD are said to be equivalent to those of non-smokers (see Chapter 4 for further information on smoking cessation).

Clinical trials have shown that a weight loss of 10 kg can reduce systolic blood pressure by 10 mmHg and diastolic blood pressure by 20 mmHg. Blood concentrations of high-density lipoprotein (HDL) cholesterol are increased and those of low-density lipoproteins (LDL) cholesterol reduced by weight loss, although the magnitude of this effect is sometimes quite small.

| Table 8.2 Cardiovascular disease risk factors | |
|---|---|
| **Non-modifiable risk factors** | **Modifiable risk factors** |
| • Age | • High blood cholesterol concentration |
| • Sex | • Smoking |
| • Family history | • Overweight/obesity |
| • South Asian ethnicity | • Diet |
| | • Physical activity |
| | • Diabetes |
| | • Hypertension |
| | • Alcohol intake |
| | • Stress |

It has been shown that lowering blood cholesterol levels reduces the morbidity and mortality of cardiovascular disease, and this appears to be unrelated to the baseline or pre-treatment level. However, it should be noted that raised blood cholesterol levels alone do not increase the risk of cardiovascular disease in the majority of people unless there are also other risk factors. It is very important to convey this message to the public. The national service framework target in the United Kingdom for total blood cholesterol is 5.0 mmol/litre, but this does not mean that every person who has blood cholesterol above this level should be given treatment. The average total cholesterol in men in the UK is approximately 5.8 mmol/litre, and over 75% of men will have total cholesterol greater than 5.0 mmol/litre. Measurement of total cholesterol levels alone can overestimate the risk of CHD. Therefore, hospital laboratories measure LDL cholesterol and the ratio of total cholesterol to HDL cholesterol levels, which give a better estimation of risk. It should be stressed that any attempts to lower blood cholesterol levels should be made as part of a lifestyle programme to reduce all risk factors for cardiovascular disease. The signs and symptoms described in Table 8.3 can be present in individuals who have very high cholesterol levels and if these are observed the individual should be referred for medical investigation.

A raised systolic or diastolic blood pressure is a risk factor for cardiovascular disease. This risk increases with age, and treatment of a raised blood pressure, particularly in the elderly, can result in significant reductions in morbidity and mortality.

## Management options

### Exercise

A lack of exercise is a risk factor for cardiovascular disease, and it has been shown that increasing exercise is beneficial against CHD and stroke through the beneficial action of supporting weight loss, reducing blood pressure and reducing blood lipids, by small amounts. The amount of exercise required is controversial, but it may be as little as one hour's walking per week to achieve measurable benefits. Ideally 30 minutes of moderate aerobic exercise on most days is the quoted norm, and 'moderate' is often defined as breathing harder and getting warmer than normal, but one should be able to talk and be active at the same time.

### Diet

A healthy diet for disease prevention should be encouraged for all individuals, not just those with pre-existing conditions. The cardioprotective ('Mediterranean') diet is recommended in primary and secondary prevention of cardiovascular diseases and should form a central part of the management of cardiovascular disease. The diet includes moderate intakes of fish, including oily fish, reductions in saturated fat (replaced by monounsaturated or polyunsaturated fats), high intakes of fruit and vegetables (for their antioxidant properties) and legumes, nuts and whole grain foods for their high fibre content, which helps to reduce fat absorption and promote gut transit; it also includes regular meals, moderate alcohol, limited salt and processed foods, and reductions in meat and meat products.

Oily fish contains omega-3 fatty acids, believed to be beneficial in reducing cardiovascular disease, and current recommendations are one to two portions of oily fish, such as mackerel, sardines or salmon, per week.

Olive oil contains monounsaturated fatty acids and is believed to be beneficial, being a component of the Mediterranean diet. Antioxidants, for example flavonoids, such as those occurring in red wine,

| Table 8.3 | Clinical features of dyslipidaemia |
| --- | --- |
| Feature | Description |
| Corneal arcus | An opaque, greyish, ring visible around the coloured part of the eye. |
| Xanthelasma | Small, soft, yellow cholesterol deposits found on the eyelids. |
| Xanthomata | Small, soft, deposits of cholesterol, usually seen in the Achilles tendon or as nodules in the tendons of the fingers (tendon xanthomata). Palmar xanthomata may be seen as yellow lines in the palmar creases and tuberous xanthomata present in the form of masses around the elbows or knees. At very high triglyceride levels, individuals may present with eruptive xanthomata, which appears as small, yellow skin nodules. |

are believed to have a beneficial effect on atherosclerotic plaques in arteries.

Changes in the diet will usually only produce a modest reduction in total blood cholesterol (of the order of 5% in individuals), but components such as olive oil and antioxidants may have beneficial effects that are not directly related to cholesterol levels.

Plant sterols and stanols have also been found to inhibit cholesterol absorption from the gastrointestinal tract and re-absorption of cholesterol from bile acids, showing a dose–response on cholesterol levels. At an optimal intake of 2.0–2.5 g/day, plant sterols or stanols have been shown to reduce LDL cholesterol by approximately 10% within 2–3 weeks. These are currently available in the form of supplemented spreads, yoghurts and milks, and are generally a well tolerated adjunctive therapy to dietary measures and statins. However, in those individuals with a limited food budget, the focus should be placed on other cardioprotective foods.

A moderate intake of alcohol is beneficial, but ingestion of more than 2–3 units per day is detrimental to health and causes increases in blood pressure, body weight and blood triglyceride levels, and an increased risk of CHD and liver disease.

Clinical trials have shown that reducing salt intake reduces blood pressure. Although these reductions will be small in the majority of people, a reduction of 5 mmHg can be critical for someone whose blood pressure lies around a critical threshold for treatment. The public should be educated that salt is present in many convenience and tinned foods, for example crisps, nuts, tinned meats and soups, and ready-made meals, although manufacturers have made significant advances in reducing the salt content of their products. Reducing the intake of these types of food as well as modest reductions in adding salt in cooking or at the table may be beneficial. As an alternative, individuals can be advised to try using more herbs and spices for flavouring food.

### Lipid-regulating drugs (BNF section 2.12)

Statins inhibit the enzyme 3-hydroxy-3-methylglutaryl coenzyme A (HMG-CoA) reductase which catalyses the conversion of HMG-CoA in the biosynthetic pathway of cholesterol in the liver. This results in an increase in the number of low-density lipoprotein (LDL) receptors and thus lowers the levels of LDL cholesterol and increases high-density lipoprotein (HDL) cholesterol levels in the blood.

It is claimed that 10 mg of simvastatin daily reduces LDL cholesterol by about 25%, and this equates to a fall of one-third in cardiovascular events such as angina attacks and myocardial infarctions. There may be other beneficial effects besides their cholesterol-modifying activity exerted by statins that contribute to the reduction in cardiovascular risk, for example an effect on smooth muscle proliferation in the arterial wall, or on platelet function.

Simvastatin 10 mg tablets can be supplied from pharmacies without prescription for primary prevention (i.e. reducing the risk of first coronary event) in individuals at moderate risk of coronary heart disease (approximately 10–15% risk of major events in 10 years).

In the United Kingdom, the National Institute for Health and Clinical Excellence (NICE) has recommended that statins be used for the primary prevention of cardiovascular disease in people with a 10-year risk of cardiovascular disease greater than 20% and for secondary prevention in those who have already had a coronary event. However, in these situations, NICE recommends a starting dose of 40 mg daily in comparison to the 10 mg maximum daily dose of simvastatin supplied as a P medicine.

Without measurement of blood cholesterol concentration, which is not a requirement for supplying simvastatin as a P medicine, the dose used in this product is arbitrary, and the benefit gained may be considerably less than optimal. The use of long-term or even lifelong self-medication must be carefully considered and the risks weighed against the potential benefits, including compliance, cost, side effects and interactions.

There is a cardinal rule that should not be forgotten when using statins: that they only modify one risk factor for cardiovascular disease, that of raised lipids. Other risk factors should not be forgotten, however, and the approach should be to modify all risk factors.

Statins generally have a high benefit-to-risk ratio. The most serious (although rare) adverse effects are myositis and rhabdomyolysis, which will manifest as muscle pain. These will be rare at a daily dose of 10 mg of simvastatin and are more common in higher doses. Other side effects complained of may be abdominal pain, constipation or diarrhoea, nausea and vomiting, flatulence, headache and peripheral neuropathy (such as a sensation of pins and needles).

Individuals should be cautioned to avoid grapefruit juice while taking some statins (e.g. simvastatin and atorvastatin) as it contains compounds that interfere with the enzymes involved in the drug metabolism and can result in a higher quantity of non-metabolised drug reaching the circulation, causing greater risk of side effects and toxicity. In common with all drugs there are individuals who should not be given simvastatin as a P medicine and who must first consult their GP before commencing any lipid lowering drugs; these are detailed in Box 8.3.

---

**Box 8.3  Cautions and contraindications for the use of simvastatin as a P medicine**

- Individuals who have cardiovascular disease
- Individuals who have diabetes
- Those who have a risk of CHD greater than 15% over 10 years
- Men over 70 years or women over 55 with a family history of CHD plus one other risk factor
- Those with familial hyperlipidaemia
- Those with high blood pressure (140/90), or any anyone who is being treated for hypertension by their doctor
- Women who are pregnant
- Those with liver or kidney disease
- Those with hypothyroidism
- Those with a family history of muscle disorders
- Those with unexplained chest pain
- People who have a high alcohol intake

---

**Re-consider the case**

Before reading further, re-consider the following questions and your initial thoughts on this case.

**Trigger questions**

- What additional information would you need before considering the appropriate management options in this case?
- What issues concern you about this case?
- What health promotion issues affect this case?

**Case study**

A 47-year-old Caucasian man comes in to your pharmacy concerned about his cholesterol level. His older brother recently died of a myocardial infarction, at the age of 50, and he is concerned about his own cardiovascular disease risk. He reports that his GP measured his cholesterol about 6 months ago and it was slightly raised. He was advised to stop smoking, cut down his fat intake and lose a little weight, but unfortunately he has not been very successful with these targets. You measure his weight and height at 102 kg and 1.79 m respectively.

Dietitian opinion

This man has a BMI of 31.8 kg/m², classifying him as obese. He also has a number of non-modifiable risk factors for cardiovascular disease such as being over 45 years old, being male, and having a family history of fatal myocardial infarction. Owing to the death of his brother recently, his motivation for improving his cholesterol levels, and reducing his cardiovascular disease risk, has increased and therefore he is likely to be much more receptive to dietary and lifestyle interventions. Clear dietary advice regarding reducing saturated fats and increasing antioxidant vitamins, soluble fibre and omega-3 fatty acids, together with supporting literature, should be provided. It is important that this gentleman understands that cholesterol reduction is only one risk factor and therefore he should also be encouraged to lose weight and strategies to support smoking cessation should be recommended to reduce his overall cardiovascular disease risk.

Pharmacist opinion

Individuals must be educated about the nature of their risk and encouraged to take measures themselves to reduce it. This means following a healthy lifestyle. However, this should not be misinterpreted as spartan, nor as anything requiring hard work except for the effort involved in making some adjustments to daily routines. Any changes made will in the end make an individual healthier, both now and, more importantly, in 10–20 years' time, when age-related illnesses begin to take their toll.

It is clear that this man is aware that he needs to make changes to his lifestyle in order to reduce his CHD risk, and he has made some effort to implement these changes. It would be important to spend time with this man and establish why he thinks he has been unsuccessful and to address these issues so that he feels supported in making these changes.

This man does fit the criteria for making a supply of simvastatin 10 mg daily from the pharmacy as he is over the age of 45 and has three risk factors for CHD, i.e. he is a smoker, has a family history of CHD, and currently has a BMI that classifies him as obese. While he reports that his GP has measured his cholesterol and informed him it was 'slightly raised', it is not known what the actual figure was and whether this was a measure of HDL, LDL or total cholesterol. If the man is particularly concerned about this, he should be referred to his GP to have these measured again. This highlights the importance of why pharmacists and general practitioners should agree a protocol for recommendations about supplying simvastatin as a P medicine and lifestyle advice given to individuals with a moderate risk of cardiovascular disease.

It is important to remember that the benefits of statins come only after long-term use (at least 3 years), but they need to be taken consistently for a lifetime and this requires great commitment and compliance. Statins are very effective, as many clinical trials and years of clinical use have shown; however, it may be more prudent for some individuals with limited finances to spend their money on supporting healthier food choices.

## Summary of key points

| Condition | Management |
|---|---|
| Iron deficiency | Needs investigation to establish cause and exact nature of deficiency.<br>Can be addressed by eating foods high in iron, e.g. red meats, fortified breakfasts cereals, green leafy vegetables.<br>Can be supplemented by oral iron supplements such as ferrous sulphate, fumarate or gluconate. |
| Calcium deficiency | Calcium is required for bone growth.<br>Calcium is found in dairy products and in non-dairy products such as fish with soft bones, green leafy vegetables.<br>Can be supplemented by oral calcium supplements such as calcium carbonate. |
| Folate deficiency | It is important to take folic acid prophylactically if planning to conceive a child.<br>Pre-conception folic acid supplementation reduces risk of neural tube defects.<br>Folic acid tablets are available as a P medicine (400 microgram tablets) and prescription-only medicine (5 milligram tablets). |
| Hyperlipidaemia | Is only one modifiable risk factor for coronary heart disease.<br>Lifestyle changes are required to reduce the risk of coronary heart disease.<br>Simvastatin can be supplied from pharmacies for the primary prevention of coronary heart disease. |

# Bibliography

BAPEN (2011). *Malnutrition Universal Screening Tool.* Redditch: BAPEN Available from http://www.bapen.org.uk/pdfs/must/must_full.pdf (accessed 4 April 2011).

Complan (2011). *Complan Product Overview.* London: Complan Foods Limited. Available from: http://www.complanfoods.com/complan_overview.php (accessed 4 April 2011).

Food Standards Agency (2009). *Growth from Knowledge: Public Attitudes to Food Issues.* London: Food Standards Agency. Available from: http://www.food.gov.uk/multimedia/pdfs/publicattitudestofood.pdf (accessed 04 April 2011).

Katan MB *et al.* (2003). Efficacy and safety of plant stanols and sterols in the management of blood cholesterol levels. *Mayo Clin Proc* 78: 965–978.

Morgan JF *et al.* (2000). The SCOFF questionnaire: a new screening tool for eating disorders. *West J Med* 172(3): 164–165.

National Institute for Health and Clinical Excellence (2010). *Lipid Modification: Cardiovascular Risk Assessment and the Modification of Blood Lipids for the Primary and Secondary Prevention of Cardiovascular Disease.* London: NICE.

National Prescribing Centre (2004). *Updating Local Policies for Reducing the Impact of Cardiovascular Disease: Where does OTC Simvastatin Fit In?* Available from: http://www.npc.nhs.uk/resources/simvastatin.pdf (accessed 5 April 2011).

Nestlé Nutrition (2011). *Build Up® Shakes and Build Up® Soups.* Available from: http://www.nestlenutrition.co.uk/healthcare/gb/healthcare_home/Pages/home.aspx (accessed 04 April 2011).

Practice guidance (2004). OTC Simvastatin 10 mg. *Pharm J* 273: 169–170.

Schoeller DA (1988). Measurement of energy expenditure in free-living humans by using doubly labeled water. *J Nutr* 118(11): 1278–1289.

Todorovic VE, Micklewright A, eds. (2007). *A Pocket Guide to Clinical Nutrition.* 3rd edn updated. Birmingham: British Dietetic Association, PEN Group Publications.

# Self-assessment questions

The following questions are provided to test the information presented in this chapter.

*For questions 1–7 select the best answer in each case.*

1. Select which body mass index would be classified as 'undernutrition':
   a. $\leq 16.5 \, \text{kg/m}^2$
   b. $\leq 18.5 \, \text{kg/m}^2$
   c. $\leq 20 \, \text{kg/m}^2$
   d. $\geq 18.5 \, \text{kg/m}^2$
   e. $\geq 20 \, \text{kg/m}^2$

2. Red meat is a good source of which vitamin/mineral:
   a. Folate
   b. Vitamin C
   c. Calcium
   d. Haem iron
   e. Non-haem iron

3. Select which vitamin enhances the absorption of calcium:
   a. Vitamin A
   b. Vitamin C
   c. Vitamin D
   d. Vitamin E
   e. Vitamin K

4. Select which type of juice individuals should avoid while taking statins:
   a. Cranberry juice
   b. Tomato juice
   c. Pineapple juice
   d. Apple juice
   e. Grapefruit juice

5. Select which of the following foods contains high quantities of omega-3 fatty acids, believed to be beneficial in reducing cardiovascular disease:
   a. Olive oil
   b. Beef
   c. Broccoli
   d. Mackerel
   e. Grapefruit

6. Select which of the following is the correct recommendation for exercise levels in the general population:
   a. 30 minutes of moderate aerobic exercise, most days
   b. 30 minutes of high intensity aerobic exercise, most days
   c. 60 minutes of moderate aerobic exercise, 3 days per week
   d. 45 minutes of light aerobic exercise, 3 days per week
   e. 60 minutes of light intensity exercise, most days

7. Select which of the following are modifiable risk factors for cardiovascular disease:
   a. Age
   b. Sex
   c. Family history
   d. Alcohol intake
   e. Ethnicity

*For questions 8–10 select from the list below one lettered option that is most closely related to it. Each lettered option may be used once, more than once, or not at all.*
   a. folate
   b. iron
   c. phosphate
   d. cobalamin
   e. vitamin A

8. Vitamin C enhances the absorption of which mineral?

9. Pregnant women should not take supplements of which micronutrient?

10. Should be taken by women who are planning on conceiving a child.

*For questions 11 and 12 select from the list below one lettered option that is most closely related to it. Each lettered option may be used once, more than once, or not at all.*
   a. <5% weight loss
   b. 5–9% weight loss
   c. 10–20% weight loss
   d. >20% weight loss
   e. >30% weight loss

11. Is not significant unless likely to be on-going.

12. Is clinically significant requiring nutritional support.

*Questions 13–16: Each of the questions or incomplete statements in this section is followed by three responses. For each question one or more of the responses is/are correct. Decide which of the responses is/are correct and then choose a–e as indicated in the table below.*

| Directions summarised | | | | |
|---|---|---|---|---|
| **a** | **b** | **c** | **d** | **e** |
| If 1, 2 and 3 are correct | If 1 and 2 only are correct | If 2 and 3 only are correct | If 1 only is correct | If 3 only is correct |

13. The following are situations where simvastatin should not be supplied as a P medicine:
    1 – individuals who have diabetes
    2 – individuals who have cardiovascular disease
    3 – those with familial hyperlipidaemia

14. The following predispose women to conceiving a child with a neural tube defect:
    1 – asthma
    2 – coeliac disease
    3 – prescribed antiepileptic drugs

15. The following are non-modifiable risk factors for cardiovascular disease:
    1 – age
    2 – high blood cholesterol
    3 – smoking

16. The following are non-dairy sources of calcium:
    1 – tinned sardines
    2 – cereal products
    3 – spinach

*Questions 17–20 consist of two statements linked by the word* because; *decide whether each statement is true or false. If both statements are true then decide whether the second statement is a correct explanation of the first statement. Choose a–e as your answer as indicated in the table below.*

| Directions summarised | | | |
| --- | --- | --- | --- |
| | **First statement** | **Second statement** | |
| a | True | True | Second statement is a correct explanation of the first statement |
| b | True | True | Second statement is not a correct explanation of the first statement |
| c | True | False | |
| d | False | True | |
| e | False | False | |

**17.**

| Calcium needs are lower in adolescents than in adults | BECAUSE | Children have higher skeletal growth rates than adults |
| --- | --- | --- |

**18.**

| Lactating women should consume an additional 400 micrograms/day folic acid | BECAUSE | Folate reduces the risk of neural tube defects |
| --- | --- | --- |

**19.**

| An individual with iron deficiency anaemia can be treated with ferrous sulphate tablets | BECAUSE | Iron stores are primarily regulated by absorption of iron from the diet |
| --- | --- | --- |

**20.**

| A person with coeliac disease may benefit from taking calcium supplements | BECAUSE | People with coeliac disease have a higher requirement for calcium |
| --- | --- | --- |

## Answers

1-b; 2-d; 3-c; 4-e; 5-d; 6-a; 7-d; 8-b; 9-e; 10-a; 11-a; 12-c; 13-a; 14-c; 15-d; 16-b; 17-d; 18-d; 19-b; 20-a

# 9

# Dermatology

*Gwen Gray*

| This chapter will cover the following conditions: | This chapter will cover the following range of medicines: |
|---|---|
| • Scabies<br>• Head lice<br>• Eczema<br>• Napkin rash<br>• Molluscum contagiosum<br>• Seborrhoeic eczema<br>• Acne | • Salicylic acid<br>• Imidazoles<br>• Amorolfine<br>• Emollients<br>• Topical steroids<br>• Benzoyl peroxide<br>• Ketoconazole<br>• Antipruritics |

In this chapter common minor illnesses of the skin that are encountered in pharmacies will be considered. When dealing with illnesses of the skin it is important to consider differential diagnosis to determine whether major disease, which cannot be managed by a non-prescription medicine, is present. This may include situations where the presenting condition is not an actual skin condition but rather a systemic condition in which skin involvement is a symptom. Treatment of minor skin conditions will also be considered in this chapter.

The skin consists of two layers, the epidermis and the dermis. The epidermis is the outer layer and the dermis, which consists of connective tissue, lies beneath the outer layer. Normal healthy skin prevents water loss and protects underlying tissues from irritants. When the barrier is impaired, water is lost and irritants penetrate, resulting in damage to the skin. Genetic changes may also lead to defects in the epidermal barrier that result in conditions such as atopic eczema and psoriasis.

Many skin conditions are chronic, and the sufferer will report a long-standing lesion or rash. Examples of such conditions are acne vulgaris and acne rosacea, seborrhoea, most cases of eczema and psoriasis. In such cases even if referral to a doctor for treatment is thought to be appropriate it can in most cases be arranged at the sufferer's convenience. Some skin lesions will recur after a relatively symptom-free interval. This may represent a chronic condition that spontaneously resolves and relapses (e.g. seborrhoeic eczema or atopic eczema) or repeated exposure to the chemical irritant or allergen, as may occur in contact irritant or allergic eczema. The onset of a skin rash can often be related in time to likely causative factors, such as the use of a hair colorant or cosmetics, or concomitant drug therapy.

Table 9.1 provides a summary of some common terms used in dermatology.

## Acne and eczema

Before reading further, consider the following case and note your initial thoughts.

| Table 9.1 | Descriptive terms used in dermatology |
|---|---|
| **Term** | **Description** |
| Erythema | Redness due to inflammation |
| Excoriation | Marks on the skin caused by scratching |
| Lichenification | A thickening of the skin, often a result of rubbing in localised areas in eczema |
| Macule | A well-defined mark on the skin, which is flat and not raised (e.g. freckle) |
| Papule | A small, raised lesion – a large papule is termed a nodule |
| Plaque | A well-defined, raised patch of tissue (commonly seen in psoriasis) |
| Pustule | A small blister containing pus |
| Vesicle | A small blister containing serum (i.e. non-purulent) |

 **Case study**

A young father comes into the pharmacy and asks for something to treat the rash on his son's face. The child's cheeks are red and the skin is very dry and flaky. The rash has been present for about a week and no other areas of the body are affected. The child is 1 year old. The father suffers from asthma.

**Trigger questions**

- What additional information would you need before considering the appropriate management options in this case?
- What issues concern you about this case?
- Are any alarm symptoms being exhibited that require more urgent treatment or referral?

## Assessing symptoms

### Rash on face

Rash is characteristic of a variety of skin disorders. Rash on the face is usually relatively easy to diagnose and classify by observing the lesion and collecting

**Box 9.1    Face lesions**

- Acne vulgaris
- Acne rosacea
- Systemic lupus erythematosus
- Furuncles
- Rodent ulcer
- Sebaceous cyst
- Photosensitivity
- Shingles
- Atopic eczema
- Seborrhoeic eczema
- Contact eczema

**Box 9.2    Examples of drugs causing acne**

- Isoniazid
- Lithium
- Oral contraceptives
- Phenobarbital
- Phenytoin
- Steroids

information from the history. There are a range of disorders in which rash on the face will occur and this can vary according to age, with some disorders being more common in children and others more so in adults. The lesions found on the face that are discussed in this chapter are shown in Box 9.1.

The appearance of acne vulgaris is well known, with the characteristic red papular lesions, pustules and blackheads. These are located particularly on the skin of the forehead, nose, chin and beard area, but can affect any part of the face. Acne may also appear on the nape of the neck, the shoulders and the upper trunk. In severe cases scarring may result. The skin is generally greasy in appearance. There is no pruritus, but the rash causes embarrassment and self-consciousness in young people. Acne (Figure 9.1)

is caused by inflammation and blockage of the sebaceous glands and hair follicles. It is associated with the bacterium *Propionibacterium acnes*, which is thought to split the triglycerides in sebum into fatty acids, which are irritant to the pilosebaceous unit.

Acne usually appears during adolescence, classically appearing around the time of puberty, and gradually disappears in young adulthood, but in some cases it may persist into adulthood. The condition can be caused by drugs (Box 9.2).

By contrast, an acneform rash appearing during middle age may be acne rosacea (Figure 9.2). This starts as a red rash or flushing, particularly over the cheeks and bridge of the nose. It often progresses to a papular acne-like rash. The rash may appear symmetrically and is often described as a butterfly rash because of its shape and distribution. If this condition is suspected, the individual should be referred to a doctor for appropriate antibiotic treatment.

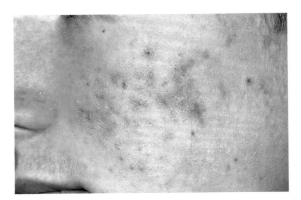

**Figure 9.1**    Adolescent acne vulgaris.

(Reproduced with permission from Dr P Marazzi/Science Photo Library, SPL M108/367.)

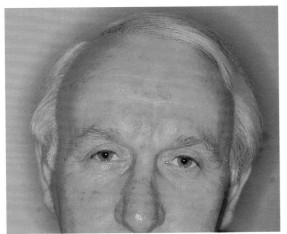

**Figure 9.2**    Rosacea.

(Reproduced by permission from the Science Photo Library, SPL C0015427.)

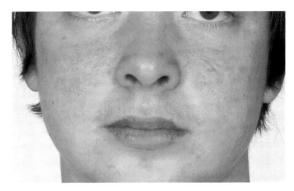

**Figure 9.3** Systemic lupus erythematosus.

(Reproduced with permission from the Wellcome Trust Medical Photographic Library.)

Another rash that causes a butterfly appearance over the nose and cheeks is that of systemic lupus erythematosus (Figure 9.3). This is a relatively rare condition and the lesions are more scaly than those of rosacea. It is sometimes precipitated by drugs such as beta-blockers, chlorpromazine, hydralazine, isoniazid, lithium, methyldopa, penicillamine, phenytoin, procainamide, sulfasalazine and thiouracils. Systemic lupus erythematosus should be referred for a medical opinion.

Boils (furuncles) are commonly seen on the nose or chin, but can also occur on the nape of the neck, particularly in adolescent males. A boil is an abscess with a single pus-filled or discharging centre. A tender, red swollen area of skin may herald a boil or sometimes such a red area may be the result of an insect bite.

A small, discrete, raised nodular lesion that eventually ruptures to form a small, red or purple wart-like ulcer should be viewed with suspicion, as this is how rodent ulcers (basal cell carcinoma) present (Figure 9.4). They can occur anywhere on the face,

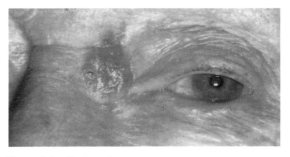

**Figure 9.4** Rodent ulcer.

(Reproduced with permission from the Royal Victoria Infirmary, Newcastle upon Tyne.)

| Box 9.3 Examples of photosensitising drugs |
| --- |
| ● Amiodarone |
| ● Chlorpromazine |
| ● Nalidixic acid |
| ● NSAIDs |
| ● Quinolones |
| ● Sulphonamides |
| ● Tetracyclines |
| ● Thiazides |
| ● Tricyclic antidepressants |

but are most common on the nose, cheeks and pinna of the ear. If a rodent ulcer is suspected, referral for medical opinion is essential.

A raised cystic lump of epidermis may be due to a sebaceous cyst, which is most commonly found on the face, ears or neck. It appears as a pale, non-pigmented firm swelling and is painless, but requires referral to a doctor to confirm the diagnosis. If the lesion is upsetting to the sufferer, the only remedy is surgery.

A facial rash resembling sunburn that is limited to exposed skin on the face, neck, and possibly the backs of the hands suggests a photosensitive rash. This is often caused by drugs (Box 9.3). A striking slate-blue or grey discoloration of the face is characteristically caused by amiodarone. It is therefore important to ask about current medications. Although the use of a sunblock and advice to cover the skin are helpful, anyone in this situation should be referred for medical opinion initially.

A rash occurring unilaterally over the scalp and forehead, extending to the eye, should be suspected as shingles (Figure 9.5). The rash may be macular at first, changing to vesicles and it eventually forms crusts. Sufferers should be referred to a doctor for treatment immediately. Shingles is a herpes zoster infection that follows the course of a nerve tract. It is caused by reactivation of the herpes zoster (chickenpox) virus that has lain dormant in a sensory root ganglion. The rash may run from the back across the chest, along the course of an intercostal nerve or around the abdomen, always stopping at the midline (Figure 9.6). The condition can be very painful, both before the rash appears and after it has gone.

The infection is most contagious during the period before the rash appears. There may be fever,

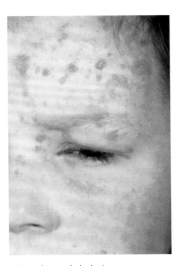

**Figure 9.5**  Shingles, ophthalmic.
(Reproduced with permission from the Wellcome Trust Medical Photographic Library.)

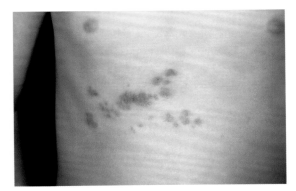

**Figure 9.6**  Shingles.
(Reproduced with permission of Dr P. Marazzi/Science Photo Library, SPL M260/292.)

malaise and anorexia before the rash appears. There is often a painful neuralgia that persists for many weeks after the rash has disappeared.

Seborrhoeic eczema presents as a scaly rash with mild erythema affecting the scalp and forehead, eyebrows, nose and pinna of the ear. (Figure 9.7). It may also be associated with scaling on the edge of the eyelids (blepharitis), sometimes with loss of eyelashes. Seborrhoea is a marked increase in the activity of the sebaceous glands. The yeast *Pityrosporum* has been implicated as a causative agent.

Dandruff is considered as a mild form of seborrhoeic eczema. In babies during the first few months of life it may present as cradle cap, producing yel-

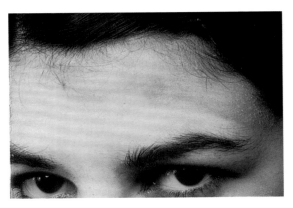

**Figure 9.7**  Seborrhoeic eczema.
(Reproduced with permission from the Wellcome Trust Medical Photographic Library.)

lowish crusts, chiefly on the scalp but sometimes also on the ears and eyebrows (Figure 9.8).

A red, dry scaly rash appearing on the cheeks of babies may be seen in atopic eczema (Figure 9.9). Atopic eczema is a constitutional eczema that usually occurs in people with a family history of atopy. The chance of developing the condition is increased if one or both parents suffer from eczema, hay fever or asthma. However, children can become atopic in the absence of an obvious family history. Atopic eczema commonly begins after the first few months of life, and although it often resolves spontaneously

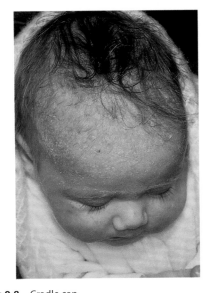

**Figure 9.8**  Cradle cap.
(Reproduced with permission from the Wellcome Trust Medical Photographic Library.)

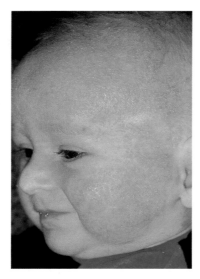

**Figure 9.9**  Atopic eczema.

(Reproduced with permission from Dr P. Marazzi/Science Photo Library, SPL M150/132.)

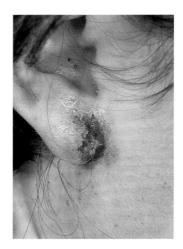

**Figure 9.10**  Reaction to nickel.

(Reproduced with permission from the Wellcome Trust Medical Photographic Library.)

it can persist into adulthood. The lesions are erythematous, papular, and either dry or weeping. It often spreads to flexures in the neck, wrists, elbows, and behind the knees. It is very irritant and the scratching that ensues can cause marked excoriation of the skin and increases the risk of infection. About 75% of children outgrow their eczema by the early teenage years, but in a few cases the condition persists into adulthood as a chronic eczema. In older children and adults, atopic eczema appears as lichenification, which is a dry, crusty thickening of the skin that often becomes cracked.

Contact eczema occurs as a result of contact with allergens or irritants. Contact eczema on the face most commonly occurs around the eyes and is often caused by allergens in cosmetics. It may, however, be seen anywhere on the face, according to the irritant or sensitising agent used. Common irritants include soaps, shampoos and detergents. It occurs as an erythematous rash, with inflammation. An allergy to nickel in earrings can result in contact eczema of the pinna of the ears. On the ears, in particular, weeping vesicles are often seen that eventually produce crusting lesions (Figure 9.10).

### Dry, flaky skin

Dry, flaky skin can be seen in atopic eczema (see above), although the presentation will vary

depending on the age of the sufferer and the location of the eczema.

Seborrhoeic eczema is characterised by scaling of the skin. The appearance of this will vary depending on the age of the sufferer (see above).

Psoriasis occurs usually as individual plaques of scaly, silvery lesions, particularly on the knees, elbows and forearms. The outside of the elbow is a common site for the characteristic appearance of psoriasis (Figure 9.11).

Severe scaling of the scalp may be due to psoriasis but it rarely affects the face. On the scalp it

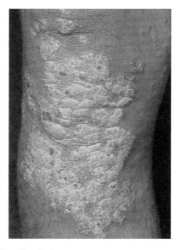

**Figure 9.11**  Psoriasis.

(Reproduced with permission from Glaxo Wellcome.)

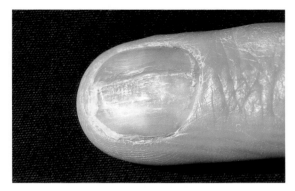

**Figure 9.12**  Psoriasis of the nail.

(Reproduced with permission from Dr P. Marazzi/Science Photo Library, SPL M240/280.)

usually appears as a scaly or red rash and there may be some loss of hair. Psoriasis may occur as red lesions on the palms of the hands and can affect the fingernails, producing characteristic pitting or denting on the surface of the nail (Figure 9.12). Psoriasis is a chronic recurrent disorder and must be referred to a doctor for management.

Ringworm infection of the trunk or limbs (tinea corporis) may be contracted from animals or humans. Typically there are isolated erythematous and scaly lesions, often round or oval in shape (Figure 9.13).

## Accompanying symptoms

A skin rash may be accompanied by other symptoms. It is important to distinguish between a rash of systemic disease and that of a skin disease. Some symptoms may require immediate medical attention.

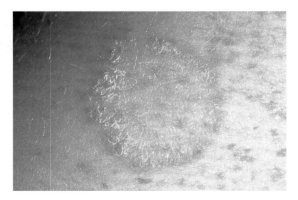

**Figure 9.13**  Tinea corporis (ringworm rash) on an arm.

(Reproduced with permission from Dr P. Marazzi/Science Photo Library, SPL M270/050.)

### Itching

Itching (pruritus) is a common accompaniment to eczema, and also to scalp infections and infestations. Generalised itching over most of the body without the appearance of a rash may be a sign of systemic disease, such as liver or kidney disease, and therefore requires referral.

### Headache, fever and malaise

Headache, fever, malaise and lymphadenopathy (swollen glands, seen or easily felt in the neck) suggest systemic disease or infection and require referral for medical attention.

### Swelling

Swelling of the lips or tongue, especially in the case of an urticarial rash, requires immediate medical attention.

## Management options

People suffering from eczema should be discouraged from using perfumed soap and bath additives, as these may cause sensitisation as well as having a degreasing effect on the skin, causing it to dry out after bathing. If irritants or sensitising agents are thought to be the cause of an eczematous reaction, it is obvious that these should be removed or the skin protected from them before any treatment can be successful. Other trigger factors for atopic eczema such as clothing or heat should be avoided. Also scratching should be avoided and nails should be kept short.

Acne sufferers should be advised that it is not caused by poor hygiene and there is no evidence to suggest that frequent washing and degreasing improves the condition. They should be advised to wash no more than twice a day with a mild soap or cleanser and be made aware that treatments available for acne are effective but that they will take time to work and may cause some irritation when treatment is commenced. Diet has little effect on acne but if a particular food seems to aggravate the condition then it should be avoided if possible. Excessive use of make-ups and cosmetics should be avoided, but if this is not possible then water-based preparations should be selected. Sunlight appears to have little benefit in acne.

Sufferers of seborrhoeic eczema should be advised that it is not caused by poor cleanliness. Treatment is available to control the symptoms but it is not a cure as symptoms often recur after treatment is stopped. Thick crusts or scales should be removed from the scalp before the use of antifungal shampoo. This can be achieved by applying olive oil to the scalp and leaving it on for several hours before washing with a detergent. Parents of babies suffering from cradle cap should be reassured that it is not a serious condition and it will resolve within weeks. Simple measures such as softening the scales with baby oil or olive oil, followed by gentle brushing with a soft brush then washing with baby shampoo may be effective. If this does not soften the scales then emulsifying ointment may be used to loosen the scales, followed by shampooing.

### Emollients (BNF section 13.2.1)

Emollients are indicated for the treatment of dry or scaling skin disorders. They maintain hydration of the stratum corneum and are effective in preventing drying and cracking of the skin, which can be very painful. They should be applied after washing or bathing, when the skin is still moist. Emollients should be applied liberally and frequently.

Non-proprietary preparations are suitable, and there is also an array of proprietary emollient products. The choice between the different products available is largely one of cosmetic acceptability. Ointments such as emulsifying ointment tend to be most effective, but creams are less greasy and more acceptable. Emulsifying ointment forms a protective layer that prevents evaporation of moisture from dry skin, as occurs in eczema when the hydrolipid layer is not functioning properly and abnormal water loss from the epidermis occurs. An appropriate treatment regimen would be to use a greasy ointment at night and a more cosmetically acceptable cream by day.

For an enhanced effect, the use of preparations containing a humectant such as urea may be appropriate. Urea absorbs water from the dermis into the epidermis, thereby helping to maximise the water-retaining properties of occlusive ingredients such as soft paraffin. Ingredients such as wool fat (lanolin) and wool alcohols also act as moisture absorbents.

Aqueous cream has fallen from favour because of its irritant properties, which make dry skin conditions worse and it should only be used as a wash-off soap substitute, not as an emollient. Bath emollients may also be helpful. Most bath emollients contain light liquid paraffin as the active constituent, and although their effectiveness is matched by emulsifying ointment they tend to be more cosmetically acceptable, despite their higher cost.

### Topical corticosteroids (BNF section 13.4)

Topical corticosteroids are used to treat skin conditions where inflammation is present such as eczema. Corticosteroids suppress inflammation and are used to relieve symptoms, but rebound of the condition may occur when use of the corticosteroid is stopped.

Topical hydrocortisone 1% is available as a P medicine and is licensed for short-term use in the treatment of mild to moderate eczema flare-ups in known sufferers, as well as for contact eczema and insect bites. It is effective for mild, uncomplicated contact eczemas. It cannot be sold for use on the face, or on broken or infected skin and should not be sold for children under 10 years of age without medical advice.

Clobetasone 0.05% is a more potent steroid than 1% hydrocortisone and is more suitable for the short-term treatment of flare-ups of eczema of a more severe nature in adults and children over 12 years of age. Where the skin is thickened and lichenified, referral to a doctor is probably best so that consideration can be given to the prescription of more potent topical steroids.

In contrast to the liberal use of emollients, users of topical steroids should be instructed to apply these preparations more carefully and economically. The fingertip unit is an arbitrary but convenient measurement for providing instruction on how much to apply. The unit is the amount of product that can be squeezed out from the tip of the finger to the first crease (Figure 9.14). For example, half a unit will be sufficient to apply to an area the same size as the palm of one hand.

### Topical preparations for acne (BNF section 13.6.1)

The most common constituent of proprietary creams and gels for acne treatment is benzoyl peroxide. It has been shown to be effective in clinical trials for the treatment of mild to moderate facial acne. It is bactericidal to *Propionibacterium acnes*

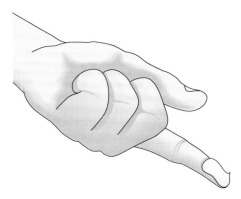

**Figure 9.14** The fingertip unit.

and is also thought to act partly by reducing the breakdown of sebum into irritant fatty acids, which cause inflammation in the sebaceous ducts. Benzoyl peroxide is also keratolytic, and is thereby thought to unplug the ducts and drain the sebum from the sebaceous glands. It thus has an action on the pre-inflammatory stage of acne (comedones) as well as the inflammatory stage (papules and pustules). It often causes an irritant dermatitis characterised by dryness, erythema, peeling and stinging after the first few applications. Users should be warned of this and advised to use products cautiously at first, perhaps just once a day. If usage proves to be too unpleasant, application should be stopped for a few days and then started again, perhaps on alternate days at first. Application should be to all

the affected area and not just to the comedones. Benzoyl peroxide is also well known for its bleaching action on clothes and hair, and this should be pointed out to users before use. In common with most acne remedies, there may be no apparent benefit for several weeks or months after starting treatment and it is wise to ensure that people using benzoyl peroxide are aware of this. Products containing a low concentration should be used at first, and if no improvement is seen after 4 weeks a higher concentration can be substituted.

Salicylic acid is an old-established keratolytic agent that is present in various proprietary products as well as in official preparations such as salicylic acid ointment. It is thought by some to have dubious efficacy in acne, and its use is falling out of favour.

### Shampoos and other preparations for scalp and hair conditions (BNF section 13.9)

Seborrhoeic eczema may be treated with an anti-dandruff shampoo, such as a product containing selenium sulphide or pyrithione zinc. Ketoconazole shampoo, which attacks the yeast *Pityrosporum ovale*, a causative factor in seborrhoea, is effective, especially in difficult cases. It can be sold from a pharmacy for both prevention and treatment of dandruff and seborrhoeic eczema and should be applied no more than once every 3 days. Tar-based shampoos may also be useful. Severe or chronic cases may need to be referred for medical opinion.

 **Re-consider the case**

Before reading further, re-consider the following questions and your initial thoughts on this case.

**Trigger questions**

- What additional information would you need before considering the appropriate management options in this case?
- What issues concern you about this case?
- Are any alarm symptoms being exhibited that require more urgent treatment or referral?

**Case study**

A young father comes into the pharmacy and asks for something to treat the rash on his son's face. The child's cheeks are red and the skin is very dry and flaky. The rash has been present for about a week and no other areas of the body are affected. The child is 1 year old. The father suffers from asthma.

Pharmacist opinion

The fact that the rash is only present on the face and no other symptoms are apparent would suggest that the child is suffering from a skin condition rather than a systemic condition.

As the father of the child suffers from asthma, this would suggest that the child has developed atopic eczema, as this usually occurs when there is a family history of atopy. The child is aged 1 year and atopic eczema commonly begins in babies. The appearance of a red, dry, flaky rash on the face also suggests atopic eczema. Although no other body areas are affected at present, atopic eczema often spreads to other areas. As atopic eczema is suspected, referral to a doctor for diagnosis and management is required, but in the meantime an emollient could be suggested for symptomatic relief.

 General practitioner opinion

It is extremely important to ascertain the social context of this child. This can be done fairly quickly and easily without making the father uncomfortable. Who first noticed the rash? Has anyone tried treating it on this occasion or on previous occasions? Does anyone in the family have particular concerns about what the rash may be? Questions of this sort are focused on the medical problem, but probe a little into the family situation. This is usually enough to place a child in its social context.

The main differential diagnoses for this rash are seborrhoeic eczema and atopic eczema, the treatments for which are quite different. It should be confirmed that the child had not been unwell. Brief examination will reveal general health and any evidence of skin infection; all other skin areas should also be examined. The age of the child, distribution of the rash and the father's history of atopy would point to the diagnosis of atopic eczema.

If there is no skin infection, the use of a steroid preparation to reduce inflammation would be appropriate. An ointment emollient would be helpful here and is easier to use on the face than other areas, so should be acceptable to the carers. It is worth spending some time emphasising the importance of appropriate emollient use and consider giving extra written information, as communication between carers needs to be clear.

It would also be appropriate to review this child again fairly soon to assess the rash and to be sure the treatment has been used appropriately. A quick follow-up will usually reassure carers and give them confidence that they can manage these problems in the future.

 Summary of key points

| Condition | Management |
| --- | --- |
| Acne vulgaris is characterised by comedones (whiteheads and blackheads), which often become pustular. | Topical preparations such as salicylic acid containing products and benzoyl peroxide may be used for mild to moderate acne. |
| Eczema is characterised by erythema, papules and either dry or weeping skin, which is accompanied by itching. It may be classified as atopic or contact (allergic or irritant). | Avoidance of triggers or irritants.<br>Emollients can be used to hydrate the skin.<br>Topical corticosteroids suppress the inflammation of eczema and may be used for mild to moderate eczema. |
| Seborrhoeic eczema is characterised by dry or greasy scales. It is known as cradle cap in babies. | Anti-dandruff shampoo such as products containing selenium sulphide or pyrithione zinc.<br>Ketoconazole shampoo may be used for prevention and treatment of seborrhoeic eczema.<br>Tar-based shampoo may also be useful.<br>Simple measures such as softening the scales with baby oil or olive oil, and gentle brushing followed by use of a baby shampoo may be effective in cradle cap. |

**When to refer**

- Any severe condition that does not respond to management with medicines purchased from a pharmacy, such as eczema, seborrhoeic eczema, dandruff and acne
- Vesicles or crusting rash indicating infection
- Butterfly distribution of erythema over the nose and cheeks
- Any newly appeared lump, even without symptoms such as itch or pain
- Abnormal facial coloration, such as yellow, blue or greyish complexion, or a sun-tanned appearance extending to the whole body when there is no history of sun exposure (as may occur in the hyperpigmentation that accompanies suppression of the adrenal glands)
- Small, discrete, red macular lesions that blanch when pressure is applied
- Small, discrete ulcer or lesion with raised edge (rodent ulcer)
- Abnormal hair loss, not related to male-pattern baldness
- Unilateral rash on the face, the scalp or the skin around the eye, especially if painful
- Acne, photosensitive rash or yellow, jaundiced skin coloration that has recently appeared or has been exacerbated in someone taking any medication that could be responsible
- Rash on the face that spreads down to the trunk
- Any skin rash, lesion or pruritus that does not respond to management with medicines purchased from a pharmacy
- Skin lesions accompanied by any of the following: malaise, fever, headache or swollen lymph glands

# Head lice, scabies, infections

Before reading further, consider the following case and note your initial thoughts.

**Case study**

A 25-year-old man comes into the pharmacy and asks to speak to the pharmacist. He wants to get something to treat his itch. He seems embarrassed to discuss his problem but eventually tells the pharmacist that the itching started between his fingers but has now spread to his palms and wrists. The itching is particularly troublesome at night. He also wonders if there is anything that will help to treat his painful fingernails. He then says that his girlfriend has spots on her feet that have black dots in the centre and wonders what these could be.

**Trigger questions**

- What additional information would you need before considering the appropriate management options in this case?
- What issues concern you about this case?
- Are any alarm symptoms being exhibited that require more urgent treatment or referral?

## Assessing symptoms

### Itching

Itching is characteristic of a variety of skin disorders. Such disorders are usually easy to diagnose and classify by gathering a detailed history. Skin disorders in which itching is a characteristic and that are discussed in this chapter are shown in Box 9.4.

One of the most common causes of an itchy scalp, especially in children, is head lice. Although head

### Box 9.4 Skin disorders with itch

- Head lice
- Scabies
- Body lice
- Tinea pedis (athlete's foot)
- Tinea cruris (jock itch)
- Tinea capitis (scalp ringworm)
- Pompholyx
- Insect bites
- Lichen planus
- Prickly heat
- Urticaria

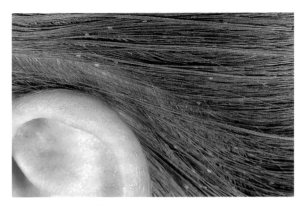

**Figure 9.16** Head louse eggs (nits).

(Reproduced with permission from Dr Chris Hale/Science Photo Library, SPL M240/283.)

lice are most commonly found in children, adults can have them too. Head lice cannot jump and they can only spread by children touching heads, usually for some time. Head lice found on pillows, hats and other locations are generally thought to be incapable of infecting a person and usually die within 24 hours. The head louse, *Pediculus capitis*, is 1–3 mm long and has three pairs of legs (Figure 9.15).

It clings to hair with its claws and feeds on blood from the host's scalp. The female lays five or six eggs per day (up to 300 eggs in her lifetime), which attach to hair shafts by means of a glandular discharge that she secretes. After 7–10 days the eggs hatch and leave white, shiny cases (nits) on the hair (Figure 9.16). Within 10 days, fully developed adult

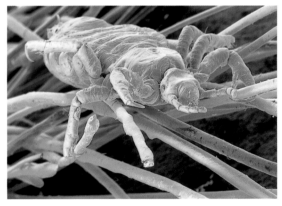

**Figure 9.15** Head louse. Scanning electron micrograph of *Pediculus humanus capitis* among hair. Actual size is approx 2-3.5 mm. The louse's three pairs of legs can be seen directly behind the head.

(Reproduced with permission from Eye of Science/Science Photo Library, SPL Z265/105.)

lice form. Lice live for 1–2 months. The eggs are laid close to the scalp and are found farther from the scalp as the hair grows.

Nowadays, most children's heads will be infected with as few as 10–20 lice. Such small numbers will be difficult to find with the naked eye. The diagnosis of head lice infection can, however, be made when lice are detected by combing dampened hair with a fine-toothed comb over a sheet of white paper. Outbreaks of head lice often occur in schools, nurseries, etc., and parents will often diagnose the condition themselves. Infection may be asymptomatic in some children, whereas in others there will be an itchy scalp, especially behind the ears. This itch can take a few weeks to develop after infection, as it is a manifestation of an allergic response to the lice, and by the same token the itch may persist for some time after successful eradication with insecticidal lotions. Box 9.5 describes the technique for detection combing.

The intense itching of scabies is caused by an allergic reaction to the excreta of the mite *Sarcoptes scabei*. The scabies mite burrows into the epidermis and leaves eggs and faeces behind it. Protein in the faeces causes an allergic reaction in the skin and it sometimes takes several weeks after infection before the pruritus begins. The pruritus is sudden in onset, severe, and worse at night. Itching occurs several weeks after infection has occurred and may not disappear until a similar period after successful eradication of the mite. Itching in the finger webs with discrete, small, red lesions is a classic symptom of scabies (Figure 9.17).

1. The hair should be wetted and dried to dampness to prevent lice moving when combed. Many sources recommend wetting the hair with a conditioner, but this can produce a foam on the hair shaft, which makes visualisation of the lice or nits difficult. The use of an oil such as olive or coconut is said to be better.
2. The hair is then combed with a normal comb to remove tangles.
3. The hair should then be combed using a plastic detection comb, starting at the roots and combing along the length of the hair. This process should be repeated several times.
4. The comb should be tapped on white paper to dislodge any lice, which can then be seen. Each louse is about the size of a pinhead.
5. Any lice found should be stuck to the paper with a piece of adhesive tape and taken to the pharmacy or nurse as proof of infection.
6. The comb should be washed under the tap.
7. Detection combing is best performed on all contacts and family members to discover who is infected. Family members should not be routinely treated unless lice have been detected.

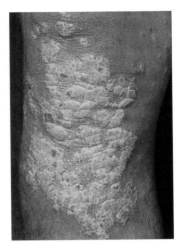

**Figure 9.17** Scabies skin infection.

(Reproduced with permission from the Wellcome Trust Medical Photographic Library.)

The rash is papular but not always obvious. The presence of a pruritic rash in other family members will provide a clue to its diagnosis. In infants and toddlers the head and neck, trunk, wrists, palms, soles and insteps are particularly affected. This distribution is slightly different from that seen in adults where the lesions may spread to the palms, wrists, armpits, genitalia, buttocks and abdomen. Burrows (tracks made by the mite burrowing through the skin) may be identified as small (up to 1 cm) grey curved lines in the skin, but it is not always possible to see them. Scabies is spread by skin contact and commonly by holding hands. Family members and any sexual contacts will sometimes be affected.

Vagrants and people with low standards of personal and domestic hygiene who present with severe itching may have body lice. These mites live in clothes and bedding, and bite the trunk, buttocks and shoulders. Questioning about the site of the initial skin irritation can sometimes help to distinguish this condition from scabies. However, the precise diagnosis is of little consequence as the treatment is similar for both conditions.

Itching commonly occurs in tinea pedis (athlete's foot). This is the most common skin condition affecting the feet that will present in the pharmacy. It usually starts between the toes, classically between the fourth and fifth digits, and can spread to the sole and upper part of the foot. It often appears red and itchy at first, and later turns white with maceration and soreness between the toes (Figure 9.18). The condition can spread to other parts of the foot and can cause considerable irritation. If the diagnosis is in doubt or the toenail is affected, referral to a doctor is required for appropriate management. Athlete's foot can be present for months and it often recurs even after treatment.

Itching is often present in tinea infection of the groin (tinea cruris), commonly known as jock itch. It is more common in men than women and it appears as a red, itchy rash on the inner thighs, adjacent to but rarely involving the scrotum. It results in a circular, scaly, erythematous lesion characterised by

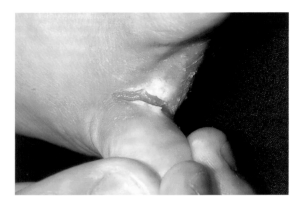

**Figure 9.18** Tinea pedis (athlete's foot.).

(Reproduced with permission from Dr P. Marazzi/Science Photo Library, SPL M270/167.)

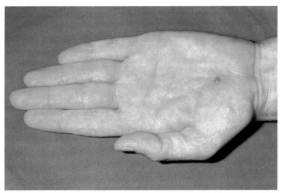

**Figure 9.20** Pompholyx.

(Reproduced with permission from Dr P. Marazzi/Science Photo Library, SPL M150/078.)

well-defined edges. The rash, which is symmetrical, appears to clear from the centre, is redder at the edges and spreads outwards. Sufferers will often also have tinea pedis.

A bald patch on the scalp may be caused by scalp ringworm (tinea capitis; Figure 9.19). It presents as scaly itching lesions and should be referred to a doctor for management.

Pompholyx is an endogenous condition that is very itchy. Lesions occur on the palms of the hands and it often affects the feet as well. Lesions appear as vesicles (Figure 9.20). The condition can be chronic or recurrent and, if the pruritus is severe, referral to a doctor is advisable for topical corticosteroids to be considered.

Itchy papules or larger lumps on the lower leg are often the result of insect bites. The diagnosis can generally be confirmed by an appropriate history.

Lichen planus is an eruption of small, itchy, papules that are often a purplish colour initially, later turning brown (Figure 9.21). Sometimes a white lace-like pattern may be seen on the papules. The condition often affects the mouth at the same time, producing characteristic white lacy streaks on the buccal mucosa. As well as the legs, this condition can also occur on the wrists, back and abdomen. It is usually symmetrical, occurring at similar sites on both legs. It is seen in young and middle-aged adults, but is rarer in older people and in children. The condition, which is of unknown aetiology, is

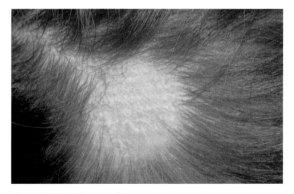

**Figure 9.19** Tinea capitis.

(Reproduced with permission from the Science Photo Library, SPL M270/085.)

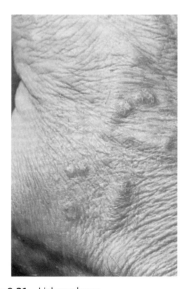

**Figure 9.21** Lichen planus.

(Reproduced with permission from Glaxo Wellcome.)

self-limiting over several months. As it subsides, post-inflammatory hyperpigmentation imparts a brown colour to the lesions, and in some cases this can appear without any obvious preceding inflammation. If the accompanying pruritus cannot be relieved with oral antihistamines, topical steroids may be required, in which case referral to a doctor is necessary.

Prickly heat, often referred to as sweat rash, is an itchy rash occurring at sites of friction from clothing or following the application of topical preparations that occlude the sweat ducts. Treatment involves avoiding tight clothing or offending materials. An urticarial rash (Figure 9.22) has characteristic weals and erythema, and pruritus is usually present. It may occur on any part of the body. It is often part of an allergic reaction to drugs, foods, preservatives and colorants, although it is sometimes triggered by changes in temperature and fever. It generally only lasts about 24 hours, and if mild can be treated with oral antihistamines. If there is considerable oedema, particularly if the oedema spreads to the eyelids and lips and occludes the upper airway (angio-oedema), the condition should be treated as a medical emergency. A tracheostomy can be life-saving in such circumstances.

### Painful fingernails

Fungal nail infection (tinea unguium or onychomycosis) may present as painful inflammation in the

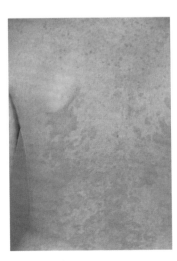

**Figure 9.22** Urticaria.

(Reproduced with permission from the Wellcome Trust Medical Photographic Library.)

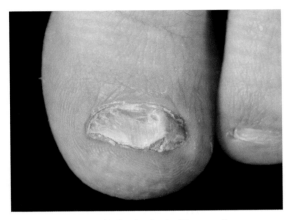

**Figure 9.23** Fungal infection in the big toenail.

(Reproduced with permission of Custom Medical Stock/Science Photo Library, SPL M270/175.)

skin around the base of the nails as well as involvement of the nail itself. It affects one or two nails initially, but can spread to involve others. It may progress so that the nail appears thickened or yellow, although this is more common in toenails.

A yellow discoloration of a toenail, often that of the big toe, indicates a fungal infection caused by the same fungus responsible for athlete's foot. The nail thickens and may crumble and become unsightly (Figure 9.23). Although judged by some doctors to be a cosmetic problem requiring no treatment, it can be treated with oral antifungals, and if it is causing distress to the sufferer it should be referred to a doctor.

Trauma to the nail bed can produce a black nail, which is a haematoma or bruise under the nail. It will clear in time, although the damaged nail may eventually separate as the new one grows. Occasionally it may be necessary for the doctor to bore a hole in the nail to drain the blood and fluid beneath if the pressure caused by the inflammatory process is causing pain that does not disappear over a few days.

A paronychia (whitlow) is similar to onychomycosis, but is usually caused by candidal infection and affects chiefly the skin around the base of the nail. Paronychias tend to be more acute and have pus in them, which may require draining.

### Spots on feet

Verrucae are viral infections caused by the wart virus (human papilloma virus), which is spread by barefoot contact. Verrucae are commonly found

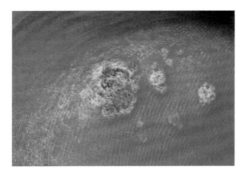

**Figure 9.24** Verrucae.

(Reproduced with permission form the Wellcome Trust Medical Photographic Library.)

on the underside of the foot mainly on the pressure areas (Figure 9.24) and can produce reactive hard pads of thickened skin around them and appear similar to corns. They can be distinguished from corns by the appearance of black dots in their core. These are blood vessels in the dermis, visible when the overlying skin is rubbed off. Verrucae are usually painless until pressure is applied on walking. They are extremely common in children, although by no means restricted to them. Verrucae that are not treated, as well as some that are, can persist for similar lengths of time. They usually resolve spontaneously within months.

### Accompanying symptoms

### Rash

The location and appearance of a rash are the principal pointers to diagnosis. Some other factors can be helpful, however, although their presence or absence should not be used as absolute criteria to exclude any conditions. Most rashes are accompanied by pruritus, and this is particularly true for most types of eczema. Sometimes psoriasis does not itch. This may be useful when differentiating between a chronic eczema and psoriasis of the palms, or between an intertriginous psoriasis (such as in the groin) and a tinea or candidal infection at the same site. It should be remembered that psoriasis can involve the scalp and nails, and inquiry should be made of someone who has a rash on the body, particularly about pitting of the nails, which the sufferer may not appreciate is due to the same condition as the psoriatic rash.

### Absence of rash

It should be remembered that pruritus may, rarely, be a sign of systemic disease, often in the absence of a rash. Someone complaining of pruritus without an obvious skin lesion should therefore be referred for medical opinion. In many cases, scratching and excoriation in response to pruritus may cause marks on the skin that can be mistaken for genuine lesions.

### Malaise, fever or other systemic symptoms

Malaise, fever or other systemic symptoms may accompany infections such as shingles and some other serious skin disorders, and such cases should be referred to a doctor for medical attention.

### Peeling of the skin

Any peeling of the skin, apart from that commonly associated with sunburn, requires referral to a doctor, as this may indicate an unusual or serious disorder. This should not be confused with the shedding of scales that may occur in some eczemas and psoriasis.

## Management options

Education of anyone who has head lice, including parents of children who have head lice, is important in managing the condition. Firstly it is important to eliminate the view that head lice are associated with a lack of hygiene or care, and that short hair is less likely to be infested than long hair. Indeed, the term 'infestation' should be replaced with 'infection' when referring to head lice, to remove the pejorative overtones that exist among the public. Often parents believe that prophylactic treatment should be applied; however, the prophylactic use of a pesticide shampoo or lotion should be discouraged, as it will be largely ineffective and may give rise to resistance. Resistance to insecticidal preparations has developed, and the former practice of rotating the use of insecticides across a district has now lost favour and a mosaic strategy is used to overcome this, whereby if one insecticide fails to cure the head lice another insecticide is used for the next course. The current maxim 'no louse, no treatment' may help to reduce the indiscriminate use of insecticides and thereby lessen the prevalence of apparent resistance.

It is also important to educate parents about the pathogenesis of the condition, pointing out particularly that the symptom of an itchy scalp is an allergic reaction to lice. The itchiness usually manifests itself several weeks after the scalp has become infected and, in similar fashion, may not disappear until several days or weeks after all lice have been removed. Before a course of treatment with two applications of insecticide is deemed to have failed, on the whim of an anxious parent who believes that a child who persists in scratching its scalp must still be infected, evidence for the continued presence of lice must be produced. Until detection combing produces such evidence, consideration cannot be given to further chemical treatment using other insecticides. Most apparent treatment failures are due to poor technique, use of inadequate quantities of lotion, or forgetting that a persistent itch is not necessarily a sign of continued infection (Box 9.6). It should also be advised that it is not necessary to wash bedding and clothing that has been in contact with lice.

Similarly to the case with head lice, it is also less stigmatising to use the word 'infection' rather than 'infestation' when discussing scabies. Sufferers should be advised that itching occurs several weeks after infection has occurred and may not disappear until a similar period after successful eradication of the mite. This is important to convey, first because symptomatic treatment for the itch may be appropriate, and second because other individuals in close contact will also probably be already infected by the time the sufferer has become symptomatic. The allergic reaction responsible for the itch may take 2 weeks to disappear, and during this time calamine lotion or crotamiton cream should be used to relieve symptoms. If a person is still symptomatic after this time, a referral to a doctor to confirm the diagnosis is advisable. Infection is spread by close physical contact, and hence it is necessary to treat all family members and sexual contacts at the same time. Close body contact should be avoided until partners and close contacts have been treated. Sufferers should be advised to wash clothes, towels and bed linen at 50°C or above on the day that the first application of treatment is applied.

Sufferers of athlete's foot should be advised on good foot hygiene measures and the importance of wearing appropriate footwear. The feet should be thoroughly dried after washing and the sharing of towels should be avoided to reduce transmission of the condition. Cotton socks should be worn and footwear that ensures the feet are kept cool and dry should also be worn. It is also important to avoid walking barefoot in communal showers and changing rooms in order to reduce transmission.

Simple hygiene measures should also be advised to anyone with fungal infection of the groin area. The affected area should be washed and thoroughly dried daily and towels should not be shared with others. Loose-fitting clothes should be worn and all clothing, bedding and towels should be washed regularly to eradicate the fungus.

Sufferers of verrucae should be advised that, although they are contagious, transmission is thought to be low. However, measures should be taken to reduce transmission such as avoiding walking barefoot in wet areas, wearing flip flops or verruca socks in swimming pools and avoiding sharing towels and socks. Children who have verrucae can still take part in sports and swimming provided measures are taken to minimise the spread of the virus. If diabetics have verrucae they should be managed by diabetic foot specialists.

### Parasiticidal preparations (BNF section 13.10.4)

Topical insecticides available from the pharmacy for the treatment of head lice include malathion, permethrin and phenothrin. Although good clinical trials are few in number, the evidence in the literature

---

**Box 9.6    Reasons for failure of head lice treatment**

- No proven initial infection (as evidenced by detection of live lice)
- Insufficient quantities of product applied to the scalp, especially in people with long hair
- Repeat application not done after 7–10 days
- Resistance to insecticide
- Short contact time of insecticide with scalp (e.g. shampoo for 10 minutes)
- Poor understanding of the need for careful application of the treatment by the parent

shows that all these agents appear to be equally effective. At the same time, resistance exists to varying extents in different regions, and patterns vary in different countries. Although these agents are effective in killing the lice, their ovicidal efficiency is unreliable and thus a second treatment is necessary 7–14 days after the first in order to kill the lice that have hatched from eggs not killed by the first application. There have been no good-quality trials comparing different formulations or vehicles, but the view is generally held that insecticidal shampoos have too short a contact time to be maximally effective, and thus lotions and liquids are to be recommended.

The liquids are aqueous preparations and are preferred in those who suffer from asthma or severe eczema. Failure to apply products properly will often result in treatment failure, which may be perceived as resistance to the agent used (Box 9.6). This may result in a second course of treatment with another chemical, which may produce the same results for the same reason that the first treatment failed. Lotions and liquids should be applied as detailed in Box 9.7.

Where there is still evidence of infection and only when the evidence is presented on a piece of paper beneath a square of adhesive tape, consideration must be given to the possibility of inadequate application before considering the use of another insecticide. Friends and family should also be investigated for infection. If a second agent fails, despite proper application, wet combing may be considered before referring to the doctor. Insecticidal products should not be used for babies under 6 months old. Adverse effects experienced with insecticides are usually minor, such as irritation and erythema of the scalp and irritation of the hands. Dimeticone may also be used in the treatment of head lice. It kills the lice by disrupting water balance in the lice and resistance to this is less likely to develop. It has a well-known safety profile but it is less active against eggs. A second application should be made 7 days after the first application.

There is now a range of proprietary products for the treatment of scabies. Benzyl benzoate is an older preparation that is irritant, is not recommended for use in children and is less effective than malathion and permethrin. Thus, a non-alcoholic lotion of malathion 0.5% or a cream containing permethrin 5% is the best recommendation.

---

**Box 9.7    Application of lotions and liquids**

1. Approximately 50–100 mL of insecticidal lotion will be needed per head, depending on the amount of hair.
2. The lotion must be applied to dry hair. This is because lice can close down their respiratory airways for a short time when immersed in water. It is thought that insecticides enter the louse, at least in part, through the respiratory airways to exert their effect. Thus the presence of water, particularly combined with the use of an insecticidal shampoo, may reduce the efficacy of the agent used. The hair should be separated with the fingers to expose the scalp, and then a small amount of lotion rubbed in until the scalp is wet. Special attention must be paid to the nape of the neck and behind the ears, where lice are usually found in greater abundance. For long hair the lotion should also be applied to the first 2–5 cm of the hair, which is the distance the lice may move from the scalp.
3. It is advisable for the child to hold a towel over the face and eyes to avoid spillage while the parent applies the insecticide.
4. The hair should be allowed to dry naturally and the lotion left on, preferably overnight.
5. The lotion should be shampooed off the next day.
6. The application should be repeated after 7 days to kill the lice that have hatched from eggs not killed by the treatment.
7. The hair can be inspected by detection combing a few days after the second application.

---

Traditionally, people were advised to take a hot bath before applying a scabicide. This is no longer deemed necessary, but the skin should be clean, cool and dry before application. The scabicide should be applied with cotton wool or a piece of sponge to the whole body, including the scalp, neck, face and ears. The scabicide penetrates the skin to kill the mite and eggs in the basal layer of the epidermis. Care should be taken to apply it between the fingers and toes and under the nails. Aqueous applications should be left on for 24 hours and creams for about 12 hours. Permethrin is more suitable for use in children because it needs to be left on the skin for only 8 hours, rather than 24 hours. Children under 2 years should be referred for treatment under medical supervision. It is important that if the hands are inadvertently washed or immersed in water during this period, the scabicide should be reapplied.

It is now recommended that malathion and permethrin be applied on two occasions, one week apart.

### Wet combing methods

The practice of 'bug busting' or wet combing has been advocated, and is especially favoured by parents who consider chemical treatment undesirable. This technique involves wet combing of the hair with a detection comb until no more lice are found. Combing is carried out first after the application of hair conditioner and then repeated on rinsed hair. Combing is done every 3 or 4 days for 2–3 weeks and continued until no further lice are found, and then for another 3–4 days. The process should take 2 hours each time. There is controversy about the effectiveness of this method, and it is generally not recommended as first-line treatment of infection. However, because it requires time and dedication on the part of parents, the reasons for failure in many cases may be due to poor methodology, and thus in particular limited circumstances it may have a role.

### Antipruritics (BNF section 13.3)

Itching is a symptom that will be reduced as the skin lesion causing it is resolved. Topical antihistamines are only slightly effective and they have a tendency to cause sensitisation. Although they should not be used in eczemas and psoriasis, they can be recommended for short-term treatment of insect bites, sunburn and urticarial eruptions, and cause problems in only a very small number of people.

Calamine lotion is a cheap, traditional antipruritic preparation and has long been used, especially for the relief of sunburn.

Preparations containing crotamiton are sometimes used for pruritis but are of uncertain value. Crotamiton may be sold from a pharmacy for use in adults and children over the age of 3 years to relieve itch. It should be applied 2–3 times daily.

Sedating oral antihistamines are also useful for pruritus. They can be taken at night to relieve night-time pruritus, as well as having a carry-over effect into the next day.

### Antifungal preparations (BNF section 13.10.2)

The imidazoles, e.g. clotrimazole, miconazole and ketoconazole, are effective topical antifungal agents and have largely superseded more traditional preparations such as Whitfield's ointment. They are effective against tinea cruris, tinea corporis and tinea pedis, as well as candidiasis. This broad spectrum of activity makes them particularly suitable for the treatment of intertriginous rashes, where the identity of the exact causative infective agent may not be clear. Where the rash is particularly irritant they may be used in a combination product with hydrocortisone. Imidazoles may occasionally cause local irritation.

Terbinafine cream is an effective treatment for tinea pedis and tinea cruris. It can only be sold to people over 16 years of age for the treatment of these conditions.

Tolnaftate is effective against tinea but has little activity against *Candida*.

Treatment for tinea and candidal infections must be continued for at least 1 week but preferably longer after symptoms have subsided to ensure complete eradication of the infection.

Topical amorolfine may be effective in treating early onychomycosis when the disease is mild and involves up to two nails. Ideally onychomycosis should be confirmed by microscopy, but dermatologists have agreed that amorolfine can be sold from a pharmacy for distal and lateral onychomycosis without having a positive diagnosis confirmed. Treatment should be applied weekly for up to 12 months, although not much improvement will be seen in the first 3 months. Topical amorolfine is not recommended for use in people under 18 years of age.

### Preparations for warts and calluses (BNF section 13.7)

Many preparations are available from the pharmacy for the treatment of verrucae. Such preparations include salicylic acid, formaldehyde, gluteraldehyde or silver nitrate. Salicylic acid is a keratolytic that is commonly used, and preparations that contain this have at least 10% salicylic acid present. Before application of the treatment, the area can be softened by soaking in warm water for 5–10 minutes; surrounding normal skin should be protected by soft paraffin or with a plaster specifically designed for this before applying the treatment. The surface of the verruca should be rubbed with a file or pumice stone to remove hard skin once weekly. It may be necessary to continue treatment for up to 3 months.

 **? Re-consider the case**

Before reading further, re-consider the following questions and your initial thoughts on this case.

**Trigger questions**

- What additional information would you need before considering the appropriate management options in this case?
- What issues concern you about this case?
- Are any alarm symptoms being exhibited that require more urgent treatment or referral?

**Case study**

A 25-year-old man comes into the pharmacy and asks to speak to the pharmacist. He wants to get something to treat his itch. He seems embarrassed to discuss his problem but eventually tells the pharmacist that the itching started between his fingers but has now spread to his palms and wrists. The itching is particularly troublesome at night. He also wonders if there is anything that will help to treat his painful fingernails. He then says that his girlfriend has spots on her feet that have black dots in the centre and wonders what these could be.

 **Pharmacist opinion**

As this man appears embarrassed about his problem, it is very important to deal with this in a sensitive manner. The information provided would suggest that this man has scabies, as it typically presents with itching in the finger webs but may also spread to other areas such as the palms and wrists and itching is worse at night. Permethrin 5% dermal cream would be an appropriate treatment for this man. It would be important to advise on the correct application of the cream, ensuring that it is applied to the whole body and washed off after 8–12 hours. If the hands are washed during this time, the treatment should be reapplied. Scabies is transferred by close physical contact so all members of the infected household should be treated. It is important that his girlfriend treats herself at the same time. The man should also be advised that the itch of scabies may persist after treatment with permethrin and symptomatic treatment of the itch may be required.

Painful fingernails may be due to onychomycosis, which could be confirmed by examining the nails. If this is the case and no more than two nails are affected, treatment with topical amorolfine could be recommended. If more than two nails are affected referral to the doctor is necessary.

From the description of the spots on his girlfriend's feet, it would appear that she has verrucae on them. It would be important to establish whether his girlfriend was diabetic before recommending treatment. If appropriate, a preparation containing salicylic acid would be recommended and advice given on how this should be applied as well as general hygiene measures to minimise the spread of infection.

General practitioner opinion

This sounds like a classic case of scabies. What causes his embarrassment? Is it the thought of having a scabies infestation or something else? Scabies is transmitted through skin-to-skin contact, which may be as brief as holding hands, but is often transmitted through sexual contact. Sensitive questioning may reveal other health needs and education.

The presence of mite burrows in the finger webs would confirm the diagnosis, although often they cannot be seen. Secondary infection is common, hence the need for careful examination. Differential diagnoses to consider are eczema and fungal skin infection.

Involvement of fingernails in scabies is unusual and may signify other underlying health problems including immunocompromised state. This would certainly require further investigation. Examination of the nails may reveal more simple explanations such as paronychia.

Careful explanation of treatment is required including treatment of contacts.

 Summary of key points

| Condition | Management |
|---|---|
| Head lice infection is characterised by an itchy scalp, although in some children it may be asymptomatic. | Parasiticidal preparations such as malathion, permethrin and phenothrin may be used in the treatment of head lice. Dimeticone may also be used. Wet combing may be favoured by parents when the use of chemical treatment is considered undesirable. |
| Scabies is characterised by intense itching, particularly at night, and a papular rash, although it is not always obvious. | Malathion and permethrin. Antipruritics may be used to relieve itch. |
| Tinea infection is generally characterised by itching and a rash or lesions, although this varies depending on location. No itch is present when the nails are affected. | Antifungal preparations such as imidazoles, terbinafine and tolnaftate. Topical amorolfine may be effective in mild onychomycosis. |
| Verrucae are characterised by hard plaques of dry skin with a small central ulcer revealing several black roots. They usually affect the pressure areas of the foot. | Preparations containing salicylic acid, formaldehyde, gluteraldehyde or silver nitrate may be used. |

 When to refer

- Any skin rash, lesion or pruritus that does not respond to management with medicines purchased from a pharmacy
- Pruritis without an obvious skin lesion
- Erythema or vesicles on the palms of the hands
- Inflamed, painful skin surrounding the nail
- Pitting of fingernails

**When to refer** *(continued)*

- Moles with two of the following characteristics:
  — Increasing in size
  — Changing shape or outline from regular to irregular
  — Changing colour or mixed colour in the same mole
  — Itching
  — Bleeding
  — Crusting
  — Inflammation
- Urticaria accompanied by swelling of the eyelids or lips, or difficulty with breathing – emergency referral to hospital
- All diabetics with foot problems (refer to either the doctor or the podiatrist)
- Athlete's foot that spreads to other areas of the foot, and if the toenails are affected
- Skin lesions accompanied by malaise and fever

# Napkin rash and molluscum contagiosum

Before reading further, consider the following case and note your initial thoughts.

**Case study**

A young mother comes into the pharmacy. She has an 18-month-old daughter and asks for advice regarding the red rash that her daughter has on the nappy area. She has had nappy rash before but it appears redder this time with small spots. Her daughter also has developed some small spots on her legs and a friend told her that they are 'water warts'. She wonders whether there is anything that she can treat this with.

**Trigger questions**

- What additional information would you need before considering the appropriate management options in this case?
- What issues concern you about this case?
- Are any alarm symptoms being exhibited that require more urgent treatment or referral?

## Assessing symptoms

### Napkin rash

Most babies develop napkin rash ('nappy rash') at some stage and it is a condition that often causes more distress to the parents than to the baby. Classically, it appears as a confluent red rash over the napkin area. In some cases it may take the form of papules or vesicles, and there may be fissuring. The condition is caused by a contact dermatitis from the ammonia released from the urine, by faecal organisms, and from other constituents of urine and faeces. It may be worsened by constant soaking of the skin in the napkin area. This contact dermatitis spares the intertriginous areas of skin (between skin folds) where there is no contact with the irritant urine, and thus it can be distinguished from candidal infection, seborrhoeic eczema and psoriasis, in which the intertriginous areas are affected.

### Water warts

Molluscum contagiosum (water warts) is a common viral infection of the skin that particularly affects infants and young children with eczema. It appears as small pearl-coloured drop-like papules, each having a small dimple in the centre. It can occur on the face, but is more common on the limbs and trunk (see Figure 9.25). The condition is not irritant and no treatment is necessary. It will resolve spontaneously

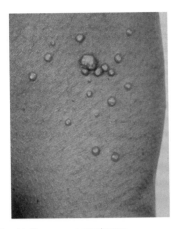

**Figure 9.25** Molluscum contagiosum.
(Reproduced with permission from the Wellcome Trust Medical Photographic Library.)

after a few months. However, referral to a doctor for management is necessary if the condition becomes infected or the child scratches the lesions.

## Accompanying symptoms

### Scaling in the napkin area

Seborrhoeic napkin dermatitis may appear as a red scaling eruption, especially in the intertriginous areas. Often the infant also has seborrhoeic eczema of the scalp (cradle cap), face, trunk, and behind the ears.

Psoriasis in the napkin area, which is rare, occurs initially as a red eruption. There may be some scaling, but not as much as is found in psoriasis that occurs elsewhere on the body. The condition may later spread to the trunk and limbs. Failure of nappy rash to resolve after several weeks of standard treatment may raise the possibility of napkin psoriasis and requires referral for medical attention.

### Pustular napkin rash

If a napkin rash appears pustular, there may be bacterial infection with *Staphylococcus*. The pustules may rupture and produce scaling. If this is suspected, then the child should be referred to a doctor for consideration of antibiotic treatment. The wet, warm environment under a napkin provides an ideal place for the growth of *Candida* and bacteria. Candidal infection of the napkin area causes a bright red eruption with pinpoint papules or pustules covering all the skin, including intertriginous areas. It may also be associated with oral candidiasis (thrush) and can be a sequela to antibiotic treatment. Candidal infection should be suspected when a napkin rash fails to respond to simple symptomatic remedies. If there is no improvement, or if the rash spreads to the trunk, referral to a doctor for management should be considered.

### Fever

If the skin in the napkin area becomes severely inflamed and fever is present, this may indicate an infection and referral to a doctor for treatment is required.

## Management options

When babies are suffering from napkin rash it is important to advise that the napkin should be changed frequently and that the area is cleansed using water or fragrance-free and alcohol-free wipes to minimise further irritation. The area should then be dried thoroughly after cleansing. Whenever possible, the skin should be exposed by removing the napkin to allow drying and healing. It should also be advised that when bathing the baby no soaps or bubble baths should be used. The use of talcum powders should also be avoided.

If babies have candidal infection of the napkin area, barrier creams should not be used until the candidal infection has settled. In napkin rash where there is inflammation present that causes discomfort to the baby, corticosteroids are useful, but these cannot be sold from the pharmacy for this purpose so referral to a doctor for treatment is required. Parents who are using corticosteroids should be advised to apply barrier preparations after the corticosteroid has been applied.

Sufferers of molluscum contagiosum should be advised that the condition is self-limiting and usually resolves spontaneously within 18 months. The lesions are contagious, however, and the sharing of towels and clothing should be discouraged. Children can continue to attend school and go swimming but should be advised to avoid scratching the lesions.

### Barrier preparations (BNF section 13.2.2)

Barrier preparations are used to protect the skin against napkin rash and should be applied at each napkin change. Such barrier agents include zinc cream, zinc ointment, zinc and castor oil ointment, and various proprietary products containing zinc, titanium and dimeticone.

### Antifungal preparations (BNF section 13.10.2)

Topical imidazoles such as clotrimazole can be used to treat candidal infection of the napkin area. A thin layer of cream should be applied to the area.

 **Re-consider the case**

Before reading further, re-consider the following questions and your initial thoughts on this case.

**Trigger questions**

- What additional information would you need before considering the appropriate management options in this case?
- What issues concern you about this case?
- Are any alarm symptoms being exhibited that require more urgent treatment or referral?

**Case study**

A young mother comes into the pharmacy. She has an 18-month-old daughter and asks for advice regarding the red rash that her daughter has on the nappy area. She has had nappy rash before but it appears redder this time with small spots. Her daughter also has developed some small spots on her legs and a friend told her that they are 'water warts'. She wonders whether there is anything that she can treat this with.

 Pharmacist opinion

It would firstly be important to gather some additional information about the history of nappy rash in this child and establish what treatment had been used in the past. It would also be necessary to inspect the nappy area to establish whether infection was present. If no infection was apparent, a barrier preparation would be recommended and the parent would be advised on the importance of frequent nappy changing, ensuring that the area is thoroughly cleaned and dried and exposed to the air as much as possible. If infection with *Candida* was suspected, an antifungal preparation would be recommended and the parent would be advised to avoid using a barrier preparation until the infected area had cleared.

The parent would also be advised that 'water warts' is a common viral infection in children that usually resolves spontaneously and no treatment is required. It is important that the warts are not scratched as they may become infected and in such circumstances referral to the doctor would be required for appropriate antibiotic treatment.

 General practitioner opinion

A quick talk through how this mother looks after her daughter's nappy area would be helpful. For example: What type of nappies does she use? How often does she change her daughter's nappy? And does she use any barrier cream? It sounds like she has managed nappy rash before – what worked previously?

General practitioner opinion (continued)

Examination of the nappy area should reveal the diagnosis of irritant dermatitis, atopic eczema, bacterial infection or candidiasis. Psoriasis is worth consideration but is very rare in this age group.

Appropriate treatment combined with the use of plenty of barrier cream should resolve the problem fairly quickly.

'Water warts' is a term sometimes used for the spots caused by molluscum contagiosum. The spots are very characteristic and examination will quickly confirm the diagnosis. Treatment is not necessary and careful explanation of the condition usually reassures parents. Occasionally, the spots can become infected and require antibiotic treatment. An information leaflet would be helpful here and is usually much appreciated.

 Summary of key points

| Condition | Management |
| --- | --- |
| Napkin rash is characterised by a red rash over the napkin area. | Barrier preparations containing zinc, titanium or dimeticone can be used to protect against napkin rash. |
| Molluscum contagiosum is characterised by small, smooth, shiny, pearl-coloured papules ('water warts'). | The condition usually resolves spontaneously. No satisfactory medical treatment is available. |

 When to refer

- Nappy rash not responding to treatment with medicines purchased from a pharmacy
- Bacterial infection suspected
- Nappy rash accompanied by fever
- Infected water warts

# Bibliography

Barnetson RC, Rogers M (2002). Childhood atopic eczema. *Br Med J* 324: 1376–1379.

Bassett I *et al.* (1990). A comparative study of tea-tree oil versus benzoylperoxide in the treatment of acne. *Med J Aust* 153(8): 455–458.

British Association for Sexual Health and HIV (2001). *National Guideline on the Management of Scabies*. Available from: www.bashh.org/guidelines/2002/scabies_0901b.pdf (accessed 1 April 2011).

Clark C (2004). How to choose a suitable emollient. *Pharm J* 273: 351–354.

Clark C (2007). Head lice treatments and advice. *Pharm J* 279: 185–188.

Cox NH (2000). Permethrin treatment in scabies infestation: importance of the correct formulation. *Br Med J* 320: 37–38.

Douglas G *et al*. eds (2005). *MacLeod's Clinical Examination*. Edinburgh: Churchill Livingstone.

Gibbs S *et al.* (2002). Local treatments for cutaneous warts: systematic review. *Br Med J* 325: 461–463.

Kumar P, Clark M, eds (2005). *Clinical Medicine*. London: Elsevier Saunders.

Mason AR *et al.* (2004). Topical treatments for chronic plaque psoriasis (protocol). *Cochrane Database of Syst Rev* 2004, Issue 1.

McGrath J, Murphy GM (1991). The control of seborrhoeic dermatitis and dandruff by antipityrosporal drugs. *Drugs* 41(2): 178–184.

Ozolins M *et al.* (2004). Comparison of five antimicrobial regimens for treatment of mild to moderate inflammatory facial acne vulgaris in the community: randomised clinical trial. *Lancet* 364: 2188–2195.

Watkins P (2003). ABC of diabetes – the diabetic foot. *Br Med J* 326: 977–979.

Webster GF (2002). Acne vulgaris. *Br Med J* 325: 475–479.

Williams HC (2003). Evening primrose oil for atopic dermatitis. *Br Med J* 327: 1358–1359.

# Self-assessment questions

The following questions are provided to test the information presented in this chapter.

*For questions 1–7 select the best answer in each case.*

1. Select which of the following drugs do not cause acne:
   a. Oral contraceptives
   b. Lithium
   c. Phenytoin
   d. Amiodarone
   e. Steroids

2. Select from the following skin conditions those where itch is not a symptom:
   a. Head lice
   b. Sebaceous cyst
   c. Insect bites
   d. Pompholyx
   e. Athlete's foot

3. Select which of the following skin conditions are not caused by a type of infection:
   a. Shingles
   b. Molluscum contagiosum
   c. Onychomycosis
   d. Scalp ringworm
   e. Systemic lupus erythematosus

4. Select which of the following would not be recommended for the treatment of seborrhoeic eczema:
   a. Ketoconazole
   b. Selenium sulphide
   c. Hydrocortisone
   d. Pyrithione zinc
   e. Olive oil

5. Select which of the following is not a feature of psoriasis:
   a. Silvery lesions
   b. Scaly rash
   c. Nail pitting
   d. Greasy rash
   e. Red rash

6. Select which of the following items of advice is not necessary when recommending an insecticide for the treatment of scabies:
   a. Take a hot bath before applying
   b. Apply to the whole body
   c. Treat all close contacts
   d. Reapply treatment if hands are washed after applying
   e. Apply on two occasions, one week apart

7. Select from the following conditions those for which hydrocortisone 1% cream cannot be sold from the pharmacy:
   a. Nappy rash
   b. Insect bites
   c. Mild to moderate eczema
   d. Irritant contact eczema
   e. Allergic contact eczema

*For questions 8–10 select from the list below one lettered option that is most closely related to it. Each lettered option may be used once, more than once, or not at all.*
   a. pink or tan-coloured lesions
   b. chronic redness and inflamed papules
   c. patchy depigmentation due to loss of melanocytes
   d. painful red papules that become pustular
   e. small papules, often purplish in colour

8. The appearance of acne rosacea.

9. The appearance of furuncles.

10. The appearance of lichen planus.

*For questions 11 and 12 select from the list below one lettered option that is most closely related to it. Each lettered option may be used once, more than once, or not at all.*
   a. clobetasone 0.05% cream
   b. benzoyl peroxide gel
   c. ketoconazole shampoo
   d. terbinafine cream
   e. crotamiton cream

11. This product can only be sold for use in people over the age of 16 years.

12. Erythema and dryness may occur with the first few applications of this product.

*Questions 13–16: Each of the questions or incomplete statements in this section is followed by three responses. For each question one or more of the responses is/are correct. Decide which of the responses is/are correct and then choose a–e as indicated in the table below.*

| **Directions summarised** | | | | |
|---|---|---|---|---|
| **a** | **b** | **c** | **d** | **e** |
| If 1, 2 and 3 are correct | If 1 and 2 only are correct | If 2 and 3 only are correct | If 1 only is correct | If 3 only is correct |

13. The following are reasons for treatment failure of head lice:
    1 – insufficient quantity applied
    2 – resistance to insecticide
    3 – too long contact time

**14.** The following preparations may be used to treat eczema:
1 – topical antihistamines
2 – topical corticosteroids
3 – emollients

**15.** The following may be treated with topical preparations containing salicylic acid:
1 – atopic eczema
2 – verrucae in a person with diabetes
3 – verrucae in a child aged 10 years

**16.** The following meet the criteria for the supply of topical amorolfine as a P medicine:
1 – no more than two nails affected
2 – proximal onychomycosis
3 – patient aged 16 years or older

*Questions 17–20 consist of two statements linked by the word* because; *decide whether each statement is true or false. If both statements are true then decide whether the second statement is a correct explanation of the first statement. Choose a–e as your answer as indicated in the table below.*

| Directions summarised | | |
|---|---|---|
| | **First statement** | **Second statement** | |
| **a** | True | True | Second statement is a correct explanation of the first statement |
| **b** | True | True | Second statement is not a correct explanation of the first statement |
| **c** | True | False | |
| **d** | False | True | |
| **e** | False | False | |

**17.**

| Intense pruritis is a symptom of scabies | BECAUSE | The mite Sarcoptes scabiei causes an allergic reaction in the skin in scabies |
|---|---|---|

**18.**

| Topical miconazole may be sold from the pharmacy to treat athlete's foot in a person with diabetes | BECAUSE | Topical imidazoles are used to treat fungal skin infections |
|---|---|---|

**19.**

| The whole family and contacts do not have to be treated with a parasiticide for head lice | BECAUSE | Resistance may occur to parasiticidal preparations used to treat head lice |
|---|---|---|

**20.**

| Clobetasone 0.05% cream may be sold from the pharmacy for short-term treatment of eczema | BECAUSE | Topical corticosteroids hydrate the skin in dry skin conditions such as eczema |
|---|---|---|

## Answers

1-d; 2-b; 3-e; 4-c; 5-d; 6-a; 7-d; 8-b; 9-d; 10-e; 11-d; 12-b; 13-b; 14-c; 15-e; 16-d; 17-a; 18-d; 19-a; 20-c

# Index

*Note: Box references are denoted b, figures f and tables t.*

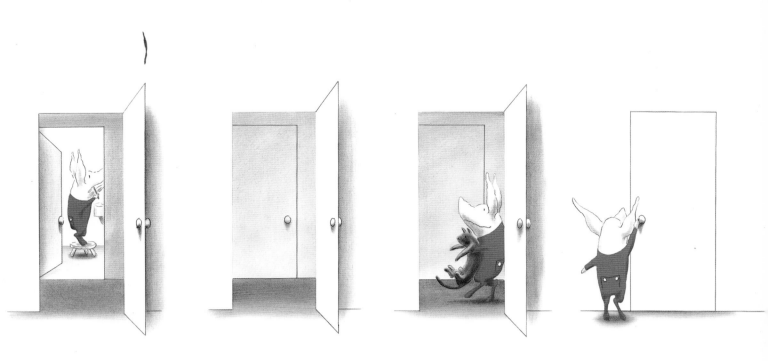

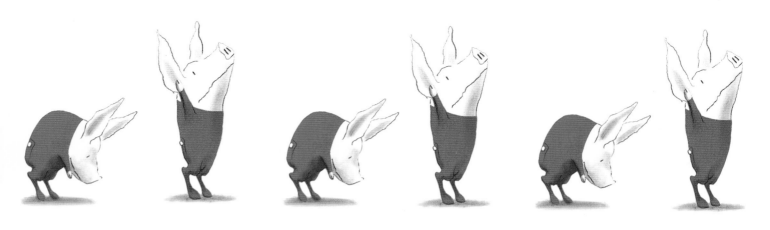

**KNOWSLEY LIBRARY SERVICE**

Knowsl@y Council

*Please return this book on or before the date shown below*

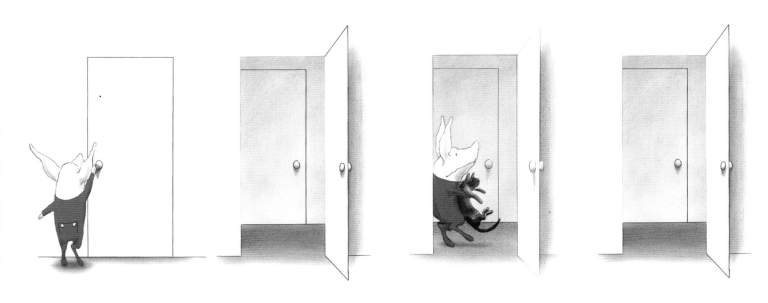

# OLIVIA
## saves the circus

written and illustrated by Ian Falconer

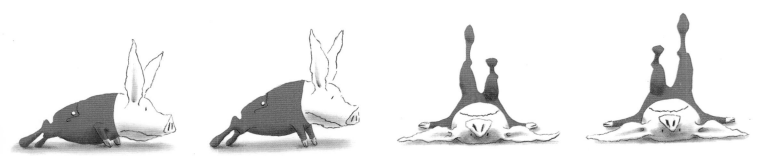

Simon & Schuster, London

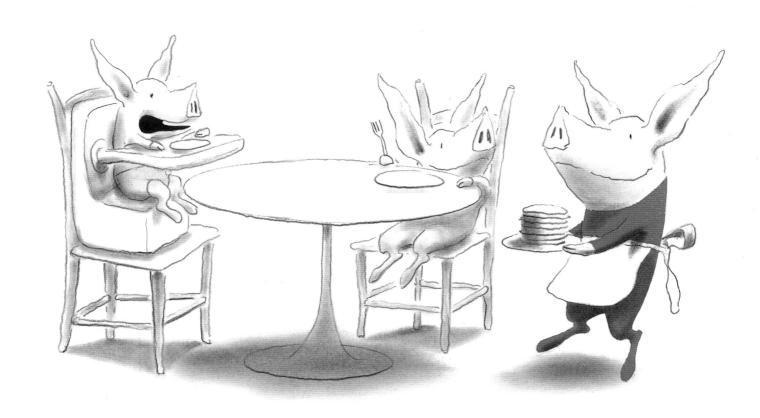

Before school, Olivia likes to make pancakes for new little brother, William, and old little brother, Ian.

This is a big help to her mother.

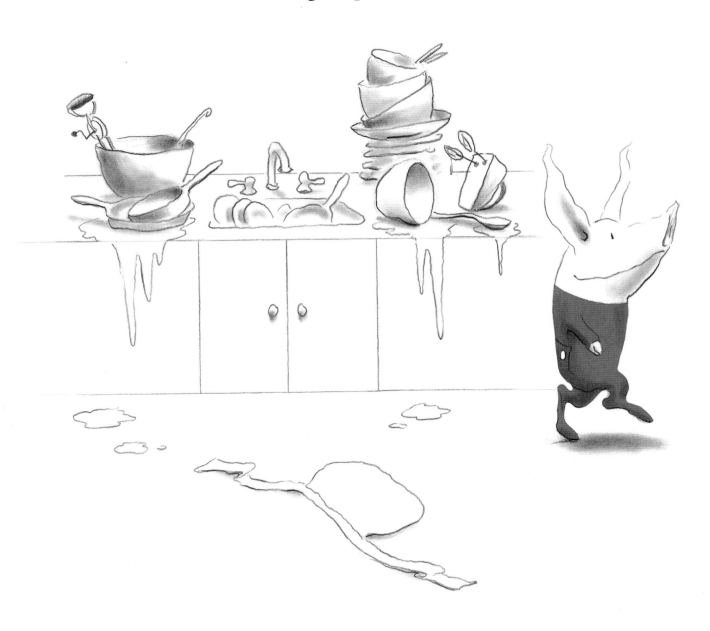

After a nice breakfast, it's time to get dressed.

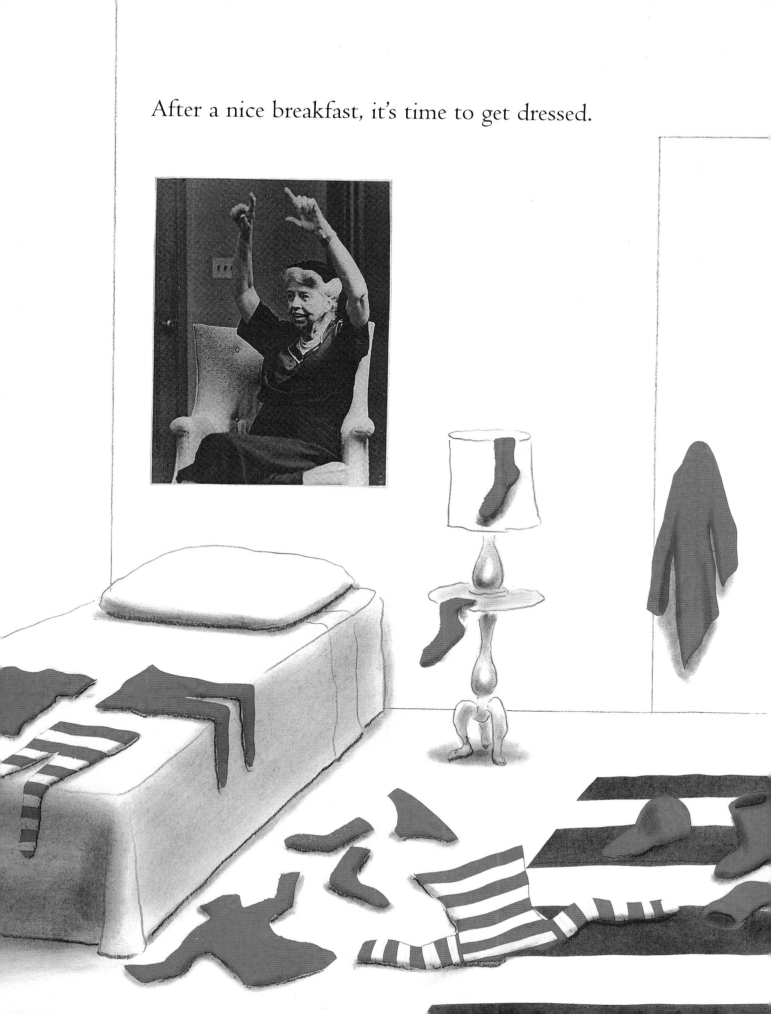

Olivia has to wear this really boring uniform.

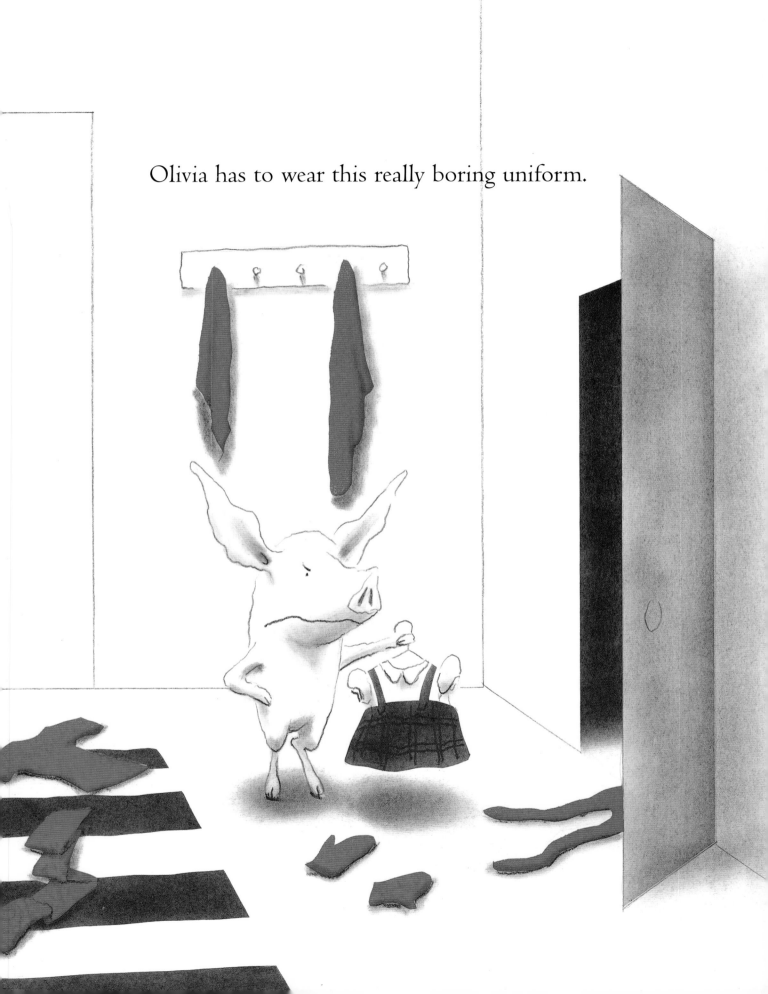

Of course you can always accessorise.

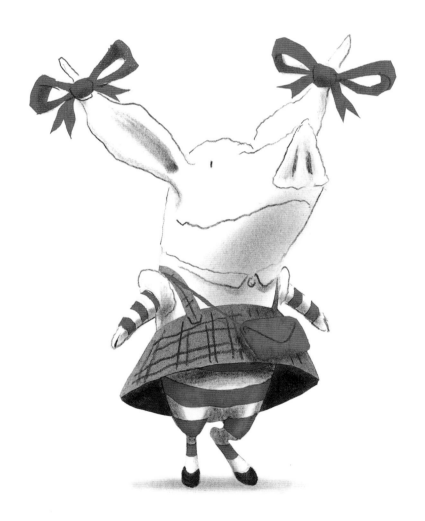

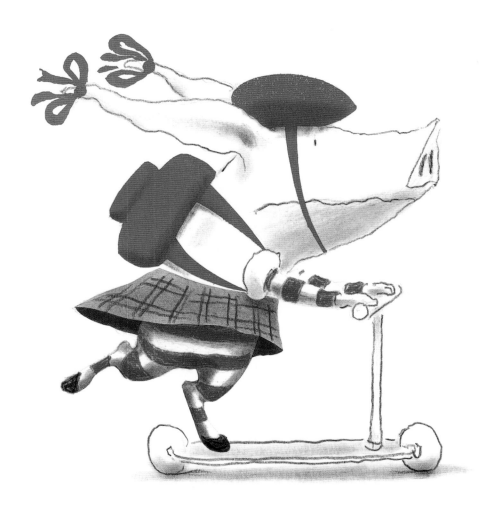

Beep, beep — coming through.

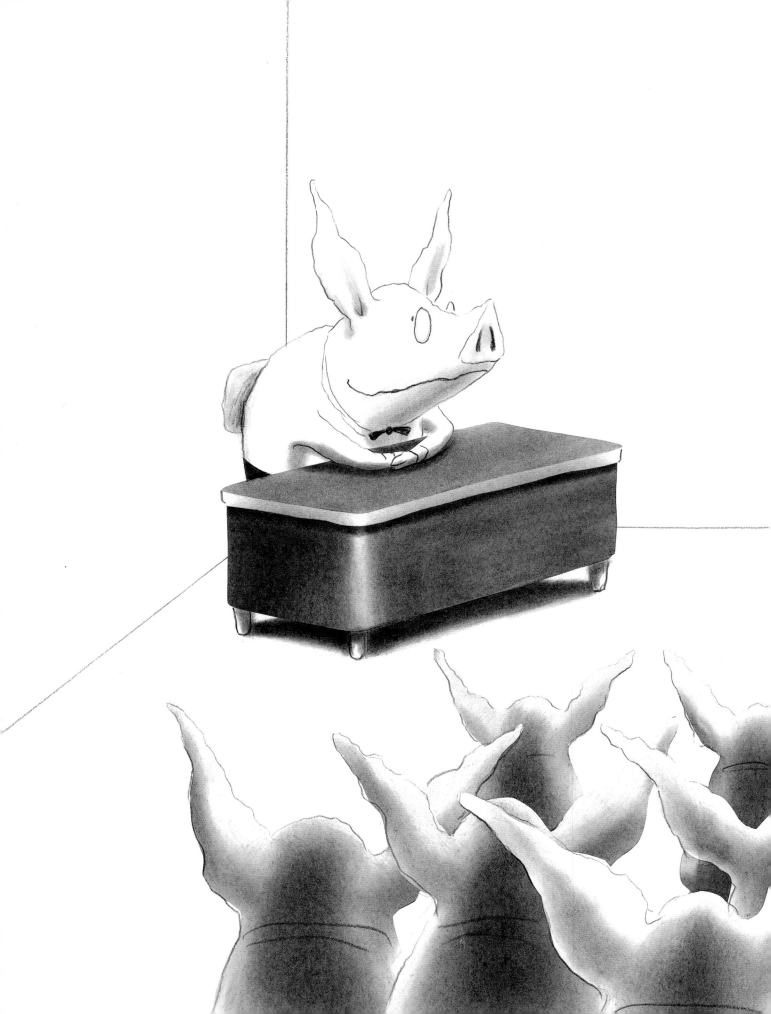

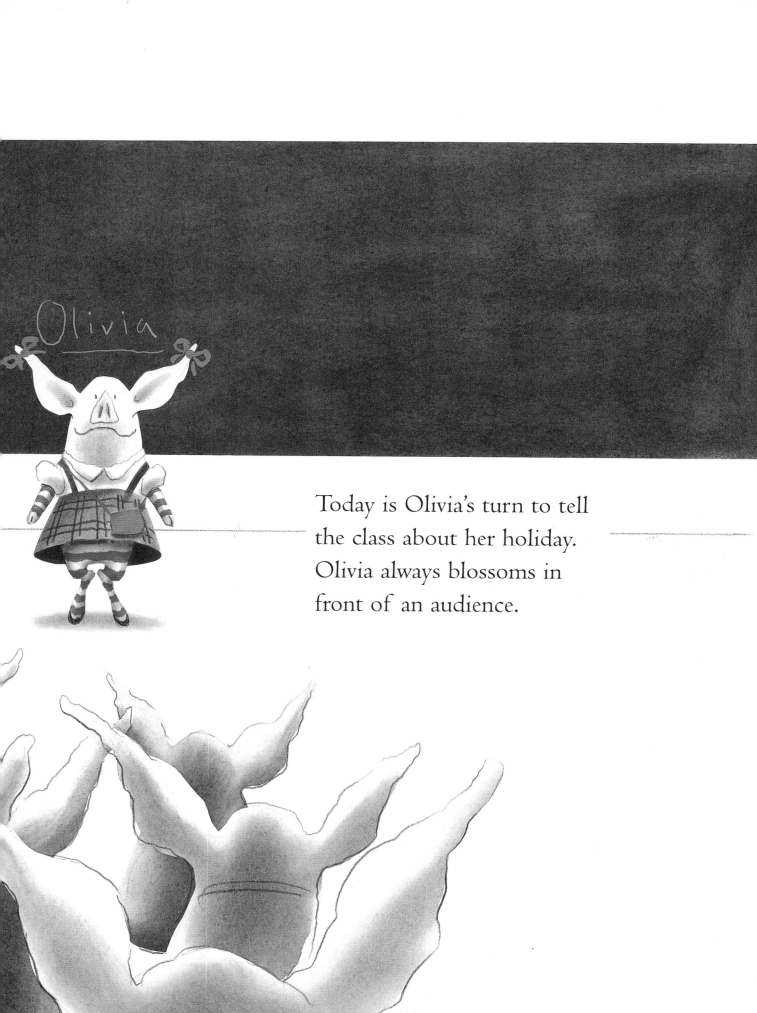

Today is Olivia's turn to tell
the class about her holiday.
Olivia always blossoms in
front of an audience.

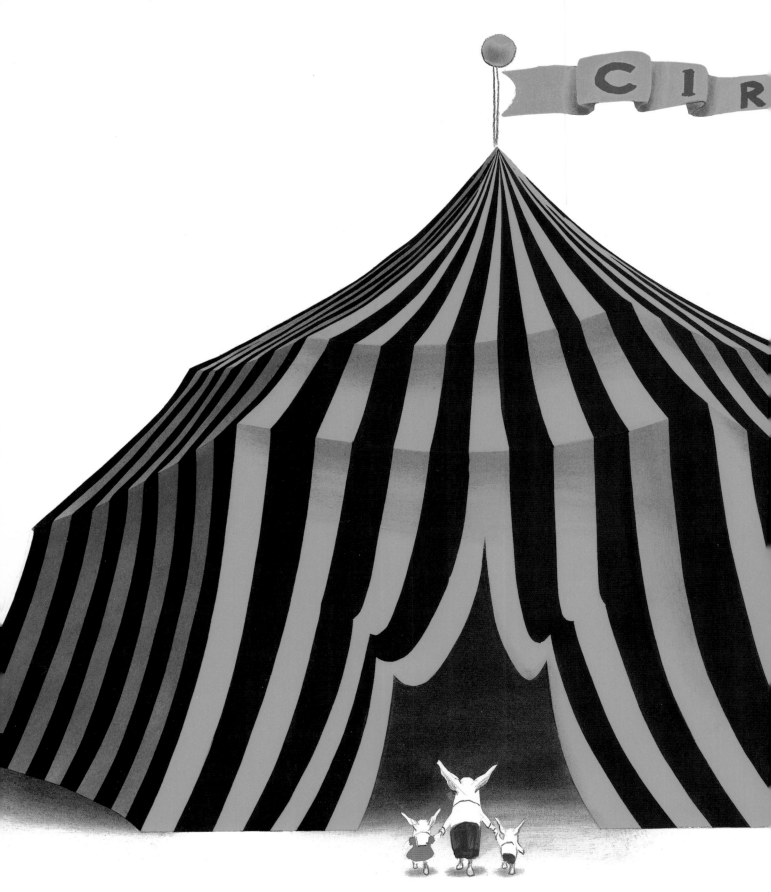

"One day my mother took Ian and me to the circus," she begins.
"William couldn't come because he still has to take a nap.

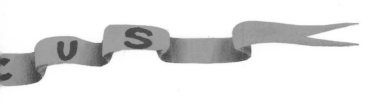

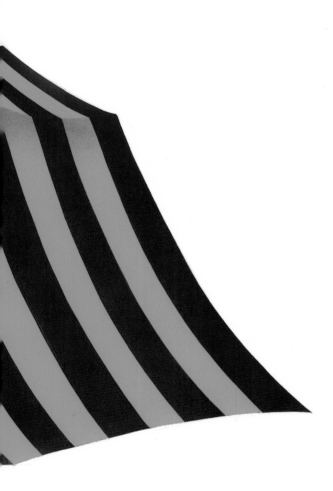

"But when we got there, all the circus people were off sick with
ear infections.

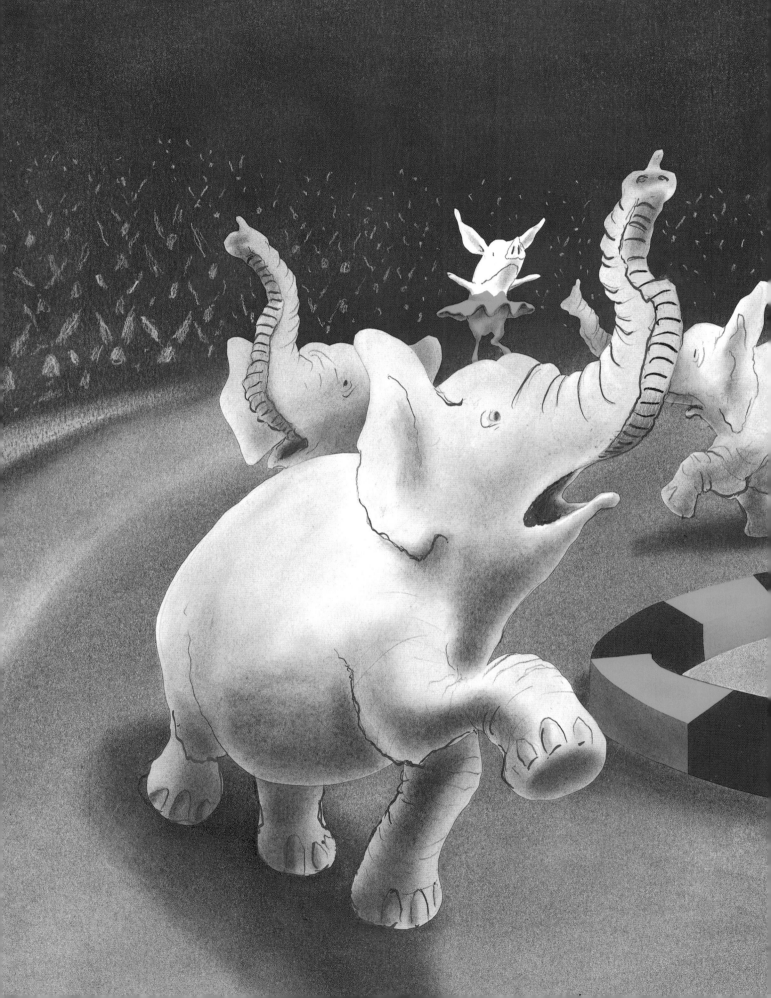

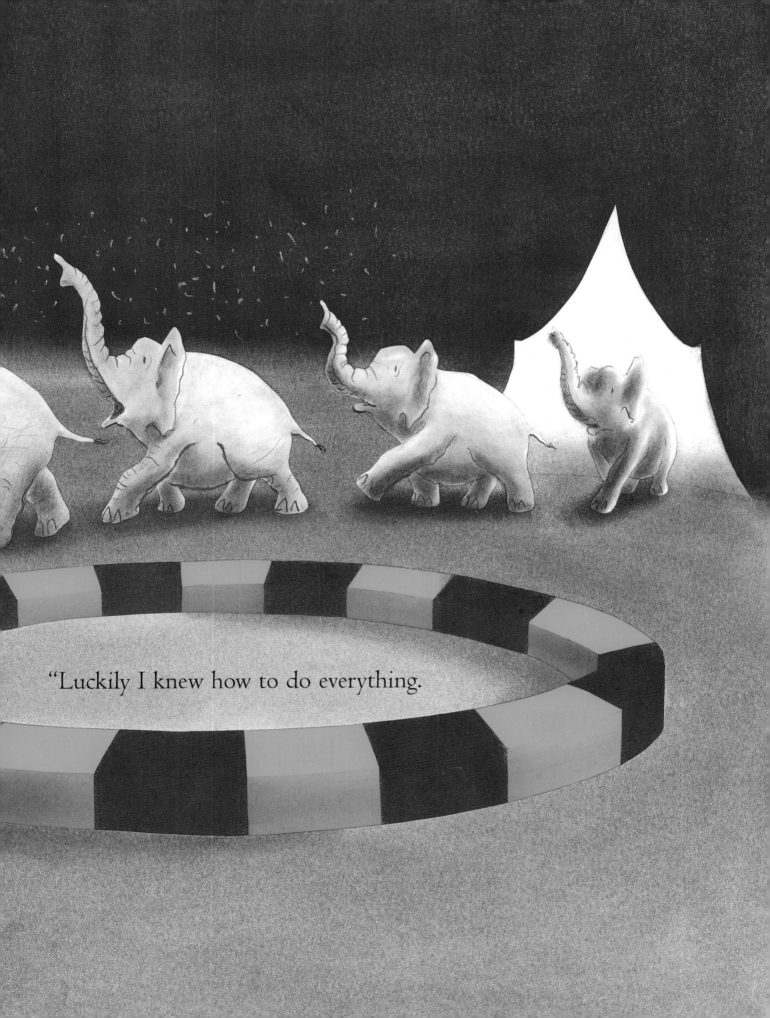

"Luckily I knew how to do everything.

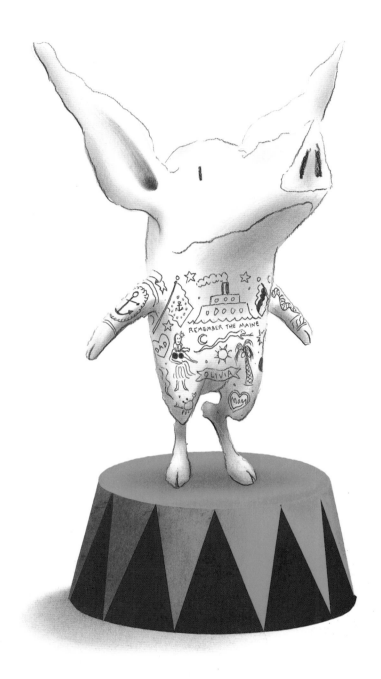

"I was Olivia the Tattooed Lady. I drew
the pictures on with marker pen.

"Then I was Olivia the Lion Tamer

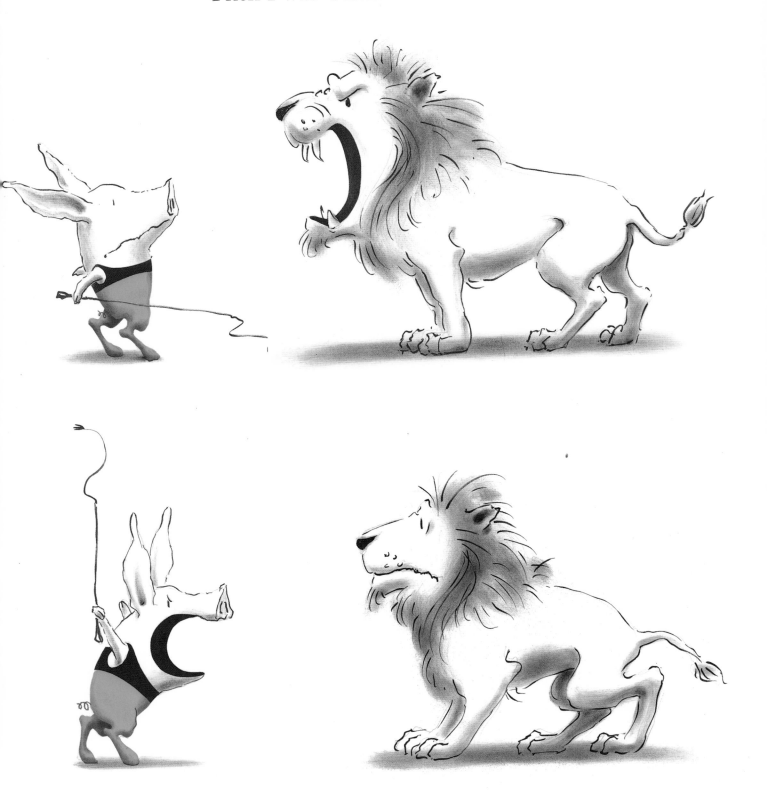

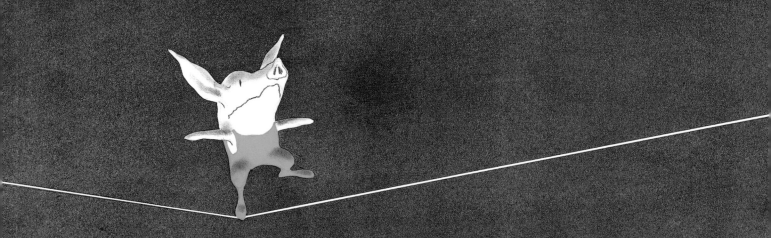

"and Olivia the Tight-rope Walker

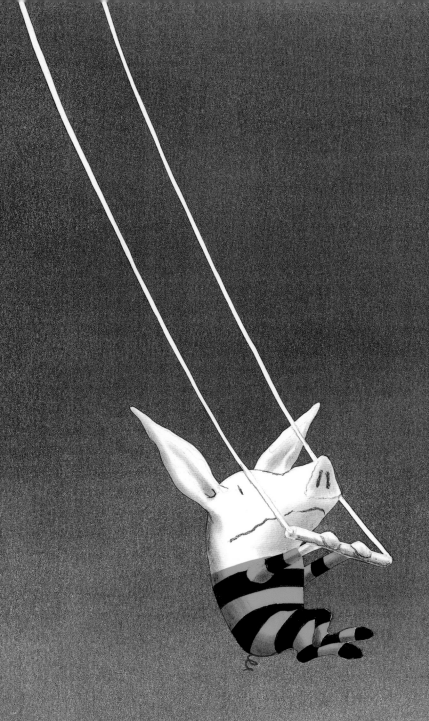

"Then I was the Flying Olivia,

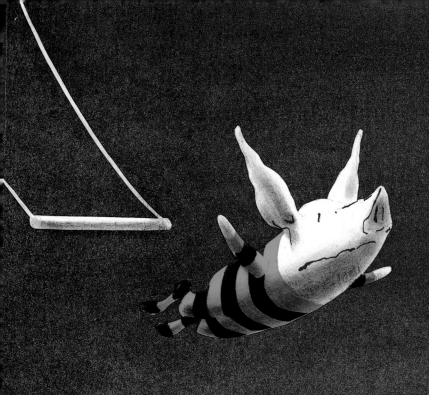

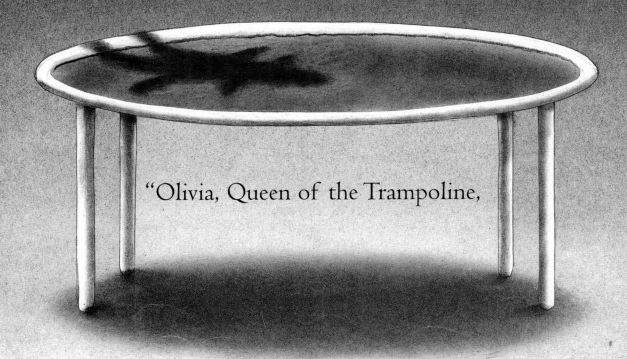

"Olivia, Queen of the Trampoline,

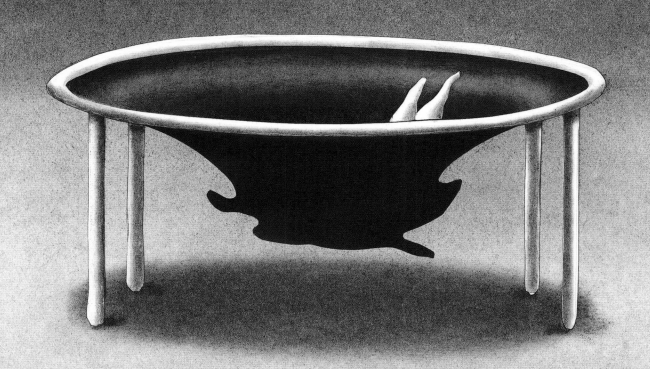

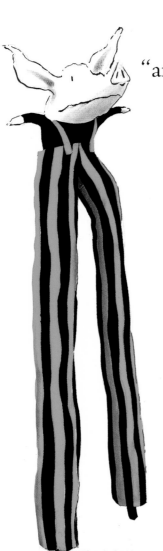

"and I balanced on stilts

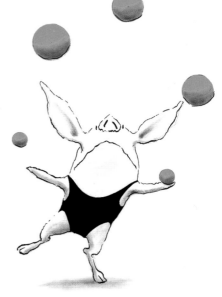

and juggled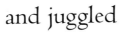

and was Olivia the Clown

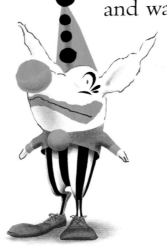

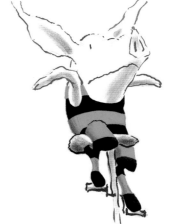

and rode a unicycle.

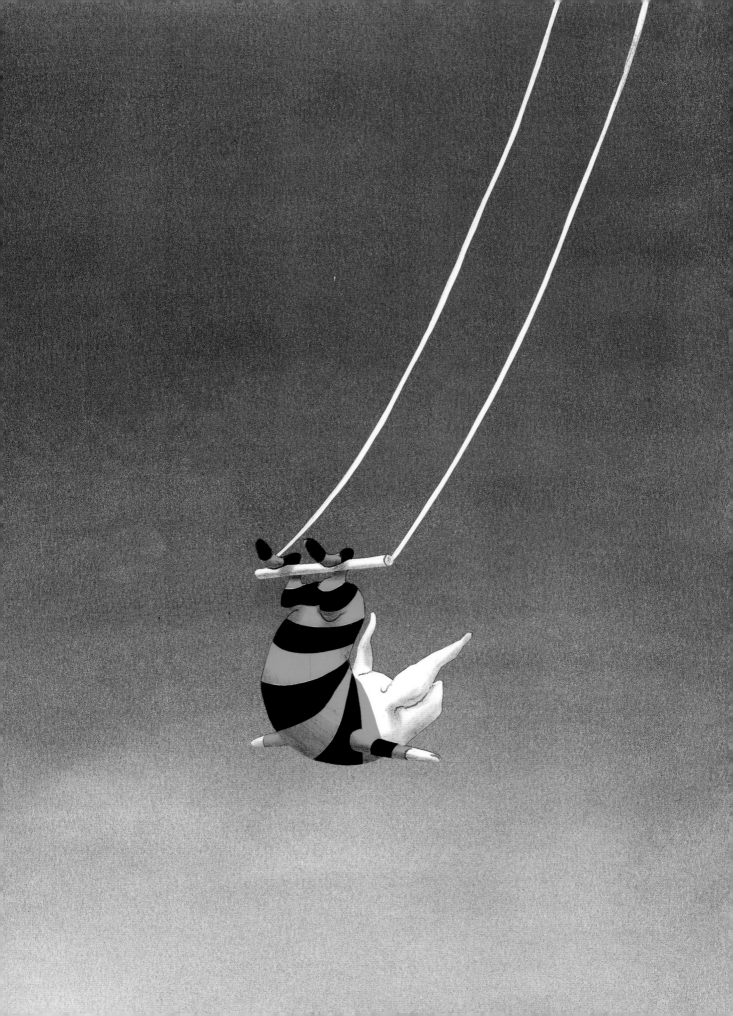

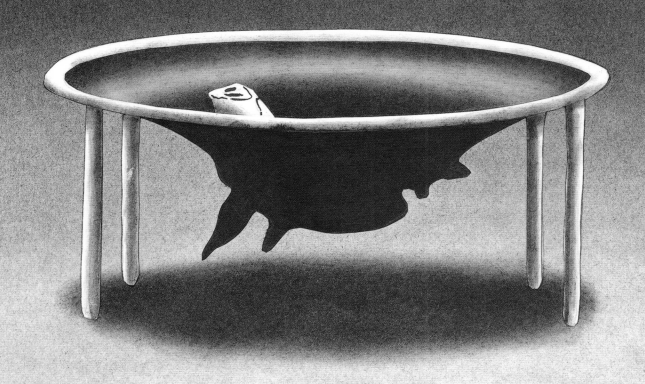

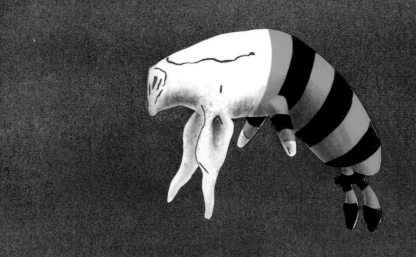
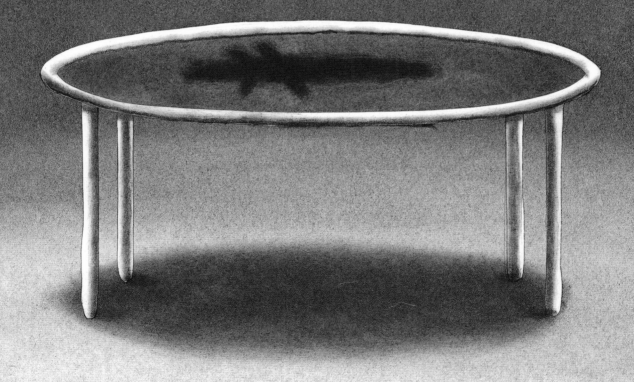

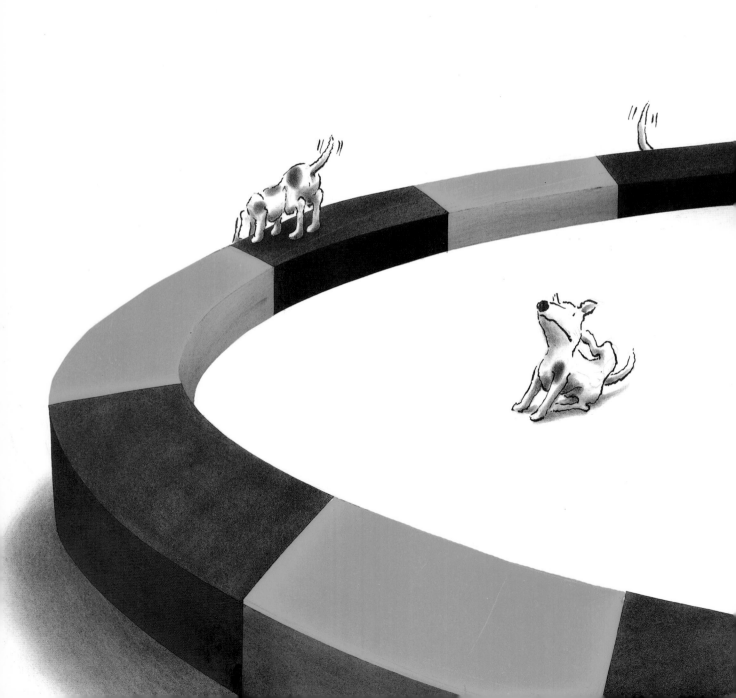

"and finally Madame Olivia and her Trained Dogs.
They weren't very trained.

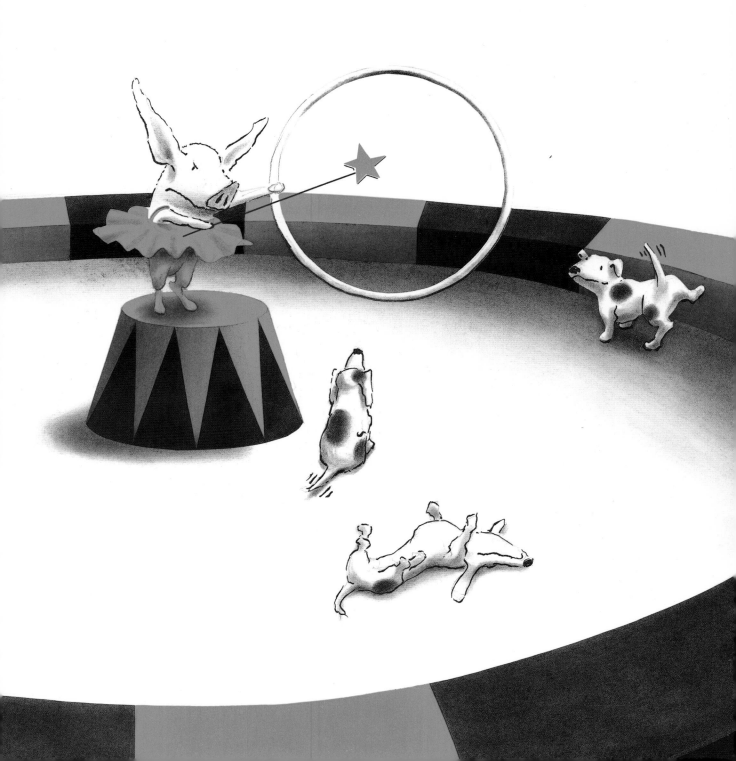

"And that's how I saved the circus.
And now I am famous.

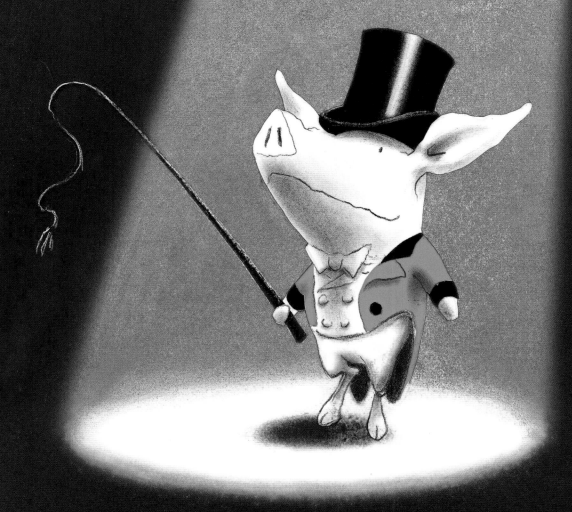

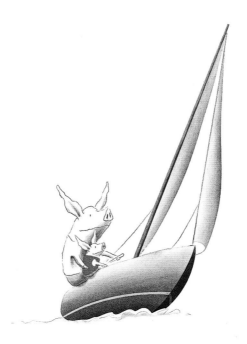

"Then one time my dad took me sailing The End."

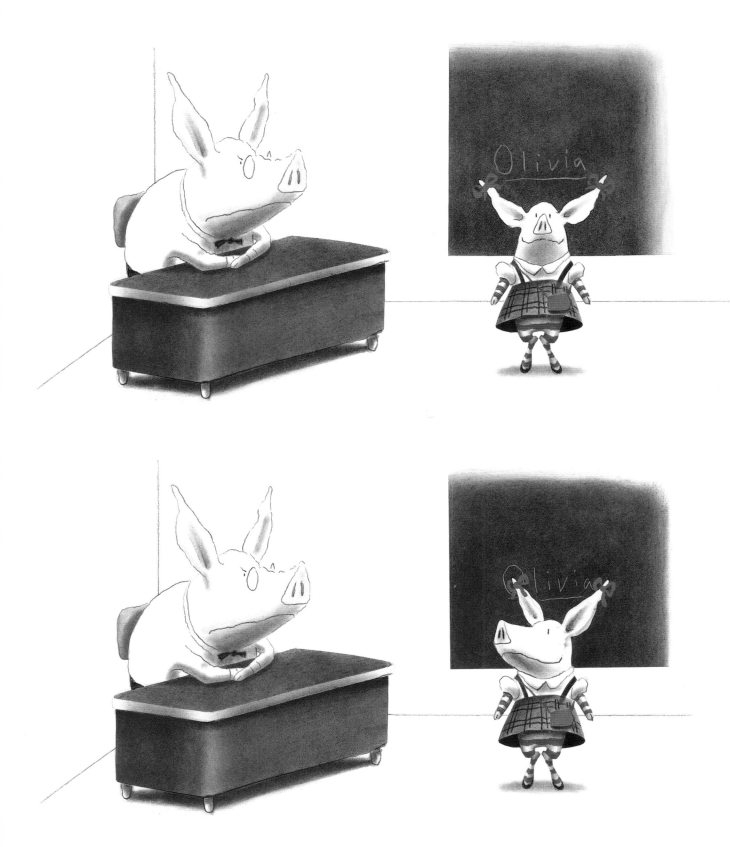

"Was that true?" Olivia's teacher asks.

"Quite true," says Olivia.

"All true?"

"Quite all true."

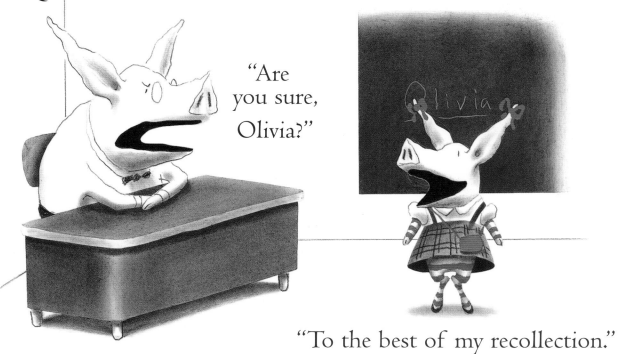

"Are you sure, Olivia?"

"To the best of my recollection."

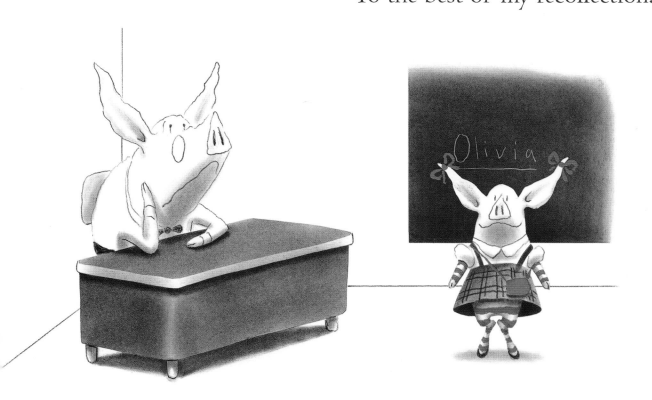

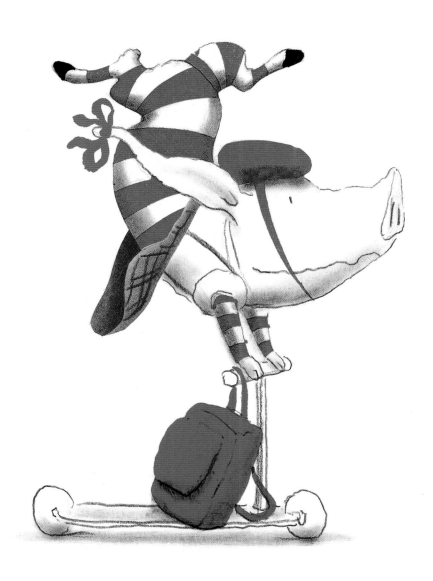

Olivia heads home gracefully.

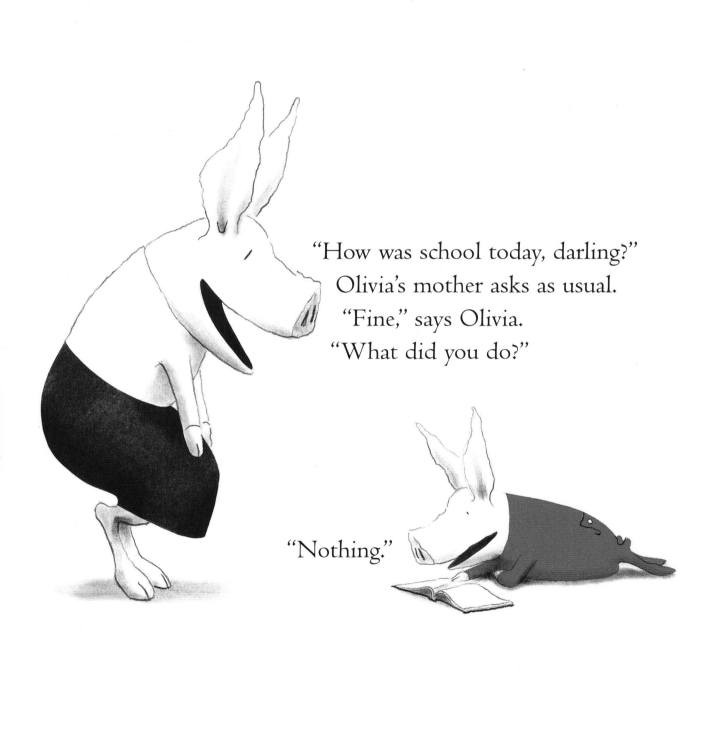

"How was school today, darling?"
Olivia's mother asks as usual.
"Fine," says Olivia.
"What did you do?"

"Nothing."

It's bedtime, but of course Olivia's not at all sleepy.

"Good night," says her mother.

"Good night, Mummy," says Olivia.

"Close your eyes."

"They are closed."

"Then go to sleep."

"I am asleep."

"And remember, no jumping."

"Okay, Mummy."

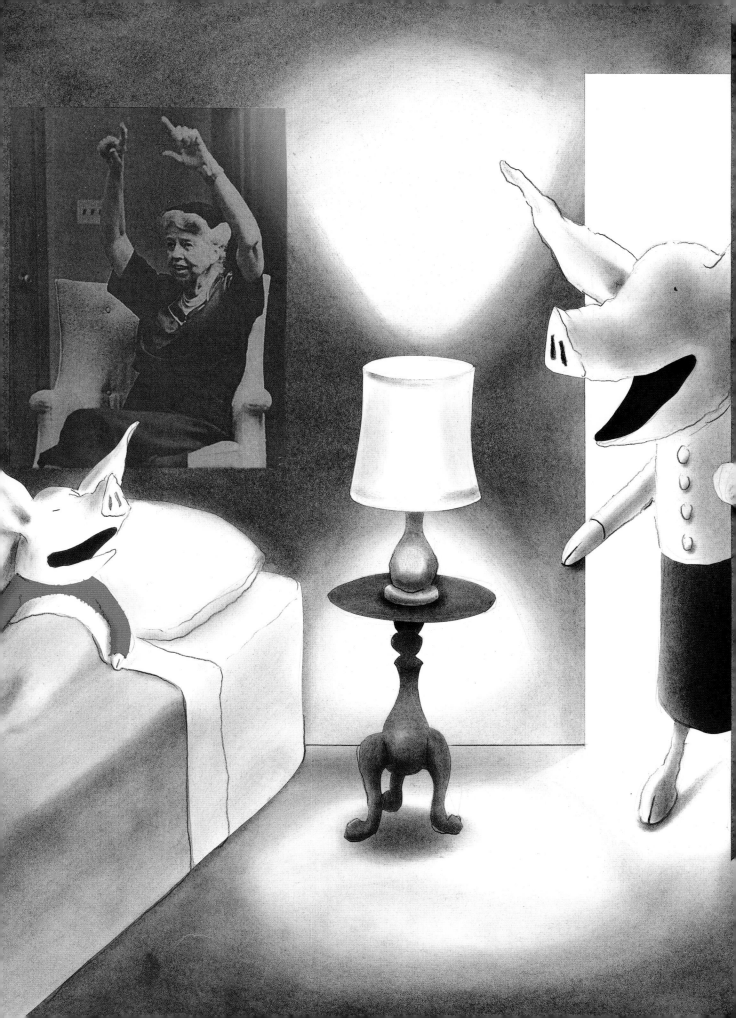

"Now, Olivia, I said, 'No jumping.'
Who do you think you are —
Olivia, Queen of the Trampoline?"

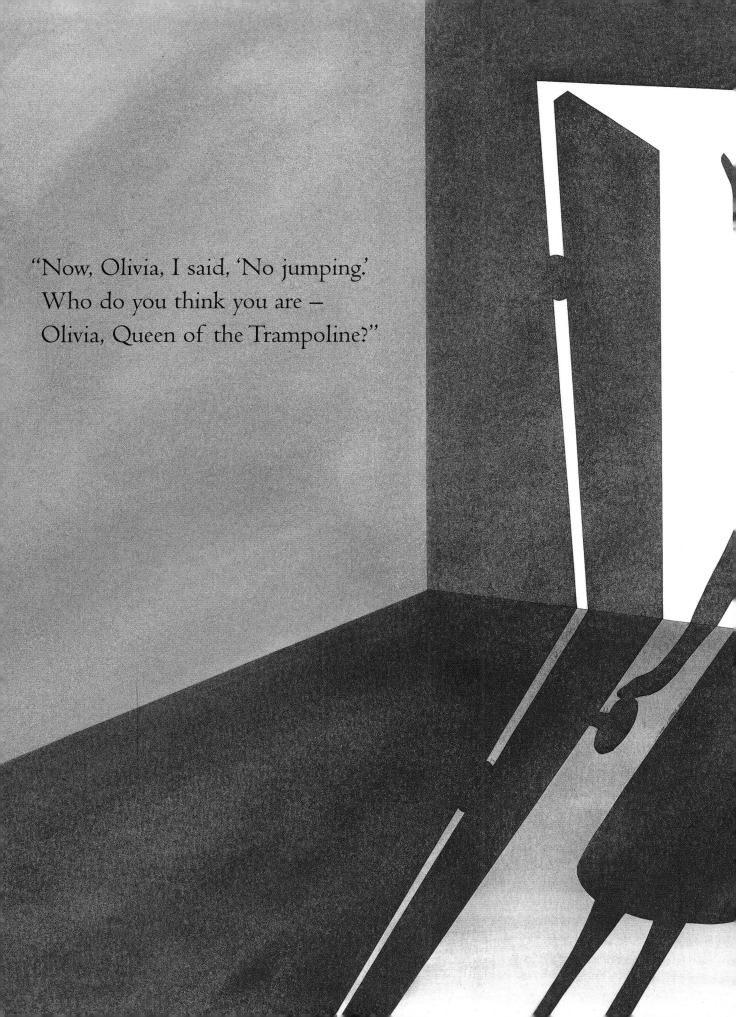

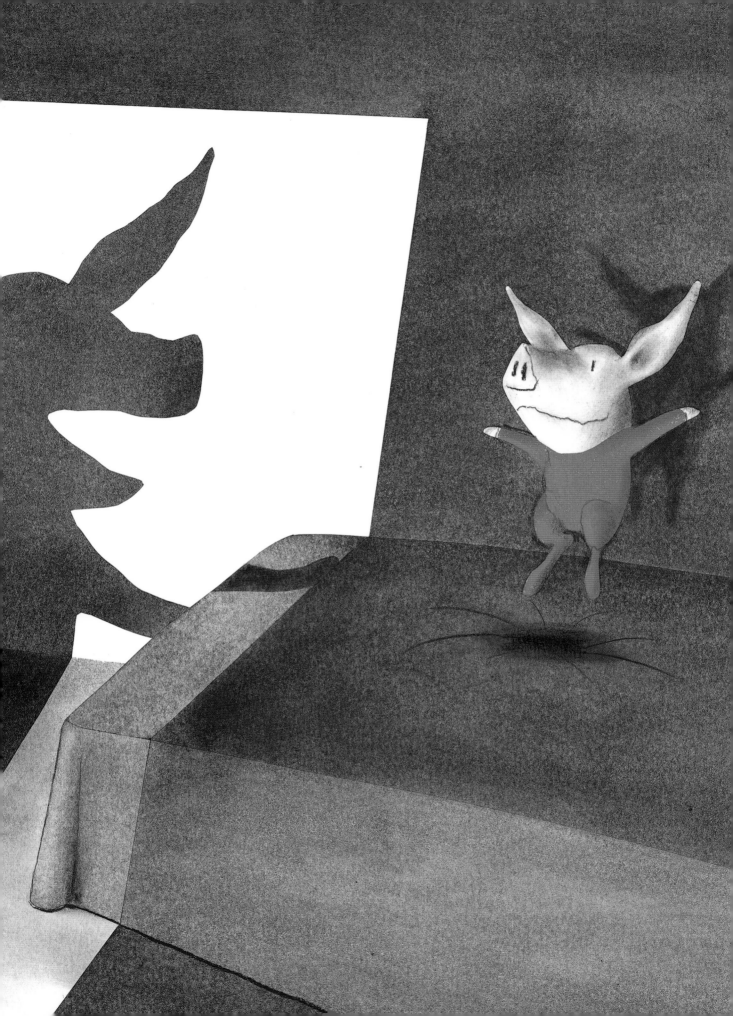

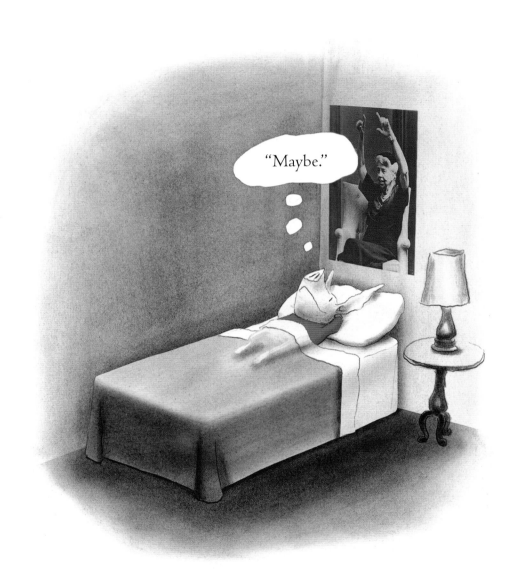

**SIMON AND SCHUSTER**

First published in Great Britain in 2001 by Simon & Schuster UK Ltd
222 Gray's Inn Road, London WC1X 8HB

This paperback edition first published in 2005

Originally published in 2001 by Simon & Schuster Books for Young Readers
an imprint of Simon & Schuster Children's Publishing Division, New York

Book design by Ann Bobco
The text for this book is set in Centaur
The illustrations for this book are rendered in charcoal and gouache on paper

A CIP catalogue record for this book is available from the British Library upon request

ISBN 978-1-41690-416-8

Printed in China

10 9 8 7 6 5 4 3

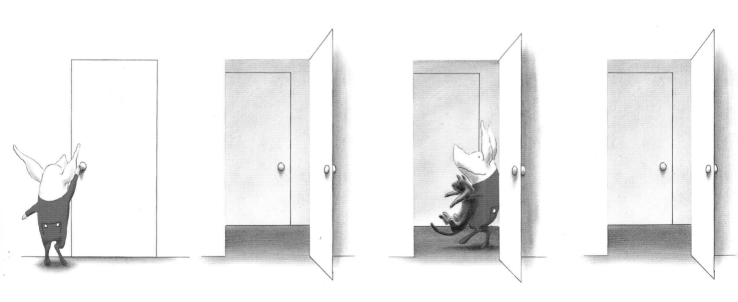

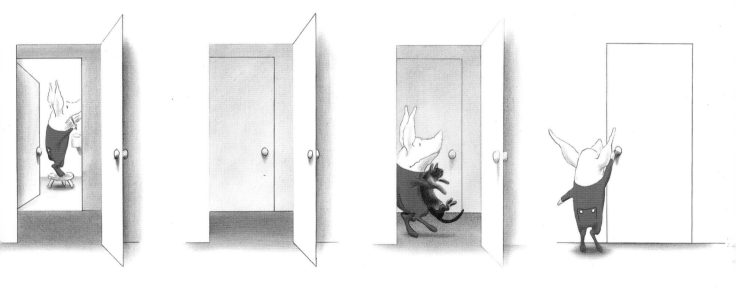